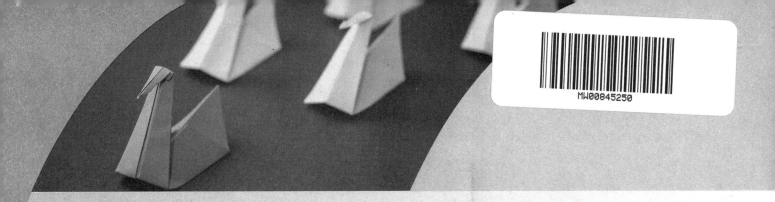

Essentials of Leadership in Public Health

Louis Rowitz, PhD

Professor Emeritus
School of Public Health
University of Illinois at Chicago

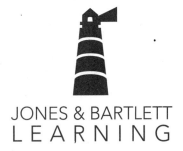

JONES & BARTLETT
LEARNING

World Headquarters
Jones & Bartlett Learning
5 Wall Street
Burlington, MA 01803
978-443-5000
info@jblearning.com
www.jblearning.com

Jones & Bartlett Learning books and products are available through most bookstores and online booksellers. To contact Jones & Bartlett Learning directly, call 800-832-0034, fax 978-443-8000, or visit our website, www.jblearning.com.

Substantial discounts on bulk quantities of Jones & Bartlett Learning publications are available to corporations, professional associations, and other qualified organizations. For details and specific discount information, contact the special sales department at Jones & Bartlett Learning via the above contact information or send an email to specialsales@jblearning.com.

12371-5

Production Credits
VP, Executive Publisher: David D. Cella
Publisher: Michael Brown
Associate Editor: Lindsey Mawhiney Sousa
Associate Editor: Danielle Bessette
Production Manager: Carolyn Rogers Pershouse
Director of Vendor Management: Amy Rose
Vendor Manager: Juna Abrams
Senior Marketing Manager: Sophie Fleck Teague
Manufacturing and Inventory Control Supervisor: Amy Bacus

Composition: Integra Software Services Pvt. Ltd.
Project Management: Integra Software Services Pvt. Ltd.
Cover Design: Timothy Dziewit
Director of Rights & Media: Joanna Gallant
Rights & Media Specialist: Merideth Tumasz
Media Development Editor: Shannon Sheehan
Cover Image: © scyther5/Shutterstock
Printing and Binding: Edwards Brothers Malloy
Cover Printing: Edwards Brothers Malloy

Library of Congress Cataloging-in-Publication Data
Names: Rowitz, Louis, author.
Title: Essentials of leadership in public health / Louis Rowitz.
Description: Burlington, MA : Jones & Bartlett Learning, [2018] | Includes bibliographical references and index.
Identifiers: LCCN 2017004818 | ISBN 9781284123715 (pbk.)
Subjects: | MESH: Public Health Administration--methods | Leadership
Classification: LCC RA410.6 | NLM WA 525 | DDC 362.1068/3--dc23 LC record available at https://lccn.loc.gov/2017004818

6048

Printed in the United States of America
21 20 19 18 17   10 9 8 7 6 5 4 3 2 1

*To Toni, my wife of 55 years, our daughters Julie and Ruth,
and our fantastic grandchildren,
Danielle, Roxanne, Noah, and Olivia*

Contents

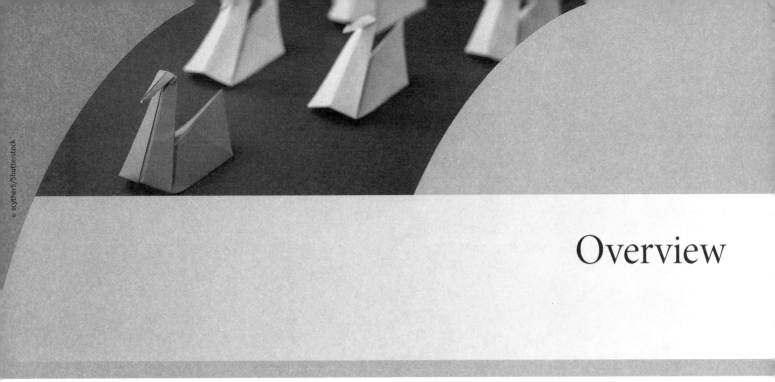

Overview

Leadership involves a shift in mindset. To be a leader requires a personal belief that the individual can live a life guided by leadership principles and practices. This book accepts that leaders are both born and made. However, leadership beliefs and practices need to be learned and then applied to the context of everyday life. Individuals who orient themselves to business will learn to be leaders within the context of business and its profit motive. Leaders who commit to public health or other human services will be guided by the social justice philosophy.

Leaders function at the personal, team, organization, community, global, and professional levels. This book provides tools and approaches to being a leader at each of these six levels of leadership. The book also explores leadership at each level in normal and not so normal situations (crises). The book includes stories of leadership heroes and villains, exercises, tools, and discussion questions. This book is written for advanced undergraduates with a public health major or as a first leadership course for master of public health students.

About the Author

Louis Rowitz, PhD, is professor emeritus at the School of Public Health, University of Illinois at Chicago, where he taught for over 40 years. In the 1980s and early 1990s, he served as associate dean of academic affairs of the school. Before that, Rowitz was a research scientist in the Illinois Department of Mental Health and Developmental Disabilities. As a social epidemiologist, Rowitz was engaged for many years in a number of research activities. He has written over 60 articles, several book chapters, and 5 books. He is the author of the blog Rowitz on Leadership since 2009. From 1992 to 2012, he was director of the Mid-America Public Health Leadership Institute. He has served as chair of the National Public Health Leadership Development Network three times. Rowitz has given numerous leadership workshops all over the United States in the last 25 years. He has also given workshops in the Czech Republic and Ireland.

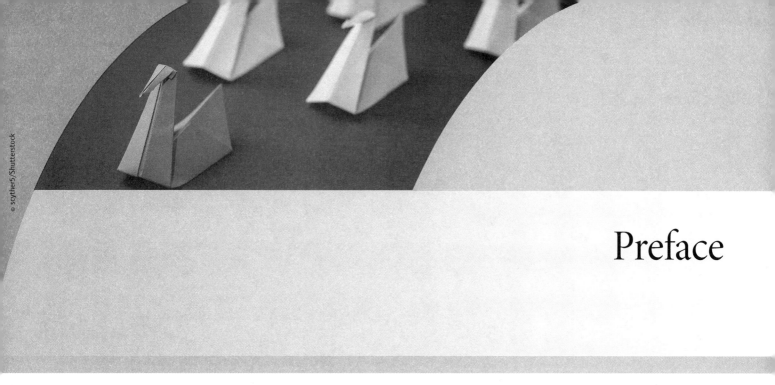

Preface

In 1988, the Institute of Medicine report on the future of public health was released. The report argued that not much energy was being spent on the training of public health leaders. Leadership would be required if public health was to advance into the future. The Public Health Practice Program Office of the Centers for Disease Control and Prevention (CDC) under Dr. Edward Baker took up the challenge to address the lack of excellent leadership in the public health profession. Tom Balderson, a public health advisor in the office, specifically took the challenge seriously. A grant proposal was initiated to fund a national public health leadership institute for directors and deputy directors of health departments around the United States. The new national institute was started in California under the directorship of Carol Woltring, who for 10 years developed a 1-year excellence program for public health leaders. I later attended the program and found the experience worthwhile. It also led to lifelong friendships with people in my leadership class.

In 1991, I met with Balderson to discuss the possibility of developing a leadership institute for state and local public health professionals who had made career commitments to public health. Many of the people in the national program were political appointees who left the field after their short tenure in public health. The Illinois Public Health Leadership Institute became the first state or regional leadership institute funded by the CDC. Parallel to the Illinois

program, the Missouri Public Health Leadership Institute was started by Dr. Kate Wright of St. Louis University and funded by the Missouri Department of Public Health. In 1994, Wright and I started the National Public Health Leadership Development Network, a collaborative organization of public health leadership development trainers from all over the United States. This organization was funded for many years by the CDC thanks to Tom Balderson and his colleague, Steve Frederick.

In 2000–2001, I talked to Mike Brown at Aspen Publishers about the fact that there was no book specific to public health leadership. I told him that I would be willing to write one based on my experiences as a director of a public health leadership institute. This led to the first edition of *Public Health Leadership: Putting Principles into Practice*, which became the first leadership book in public health. Mike Brown moved to Jones & Bartlett Learning and I followed with the publication of the second and third edition of my leadership book. This book has become more comprehensive over time. Because of the increasing need for a more foundational book on leadership for new public health leaders, this new book was written pulling essentials from the original book as well as new essential topics of interest to our new public health leaders.

Louis Rowitz
Chicago, Illinois

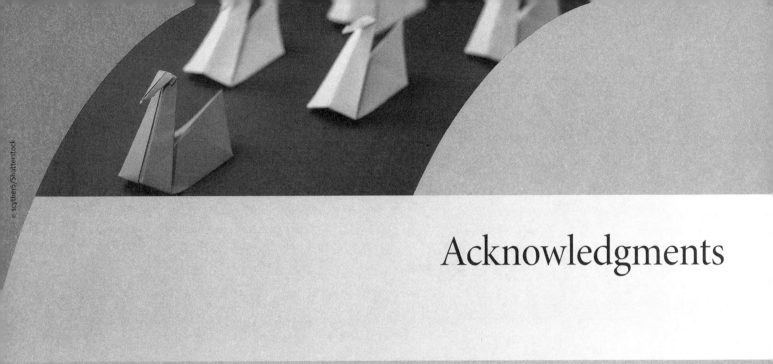

Acknowledgments

Over the past 25 years, I have been involved in the training of over a thousand public health professionals in the Mid-America Regional Public Health Leadership Institute. I have learned as much from all these leaders about public health and leadership as I have been able to teach them. I have also conducted leadership workshops for hundreds of others throughout the United States. My colleagues in leadership development can add many hundreds more to our leaders of the public health profession. Much of my writing is based on my discussions with my colleagues and the many people who have been trained. I also need to thank Ed Baker, Steve Frederick, Kate Wright, Cynthia Lamberth, Carol Woltring, Tom Balderson, Joyce Gaufin, Barney Turnock, Patrick Lenihan, Geoff Downie, Donna Dinkin, Ramon Bonzon, Judy Munson, and so many others who have strongly influenced my thinking about leadership. Thanks to my former staff at the University of Illinois School of Public Health—Rani Mishra, Sophie Naji, and Guddi Kapadia. I also need to thank Mike Brown of Jones & Bartlett Learning for encouraging my writing about leadership over the past 15 years. As always, I need to thank the love of my life, Toni, for always supporting me in all my efforts for public health leaders around the world.

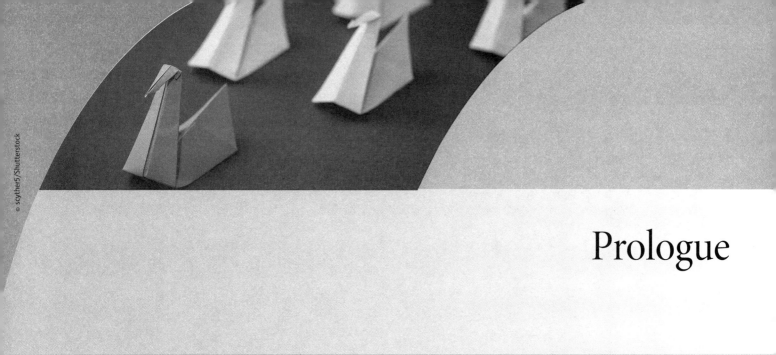

Prologue

Lou Rowitz, PhD is an internationally renowned expert in public health leadership. His previous books for advanced graduate students and public health professionals have won him a well-deserved reputation for providing practical and engaging advice on leadership.

In *Essentials of Leadership in Public Health*, Dr. Rowitz for the first time brings this approach to an introductory audience. As he writes, "The book includes stories of leadership heroes and villains, exercises, tools, and discussion questions." His engaging style including an abundance of hands-on exercises is ideally designed for all those who will take a leadership role in the future.

Essentials of Leadership in Public Health includes the full range of leadership across six levels: personal, team, organization, community, global, and professional. These levels provide a key organizing approach for the text. They also provide students with an understanding of the different forms of leadership and the skills needed for each.

I am pleased that Louis Rowitz's new book *Essentials of Leadership in Public Health* is part of our *Essential Public Health* series. I know you will be as well.

Richard Riegelman, MD, MPH, PhD
Editor, *Essential Public Health* series

Introduction

LEARNING OBJECTIVES

- Define leadership.
- Understand the importance of a culture of health.
- Comprehend the governing paradigm of public health.
- Learn why the essential services of public health are important.
- Understand the functional definition of a local health department.

It seems as though our morning newspaper has more health and public health-related articles than in times past. It seems like each day that there are articles with a public health theme. There are articles on the Zika virus, Ebola, climate change, a contaminated water supply in Michigan, influenza vaccine, terrorist activities throughout the world, gun violence, domestic violence, food-borne illness in a restaurant chain, a potential cure for schizophrenia, teenage suicides, and other public health-related issues. At the same time we are hearing about political concerns in the United States that health care costs too much and that the federal government needs to get out of the healthcare business. Regulations need to be reduced. There seems to be a disconnection between what the politicians say and what the public says it wants. Public health seems to be caught in the middle. Social services and public health services are being financially strangled at the national and state levels with a trickle-down effect at the local level. There is little or no money for training or even the belief that training will have any effect on the public health workforce.

Leadership is the important critical set of activities that must address all of these problem areas. Who and where are the leaders? For professionals in public health and human services, it will be all of us. This means that each of us needs to learn how to use our strengths with the important goal of helping to better the health of our neighbors, family, and friends. As soon as we use our public health knowledge, tools, and strategies and put them into action, we are beginning to think like a leader. Thus, leadership involves a shift in mindset to include the need to make public health real in an action sense and use our community partners to better the health of our residents.

To be a leader requires a personal belief that the health professional can live a life guided by leadership principles and practices. This book is based on the reality that leaders are both born and made. Individuals become leaders in the social arena. Leadership principles and practices need to be learned and then applied to the context of everyday life. Without application in a social context, leadership becomes only an abstract set of ideas. Individuals who orient themselves to business will learn to be leaders within the context of business organizations and their profit motive approach. Leaders who commit to public health or other human services will be guided by the social justice philosophy. Business techniques will also need to be learned but translated into processes necessary for making public health agencies more effective and efficient.

Leaders function at the personal, team, organization, community, global, and professional levels. Leaders will need to become action oriented and put their skills into practice in a community context. Action-oriented practice means leaders will need to learn adaptive leadership skills to increase the effectiveness of their work.

This book is designed to teach students new to public health and leadership about the essential knowledge, tools, and techniques for the leader new to public health practice. In this text, leaders will learn and apply the tools and techniques appropriate to the six levels of practice. At each level, leadership in normal and not-so-normal situations is explored. This book includes stories of leadership heroes and villains—vignettes of significant leadership events and people, exercises to practice leadership skills, and techniques and tools to aid the practice experience. Discussion questions are provided at the end of each chapter.

WHAT IS LEADERSHIP?

It is not an easy task to come up with a definition of leadership that satisfies everyone. Every person seems to have a definition although they tell you that they know a leader when they see one. Still, most definitions seem to have common elements. Some prerequisites to a definition of leadership are the following:

1. Ability to identify, use, and put into action the most useful information
2. Ability to motivate and work with others
3. Ability to take risks and follow through
4. Ability to communicate at many different levels
5. Understand the difference between truth and fiction
6. Ability to act as systems thinkers with an understanding of how complexity affects their work

In today's world, leaders will have to possess different skills. They will need to recognize that leading is a process in which they must pursue their vision through influencing others, the places they work, and the communities that they serve. Leaders will find that advancing the skills of their workforce will increase the chance that their vision will become a reality. Leaders will also have to break down the barriers between agency and community to create an environment in which a shared value system and a shared vision for the future will come into being. What is needed is the creation of a culture of health within the community. This concept is discussed in the next section of this chapter.

For this book, the following definition of leadership applies. Leadership is creativity in action. It is the ability to learn from our past experiences, live in the here and now, and keep our eyes focused on where we want to go. Leadership is based on respect for history and the knowledge that true growth builds on our existing strengths. Leaders are systems thinkers. They learn from their mistakes. Leadership is in part a visionary endeavor, but it requires the fortitude and flexibility necessary to put vision into action, the ability to work with others, and to become a follower when someone else is the better lead. Leaders also need to be resilient to function in normal and not-so-normal times.

Public health leadership includes a strong commitment to the community and the values for which it stands. A community perspective requires a systems thinking and complexity orientation. Community refers not only to the local community in which a person works but also to the larger global community that can affect the health of the public over time. Whatever health crises occur in other parts of the world will eventually affect the health of the public in our local communities in the future. As I write this, public health leaders are concerned about the spread of the Zika virus in the United States and other places. Cases of the possible sexual transmission of the virus are now being reported. Leadership also includes a commitment to social justice and health equity for everyone, but public health leaders must not let this commitment undermine their ability to pursue a well-designed public health agenda based on the core public health functions and essential services of public health. Although the core functions paradigm guides public health leaders in their day-to-day work, this does not mean that this governing paradigm cannot be changed or modified if necessary. Some states have added additional essential services to their governing paradigm. Leaders propose new paradigms when old ones lose their effectiveness. **Exercise I-1** presents an early chance for you to explore your leadership understanding and your leadership experiences thus far.

EXERCISE I-1 Past Leadership Experiences

Purpose: to explore past leadership experience in order to understand what leadership skills were needed

Key Concepts: experiential leadership, leadership skills

Procedure: Divide the class into dyads. Spend 15 minutes discussing past leadership experiences both positive and negative. Explore the skills used in these experiential events. Reconvene the class and list on newsprint the skills used by the individual class members. From the list of skills, come up with a class definition of leadership.

CULTURE OF HEALTH

The implementation of the Patient Protection and Affordable Care Act, commonly known as the Affordable Care Act, made the following important: an increasing acceptance of the importance of both prevention and public health preparedness, knowing that knowledge management is a good thing, a stress on informatics development, improving access to health care, an awareness of the need to bring together the multifaceted nature and parts of health and health care, and the idea of creating a national cultural orientation to health. It is not that we have to collapse all the health professions into one universal category, but rather we need to make collaboration and partnership our modus operandi. With an awareness that a move to health and a culture of health is also multifaceted, the social determinants of health were a beginning to our understanding of the values associated with

---

PUBLIC HEALTH HEROES AND VILLAINS I-1 Robert Wood Johnson Foundation Hero[1]

The Robert Wood Johnson Foundation is an organization that prides itself on its leadership role in public health. The organization includes many public health leaders who have played major roles in public health practice including direction of local and state health departments and policy roles at the national level. For over 40 years, the foundation has trained health leaders and scholars. Its mission has been to improve the health and health care of all Americans. Beginning in 2013, the foundation began to reorganize itself by removing health profession silos and replacing them with an integrated health professions model. In addition, the agency began its culture of health initiative with a community orientation and a concern with the development of leaders in the community. The new vision for the foundation is to build an American approach revolving around a culture of health paradigm to help all Americans live healthier lives for today and for the future. The foundation will put its grant and contract funds behind this initiative.

In the report on which this hero case is based, 10 underlying principles for the culture of health paradigm are given:

1. Good health flourishes across geographic, demographic, and social sectors.
2. Attaining the best health is valued by our entire society.
3. Individuals and families have the means and the opportunity to make choices that lead to the healthiest lives possible.
4. Business, government, individuals, and organizations work together to build healthy communities and lifestyles.
5. Everyone has access to affordable, high-quality health care because it is essential to maintain, or reclaim, health.
6. No one is excluded.
7. Health care is efficient and equitable.
8. The economy is less burdened by excessive and unwarranted healthcare spending.
9. Keeping everyone as healthy as possible guides public and private decision making.
10. Americans understand that we are all in this together.

These 10 principles will require important collaboration between federal, state, or local governments as well as local citizens, local leaders, and agencies. Policies will need revision. Political leaders will need to change their health priorities. The foundation will work with health professions organizations, government officials, and local communities to make the culture of health paradigm a reality. An overarching theme relates to the important issue of equity. Every American should be entitled to the healthiest life possible in every part of the United States.

The foundation is promoting a Culture of Health Action Framework to carry out this new initiative of:

1. Making health a shared value
2. Fostering cross-sector collaboration to improve well-being
3. Creating healthier, more equitable communities
4. Strengthening integration of health services and systems

The framework was developed by the foundation in collaboration with the Rand Corporation and input from 1,000 health and public health thought leaders. The outcome of using the framework should be an improvement of the health status of all citizens and the resolution of health equity issues. This improvement will ultimately help to reduce healthcare costs.

Public Health Heroes and Villains 1 is based on Robert Wood Johnson Foundation, *From Vision to Action* (Washington D.C.: 2015)

health at a community or societal level. A culture of health model is a political, economic, social, personal, family, or community set of decision points. Our immediate challenge is that it is not easy to change culture. Behavior needs to change before our cultural orientation changes.

Although leadership with a positional title is an important dimension, the creation or development of a health mindset or health cultural orientation for all Americans is the end goal. Each of us must take a leadership stance if a true culture of health is to become a reality. All must take responsibility for the change because each of us has to change our health habits. It is of course critical that our health professionals become more expert in the practice of leadership. Leadership development on the ground will be important because health challenges are often changing. The use of social media will need to increase, but in the end relationships and relationship building will be the secret weapons for bringing a new age of health into being.

To change mental models related to culture and oriented toward treatment and rehabilitation will require a culture of health model with a prevention orientation. As mentioned, leaders will need to be proficient in the skills of systems thinking, communication skills, knowledge of the sociological process of cultural systems design (understanding how mental models can be changed), psychological processes related to behavior change, policy development and advocacy, models of collaboration, informatics, and organization management. The first hero story in this book involves the Robert Wood Johnson Foundation and their initiative to support culture of health programs. Our first hero is a foundation composed of many public health leaders.

CORE FUNCTIONS OF PUBLIC HEALTH

Within the culture of health, there is the important subculture of service. The public health agency service orientation involves the core functions of public health paradigm. Many human service fields struggle with the issue of credibility. Part of the lack of credibility stems from the fact that the public often does not understand the nature of the services being provided; a paradigm can help to increase public understanding. For example, it can define the structure and parameters of public health work. The core functions of public health is such a paradigm.

A paradigm is a map with boundaries that elucidates a major area of endeavor.[2] Public health leaders, to an extent, see the world in terms of core functions. They also see it in terms of a leadership paradigm or a model for action. If the paradigm becomes effective, leaders will modify or change it. This is called a paradigm shift.[3] A paradigm shift, which

usually takes a long time to be completed, creates new set of rules, procedures, and perspectives.

The Future of Public Health first described the core functions paradigm.[4] The functions of assessment, policy development, and assurance are tied to phases of public health practice. Assessment involves the identification of health problems, policy development involves the identification of possible solutions through policy, and assurance involves the implementation of the supposed solutions (usually in the form of programs, services, or clinical interventions). Public health leaders have major responsibilities associated with each core function. It can be stated that these core functions are a universal model for understanding how human service programs work.

Policy development is seen as linking assessment to assurance. In reality, policy development is often an afterthought in the U.S. public health system—that is, assurance activities sometimes occur before policies are developed. Many public health leaders with whom I have spoken nevertheless have pointed out that leaders need to be effective in the policy development area if they are to create a comprehensive public health system.

The core functions work interactively and provide an approach to the important process of governance. Governance and public health practice are the glue that makes the entire interactive system cohere and function as it should. It is therefore a central concern for leadership at the service and community level. Governance in public health is usually a community responsibility of our elected or appointed officials. If all people involved in public health become empowered to implement a culture of health orientation, then governance as demonstrated through sound and effective public health practice will be part of the infrastructure of the entire health and public health system. In fact, governance is a major component in all aspects of public health policy and practice.

ESSENTIAL PUBLIC HEALTH SERVICES

The public health system is affected by the implementation of any proposals for a national health system (Affordable Care Act) or indeed by any substantial changes in the medical care system. Yet what the effects will be are largely a mystery, especially because the core functions paradigm is still confusing to policy makers and citizens, although the identification of essential public health services associated with the core functions helps to elucidate the paradigm. In addition, the list of essential public health services are community based rather than organization based. These services, unlike the models of public health discussed thus far, include research, enforcement of laws and regulations, and the assurance of a competent health services workforce.

Table I-1 lists not only essential services but also related leadership activities, and Table I-2 gives a brief description of each of the 10 services.[5] Leaders have key roles in the delivery of all of the essential services. The new leadership activities are associated with the three essential services. With regard to enforcement of laws, public health leaders enforce laws and regulations that protect the health of the community. With regard to development of a competent workforce, they build learning organizations based on systems thinking and support continuing education opportunities for the public health workforce. With regard to research, they use research findings to guide program development. Figure I-1, which was originally designed by the Health Resources and Services Administration, shows the relationship between the core functions and the 10 essential public health services.[6] It is presented as a circle to demonstrate that public health works in a system. Essential Service 10 is seen as research for systems management and greater understanding of how the public health system carries out its activities.

If we think of the three core functions as the trunk of a tree, each essential public health services constitute a branch that has continued to grow. The National Association of County and City Health Officials (NACCHO) put the two models together and came up with an operational definition of a functional local public health department. NACCHO was clearly aware that local health departments take many forms, but they need to support the core functions and 10 essential public health services within a public health systems approach.[7] The local public health department represents the governmental public health presence at the local level. The way they do this is to follow a set of standards as noted in Table I-3. The residents of a community hold their local public health department responsible for adhering to these standards.

Following is a list of leadership activities related to the core functions paradigm:

- Put the core functions model into practice.
- Develop leadership skills to carry out the essential public health services approach.
- Increase commitment to the model by the public health workforce and by community partners
- Use a systems perspective in implementing the essential public health services

TABLE I-1   Leadership and the Essential Public Health Services

Essential Public Health Services	Leadership Activities
1. Monitor health status to identify community problems.	Use data for decision making.
2. Diagnose and investigate health problems and health hazards in the community.	Use data for decision making.
3. Inform and educate people about health issues and empower them to deal with the issues.	Engage in mentoring and training, social marketing, and health communication activities; empower others.
4. Mobilize community partnerships to identify and solve health problems.	Build partnerships; share power; create workable action plans.
5. Develop policies and plans that support individual and community health efforts.	Clarify values; develop mission; create a vision; develop goals and objectives.
6. Enforce laws and regulations that protect health and ensure safety.	Protect laws and regulations; monitor adherence to laws.
7. Link people to needed personal health services and ensure the provision of health care when otherwise unavailable.	Stress innovation; delegate programmatic responsibility to others; oversee programs.
8. Ensure a competent public health and personal healthcare workforce.	Build a learning organization; encourage training; mentor associates.
9. Evaluate effectiveness, accessibility, and quality of personal and population-based health services.	Support program evaluation; evaluate data collected; monitor performance.
10. Do research for new insights and innovative solutions to health problems.	Use research findings to guide program development.

Modified from J. Harrell and E. Baker, *The Essential Services of Public Health*, 1997, American Public Health Association.

TABLE I-2   Essential Public Health Services

Monitor health status to identify and solve community health problems. This service includes accurate diagnosis of the community's health status; identification of threats to health and assessment of health service needs; timely collection, analysis, and publication of information on access, use, costs, and outcomes of personal health services; attention to the vital statistics and health status of specific groups that are at higher risk than the total population; and collaboration to manage integrated information systems with private providers and health benefit plans.

Diagnose and investigate health problems and health hazards in the community. This service includes epidemiologic identification of emerging health threats, public health laboratory capability using modern technology to conduct rapid screening and high-volume testing, active infectious disease epidemiology programs, and technical capacity for epidemiologic investigation of disease outbreaks and patterns of chronic disease and injury.

Inform, educate, and empower people about health issues, This service involves social marketing and targeted media public communication; providing accessible health information resources at community levels; active collaboration with personal healthcare providers to reinforce health promotion messages and programs; and joint health education programs with schools, churches, and worksites.

Mobilize community partnerships and action to identify and solve health problems, This service involves convening and facilitating community groups and associations, including those not typically considered to be health related, in undertaking defined preventive, screening, rehabilitation, and support programs; and skilled coalition-building ability in order to draw upon the full range of potential human and material resources in the cause of community health.

Develop policies and plans that support individual and community health efforts. This service requires leadership development at all levels of public health; systematic community-level and state-level planning for health improvement in all jurisdictions; development and tracking of measurable health objectives as a part of continuous quality improvement strategies; joint evaluation with the medical healthcare system to define consistent policy regarding prevention and treatment services; and development of codes, regulations, and legislation to guide the practice of public health.

Enforce laws and regulations that protect health and ensure safety. This service involves full enforcement of sanitary codes, especially in the food industry; full protection of drinking water supplies; enforcement of clean air standards; timely follow-up of hazards, preventable injuries, and exposure-related diseases identified in occupational and community settings; monitoring quality of medical services (e.g., laboratory, nursing homes, and home health care); and timely review of new drug, biologic, and medical device applications.

Link people to needed personal health services and ensure the provision of health care when otherwise unavailable. This service (often referred to as "outreach" or "enabling" services) includes ensuring effective entry for socially disadvantaged people into a coordinated system of clinical care; culturally and linguistically appropriate materials and staff to ensure linkage to services to special population groups; ongoing "care management"; transportation services; targeted health information to high-risk population groups; and technical assistance for effective worksite health promotion/disease prevention programs.

Ensure a competent public and personal healthcare workforce. This service includes education and training for personnel to meet the needs for public and personal health service; efficient processes for licensure of professionals and certification of facilities with regular verification and inspection follow-up; adoption of continuous quality improvement and lifelong learning within all licensure and certification programs; active partnerships with professional training programs to ensure community-relevant learning experiences for all students; and continuing education in management and leadership development programs for those charged with administrative/executive roles.

Evaluate effectiveness, accessibility, and quality of personal and population-based health services. This service calls for ongoing evaluation of health programs, based on analysis of health status and service use data, to assess program effectiveness and to provide information necessary for allocating resources and reshaping programs.

Research for new insights and innovative solutions to health problems. This service includes continuous linkage with appropriate institutions of higher learning and research and an internal capacity to mount timely epidemiologic and economic analyses and conduct needed health services research.

Data from J. Harrell and E. Baker, *The Essential Services of Public Health*, 1997, American Public Health Association.

FIGURE I-1 Core Functions and 10 Essential Services of Public Health

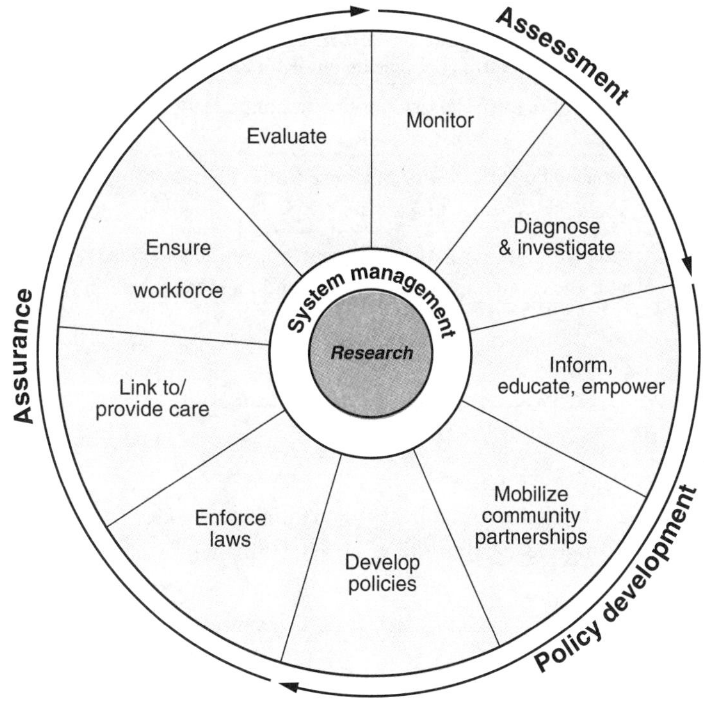

Reproduced from the U.S. Department of Health and Human Services (1999), *Public Health Functions Project.* http://www.health.gov/phfunctions/images/pubh_wh2.gif. Accessed July 30, 2012.

TABLE I-3   Standards for a Functional Local Health Department

A functional local health department:
Understands the specific health issues confronting the community, and how physical, behavioral, environmental, social, and economic conditions affect them.
Investigates health problems and health threats.
Prevents, minimizes, and contains adverse health effects from communicable diseases, disease outbreaks from unsafe food and water, chronic diseases, environmental hazards, injuries, and risky health behaviors.
Leads planning and response activities for public health emergencies.
Collaborates with other local responders and with state and federal agencies to intervene in other emergencies with public health significance (e.g., natural disasters).
Implements health promotion programs.
Engages the community to address public health issues.
Develops partnerships with public and private healthcare providers and institutions, community-based organizations, and other government agencies (e.g., housing authority, criminal justice, education) engaged in services that affect health to collectively identify, alleviate, and act on the sources of public health problems.
Coordinates the public health system's efforts in an intentional, noncompetitive, and nonduplicative manner.
Addresses health disparities.
Serves as an essential resource for local governing bodies and policy makers on up-to-date public health laws and policies.

(continued)

Provides science-based, timely, and culturally competent health information and health alerts to the media and to the community.
Provides its expertise to others who treat or address issues of public health significance.
Ensures compliance with public health laws and ordinances, using enforcement authority when appropriate.
Employs well-trained staff members who have the necessary resources to implement best practices and evidence-based programs and interventions.
Facilitates research efforts, when approached by researchers, that benefit the community.
Uses and contributes to the evidence base of public health.
Strategically plans its services and activities, evaluates performance and outcomes, and makes adjustments as needed to continually improve its effectiveness, enhance the community's health status, and meet the community's expectations.

Reproduced from National Association of County and City Health Officials, *Operational Definition of a Functional Local Health Department* (Washington, DC: NACCHO, 2005).

Exercise I-2 allows you and your classmates to address the essential public health services through leadership skills and strategies.

SUMMARY

It seems as if each day presents us with another public health crisis. Well-trained public health leaders will be required to address these crises. This book explores the essential of public health leadership. A definition of leadership was presented to guide our work. Ideally, this work will be done in a culture of health environment. A subculture within our communities will explore our public health work using the core functions and essential services of public health. Each chapter of the book also tells the stories of some of our hero leaders and public health villains. Finally, because a number of the students in the class have minimal or no public health leadership experience, exercises are presented to give you opportunities to explore leadership practice.

EXERCISE I-2 The Flood

Purpose: to practice leadership skills and strategies using the essential services of public health and the standards of a functional local health department to address a crisis situation

Key Concepts: leadership skills, essential services of public health, standards of a functional local health department

Scenario: The Mississippi River has reached flood stage again in the spring of the year. There are two adversely affected towns across the river from each other that are served by a county health department.

Procedures: Divide the class into small groups of six or seven and make half the teams County Health Department A and half the groups County Health Department B. Have all teams address how they would handle the crisis using the essential health service paradigm, leadership skills and practice, and the standards for a functional local public health department. After a half hour, pair one group from Health Department A with one group from Health Department B. Using a table, have the two groups work out a plan for working together.

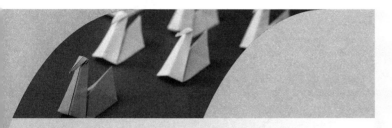

Discussion Questions

1. What are the critical public health issues of today and how might we handle them? Who should be our partners?

2. Why do we need a culture of health and how can we bring it into being?

3. What is leadership for you?

4. What are the three core functions of public health? Are any functions missing?

5. What is the relationship between the core functions and the essential services of public health?

6. What are the reasons for creating an operational definition for local health departments?

REFERENCES

1. Robert Wood Johnson Foundation, *From Vision to Action* (Washington DC: Author, 2015).
2. S. R. Covey, *The Seven Habits of Highly Effective People* (New York, NY: Simon and Schuster, 1989).
3. J. A. Barker, *Paradigm* (New York, NY: Harper Business, 1992).
4. Institute of Medicine, *The Future of Public Health* (Washington, DC: National Academies Press, 1988).
5. J. Harrell and E. Baker, *The Essential Services of Public Health* (Washington, DC: American Public Health Association, 1997).
6. www.health.gov/phfunctions/images/pubh_wh2.gif. Accessed October 14, 2003.
7. National Association of County and City Health Officials, *Operational Definition of a Functional Local Health Department* (Washington, DC: NACCHO, 2005).

CHAPTER **1**

The Management and Leadership Continuum

On the surface, it appears that management and leadership are two completely different processes. Management activity usually refers to processes related to an agency and how it is run. The expectation is that the manager/administrator is an individual or team of individuals who will run the organization effectively and efficiently. In addition to promoting a culture of health vision within the agency, the leader is the individual who works outside the agency building relationships in the community, building collaborative networks to support a culture of health system, helping develop health policies for the community, and providing a role for the public health agency in these initiatives. It is my intention to argue that management and leadership are closely related. This book argues that management and leadership are on a continuum and that leaders will often engage in both management and leadership activities. One of the important leadership heroes of the 19th century was John Snow who

took both a management and a leadership approach to a water contamination problem.

There is an interesting training exercise called the Human Likert, which has a large group line up along an imaginary continuum.[a] The general instruction is to decide how each individual defines his or her professional life. On one side of the line are individuals who define themselves as public health practitioners with a major specialty, such as an environmental health or public health preparedness professional. In the middle of the line are those who define themselves as managers or administrators, and at the end of the line are those who define themselves as public health leaders. The facilitator then goes down the line asking people why they placed themselves as they did and whether they see themselves as moving along the line as they professionally advance in their chosen public health field. What this exercise does is demonstrate how people view their professional training, their personal definitions of management, and what they perceive as leadership. When I recently used the Human Likert, one individual who defined himself as an environmental health professional said that he wanted to become an expert in his chosen field. He saw this as a demonstration of leadership without a specific designated leadership position in his organization. Those in the management position also saw that leadership could be demonstrated in a management

---

[a] I learned this exercise from Dr. Magda Peck of the University of Wisconsin-Milwaukee as she used it with a maternal and child health leadership group.

PUBLIC HEALTH HEROES AND VILLAINS 1-1 John Snow, Hero

In the 1850s, London was in the midst of a cholera epidemic. Dr. John Snow was deeply concerned about the epidemic. He believed after an investigation that the cause of the epidemic was contaminated water from the Broad Street Pump in Soho, a part of Saint James Parish. On September 7, 1854, Snow had an interview with the Board of Guardians and reported that the pump was responsible for the epidemic. Although several on the board did not agree with Snow, they let the pump handle be removed the next day. The number of new cases declined. Snow continued his research on cholera. He was clearly a leader and early epidemiologist. As a clinician, he was involved in management activities. For more information, see the John Snow website developed by UCLA: http://www.ph.ucla.edu/epi/snow.html.

EXERCISE 1-1 Problem Solving for Managers and Leaders

Purpose: to understand the difference between managers and leaders in solving problems

Key Concepts: management, leadership, problem solving

Scenario: The Harbor County Commissioners have cut the budget by 20 percent for the local health department this fiscal year.

Procedure: Divide the class into groups of six or seven. Half of the groups will be managers and develop a strategy for dealing with the deficit. The other half will solve the problem from a leadership perspective. Each of the groups will present its plans to the class as a whole. Discuss.

position as well. Thus, it is possible to move horizontally as well as vertically in an organization. Horizontally, you advance by becoming the best public health practitioner that you can or the best manager or the best leader. If you want to move to a higher administrative position in your organization—a vertical move—it is necessary to move in the direction of your strengths rather than your weaknesses.[1] What the Human Likert exercise teaches the participants is that practitioners develop expertise in their disciplinary specialty; managers maintain the organization and develop people; and leaders define the system, build relationships, and create visions for the future.

This chapter explores the connections between management and leadership. The next section examines the management issues and is followed by an example of matrix forms of organization. Next is a discussion of the starfish organizational model and the management and leadership continuum, addressing some of the connections between management and leadership and describing transactional and transformational leadership. The next section of the chapter presents a road map that begins to demonstrate how these management and leadership functions interrelate. The final section begins a discussion of the development of a personal leadership toolkit. **Exercise 1-1**

looks at potential problem-solving methods for managers and leaders dealing with the threat of a budget reduction at their public health agency.

MANAGERS AND MANAGEMENT

There are clear distinctions between managers and leaders. Managers are tied to the present and to the mission of the agencies they serve. Leaders tend to be less bound by their home agencies or their positions, although they need to be concerned about their vision for the agency and the support of the individuals who work there to move the agency into the future. Leaders in public agencies allocate much of their time to building relationships with external stakeholders in the public health enterprise.[2] Although both managers and leaders tend to be tied to a specific agency position, the manager seems to be more locked into the requirements of the job than the leader does. Leaders are more oriented to their vision and the overall public health system, whereas the manager needs to concentrate on making the agency effective and efficient. The effective manager makes the dreams and visions of the leader real.

Another reality is that a specific individual may be hired for an administrative position (management) and be expected to carry out both management and leadership activities. This may not always be an easy task. People view the world in different ways. Browning has pointed out that people have different thinking attributes.[3] There are people who tend to be linear thinkers and are intrigued with rules, regulations, and protocols. They are structured in the way they do things. They tend to be organized and to resist change. These structured thinkers can be contrasted with people who tend to be analytical in their thinking. These are the problem solvers who are very logical and like abstract thinking. They like to put facts and numbers together. If we extend this structural and analytical thinking to the organizational level, we are probably talking about many governmental agencies that like process, analyze facts, follow rules and protocols, and tend to support a status quo perspective. Many managers tend to fall into this classification of structural and analytical.

Browning stated that there are two other major thinking preferences. There are the conceptual thinkers who tend to want to view the big picture. They like change and tend to stir things up. For example, you think that you have the last draft of a technical report, and the conceptual thinker will ask if you have thought about solution X. Conceptual people tend to be creative and look at new ways to achieve their visions and goals. The fourth thinking attribute is social.

Those strong in this thinking preference tend to like to work in teams and show great concern for others. Some literature has pointed out that managers need to have strong people skills in today's environment.[4] Managers have to be able to fit people's talents into appropriate jobs that fit the needs of the organization.[5] The Browning Emergenetics Model can be seen graphically in **Figure 1-1**, where the analytical and structural half of the diagram represents left-brain thinking, and the conceptual and social half represents right-brain thinking.[6] Most people will show preference in more than one thinking attribute. All sorts of combinations are possible, from strong preference in one, two, three, or four thinking attributes. However, the thinking preferences of individuals are filtered and affected by their behavioral attributes of expressiveness, assertiveness, and flexibility.

Management takes place in the context of an agency or an organization. In 1916, Fayol defined the five elements of management as prevoyance (planning), organizing, commanding, coordinating, and controlling.[7] Planning involves a series of

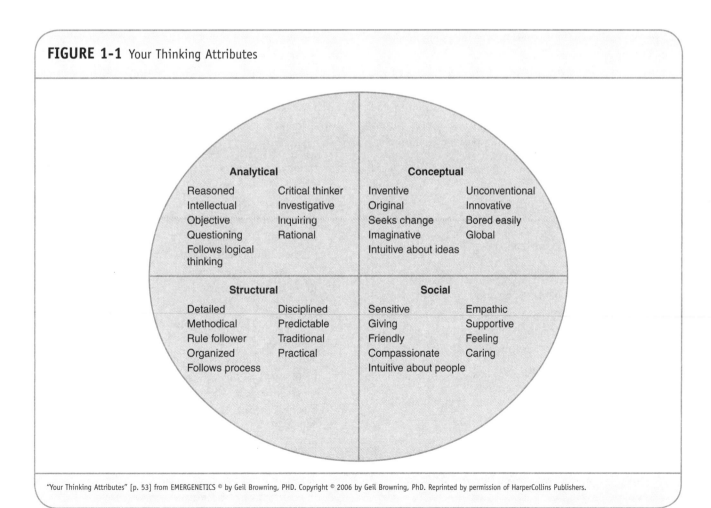

FIGURE 1-1 Your Thinking Attributes

Analytical		Conceptual	
Reasoned	Critical thinker	Inventive	Unconventional
Intellectual	Investigative	Original	Innovative
Objective	Inquiring	Seeks change	Bored easily
Questioning	Rational	Imaginative	Global
Follows logical thinking		Intuitive about ideas	

Structural		Social	
Detailed	Disciplined	Sensitive	Empathic
Methodical	Predictable	Giving	Supportive
Rule follower	Traditional	Friendly	Feeling
Organized	Practical	Compassionate	Caring
Follows process		Intuitive about people	

actions to achieve organizational goals. Organizing involves the assignment of tasks to employees, fitting assignments into the existing hierarchical structure of the organization, and tying organizational goals to these work processes. Commanding is about leadership inside the organization. Some writers discuss the issues of employee productivity, turnover and absenteeism, job satisfaction, and other human capital issues for this function.[8] Wagner and Harter of the Gallup organization strongly advocate a 12-step model for engaging employees that will be the orientation of great managers.[9] Part of the motivation of employees involves the leaders in the organization sharing their vision with the managers. The coordinating and controlling elements involve the necessity for the manager to monitor activities of the agency and make corrections and realignments as necessary. Drucker defined the three tasks of management as determining the mission of the organization, creating a work environment that is productive and leads to worker achievement, and recognizing the social impact and social responsibility of the organization's activities.[10] It is interesting to note here that businesses as well as governmental public health agencies have a social impact and social responsibility dimension that for public health is related to the philosophy of social justice.

Fayol also developed a 14-principle guide for management that is as relevant today as it was when he formulated it early in the 20th century.[11] As can be seen in **Table 1-1**, the 14 principles cover all aspects of an organization's management, from a division of work to the creation of a positive environment in which people may work. A clarification regarding management needs to be made. Management activities will differ at different levels of the organization. Robbins and Coulter point out that technical skills will be necessary at the program level of the organization, with people skills becoming more important as you move up horizontally in the organization.[12] Conceptual skills become critical for the top managers and leaders in the organization. The leaders ideally create change.

Administrators of state or local public health agencies or offices are generally appointed by elected officials or by local boards of health. New public health administrators tend to be seen as political appointees. These appointments to so-called leadership positions are in reality perceived to be high-level management positions. The job of these appointees is to manage the official public health agency. The new administrators face all types of organizational challenges during the early part of their tenure. As they accommodate to their new positions, demands from external community stakeholders need to be addressed. As community issues take precedence, the administrator may need to delegate managerial responsibilities to other people in the department.

Working in government is not the same as working in business. It is not that the tools or skills necessary to work in these two sectors are very different but rather that the public health leader needs to adapt these tools and skills to the public sector. There are at least four challenges for leaders who work in the public sector:[13]

1. The public sector administrator has to work within the framework of laws, rules, regulations, and procedures defined by governmental entities. These laws, rules, regulations, and procedures put limits and restrictions on the public agency executive, which can affect mission, vision, performance, and progress at addressing public health issues.

2. The performance of the agency is extremely visible to the outside world through legislative oversight and media scrutiny. Moore has stated that performance is affected by the challenge of creating public value for public sector issues.[14]

3. The internal and external stakeholders that are affected by the work of public agencies are more numerous and representative of diverse value perspectives than in the business world. Each stakeholder has unique issues. There are multiple and diverse demands and levels of influence on the work of the agency.

4. The realities of bureaucracy often impede or delay the ability of administrators to carry out the public's work in an effective, efficient, and timely manner.

TABLE 1-1   Henri Fayol's 14 Principles of Management

1. Division of work (specialization)
2. Authority
3. Discipline
4. Unity of command (one supervisor)
5. Unity of direction
6. Subordination of individual interest
7. Remuneration
8. Centralization (or decentralization)
9. Scalar chain (organizational hierarchy)
10. Order
11. Equity
12. Stability of tenure of personnel
13. Initiative
14. Esprit de corps

Modified from H. Fayol, *General and Industrial Management* (Paris: Dunod, 1916).

Even though we live in a democratic society, people who work in government often seem to feel limited in their ability to move their agency agendas forward because of external scrutiny as well as political agendas.

It is incorrect to assume that all agencies are the same. Different agencies require different types of administrators to address these differences. There are at least five different organizational settings for the new administrator. Daly and Watkins define these settings as a start-up situation, turn-around, realignment or shift in priorities, accelerated growth, and maintaining a successful organizational strategy.[15,16] In start-up and turnaround situations, the new administrator needs to make changes quickly and does not have the leisure to learn about the organization and its staff, as in realignment and success-sustaining situations. Accelerated growth refers to organizations going through a major growth spurt.

During 2007, the National Association of County and City Health Officials (NACCHO) undertook a process of developing a plan for a new local health official orientation program that lasted several years. In concert with a NACCHO committee, the staff of the association began an interactive process of developing this program. The committee, NACCHO staff, and curriculum design consultants developed the curriculum.[17] It became clear early that the program needed to be strong on management issues because the committee, composed of several seasoned health administrators, strongly argued that new administrators needed to spend time on management issues. Five specific competency expectations for new health officials were determined.[18] New health officials should:

1. Clearly describe to their staff and variety of public audiences the roles and responsibilities of the new administrator within local health departments (LHDs) and the LHD's roles and responsibilities within the local health system.
2. Effectively engage elected officials, governing boards, and the state health department in carrying out the roles and responsibilities of the LHDs.
3. Effectively manage their LHDs, including providing insight and direction of strategic planning and the agency's human, financial, and information resources.
4. Effectively engage community partners in developing local public health systems for community health improvement and community preparedness initiatives. Rapidly access peer and coaching resources that may assist in developing leadership skills for addressing and resolving problems and issues that challenge local health official.

Competency 3 clearly involves management competencies. Competencies 1 and 2 require both management and leadership activities. Competencies 4 and 5 are leadership competencies. What this means is that public health administrators have to do both management and leadership activities to carry out their jobs effectively. The cautionary consideration is that some people are great managers and some are great leaders. Bringing the two sets of talents and skills together may not always be possible.

MATRIX ORGANIZATIONS IN PUBLIC HEALTH

In recent years, there have been discussions about the difficulties of working in traditional hierarchical organizations. The concept of a silo has been used to reflect what goes on in vertical organizations when programmatic units become insulated from other programs in an organization or agency. There have also been discussions about changes in the way work is done in the public sector. Goldsmith and Eggers have discussed these issues in a governance by network model.[19] We are seeing the rise of third-party government where agencies contract with private firms and nonprofit organizations to do the work of government. There are also linked government activities where partnerships are created between two or more governmental entities to provide an integrated approach to delivering public programs. Changes in technology are also affecting our work relations in that it is possible to work on common projects from great distances using the Internet. Friedman described this process as evidence of a flattening world.[20] Goldsmith and Eggers also described consumer demand and the possibilities of customized service models in the future. Governmental employees involved in these new initiatives will find that the way they work will change. Instead of supervising employees in the agency, these new managers will find themselves managing portfolios of projects being done outside their home agency.

With these changes possible, it becomes necessary to change our agencies as well. One model builds on the matrix form of management with the goal of leveling the organization to be more project or goal focused using techniques for coordinating activities across projects. Robbins and Coulter have defined a horizontal matrix structure as a form of organizational model involving program specialists from various functional units in an organization to work on a multidisciplinary team to carry out a project- or goal-based program.[21] Both management and leadership activities take place in a matrix form of organization. **Figure 1-2** graphically shows a sample matrix structure model. The model labels each unit as a portfolio to reflect that the project or goal approach will allow the individual unit to manage all parts of a project or

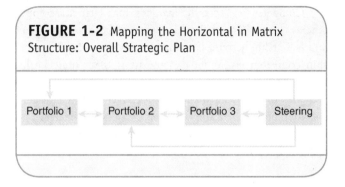

FIGURE 1-2 Mapping the Horizontal in Matrix Structure: Overall Strategic Plan

projects related to the unit program. The role of the steering committee is to be a group that includes a representative of each project or goal unit to supervise the whole project and to prioritize all the projects and goals of the organization.[22] The steering committee can also be the manager of the overall strategic plan of the organization.

On the positive side, this organizational model is flexible and allows for projects and goals to be added or subtracted as appropriate. This model also allows new projects to draw on the talents and strengths of people in the agency who will help benefit a specific project. Each unit staff also requires that both management and leadership processes happen. Creativity in the developing of new projects or subprojects will also be encouraged. There are also difficulties with the design. First, the matrix model is often superimposed on a traditional vertical organization. What this does is complicate the processes and work of the organization. On the one hand, the programmatic silos continue to exist at the same time as the matrix units are developed. The challenge then becomes how to have the silo teams buy into the matrix units' projects and goals. Marketing within the organization needs to be done to support the matrix structures.

There may also be control and communication difficulties with the model as well as resistance to the design by the established vertical organization. Some staff of the agency sometimes believe that they have two bosses and have to report to their silo supervisor as well as the team leader of the matrix unit. There is also the issue of power and the difficulty to share power. Credibility and trust issues also have to be addressed. There are possible methods for addressing some of these silo concerns. Lencioni has delineated a four-part model for this.[23] The model, if addressed early, may prevent some of the resistance to a project- or goal-based horizontal matrix model. There needs to be a clear vision for the agency that is shared by all of the silo directors serving as a leadership team for the agency. Agency goals also need to be determined. These goals are then translated into clearly defined objectives or projects that can evolve into matrix units

around these objectives or projects. These objectives then need to be aligned to standard operational requirements. Finally, there needs to be a methodology for measuring the results of the agency's activities and programs.

STARFISH ORGANIZATIONS IN PUBLIC HEALTH

In traditional organizations, an organization dies if its major reason for existence is gone. Brafman and Beckstrom use the analogy of a spider when you cut off its head.[24] However, when you cut off one of the limbs of a starfish, it grows a new limb. The starfish model is an example of a completely decentralized organization where no specific person is in charge. Rather, all the participants share in the leadership of the organization. Offices may exist in different places, depending on the project, which means that information and knowledge management may also be decentralized. Power is also distributed. Funding is mostly project or program based. Roles and responsibilities change as projects diversify. All people are equal in the core. Decisions about the organization as a whole are made by all participants as core members of the organization. Individuals may be hired for a specific project or program and leave when the project is over.

Figure 1-3 depicts the starfish model. Some public health academic units, such as research, academic, or satellite

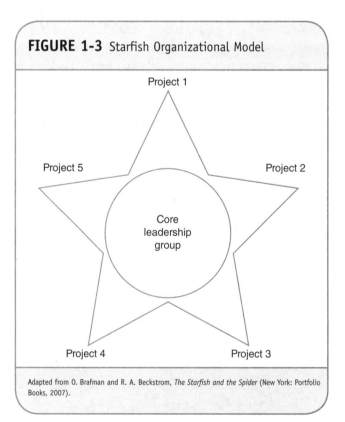

FIGURE 1-3 Starfish Organizational Model

Project 1

Project 5

Project 2

Core leadership group

Project 4

Project 3

Adapted from O. Brafman and R. A. Beckstrom, *The Starfish and the Spider* (New York: Portfolio Books, 2007).

agency centers, may use this organizational model. The core leadership group may be a group of researchers with a common multidisciplinary research perspective like public health systems research or center for public health practice. Because the center is probably funded primarily through grants and contracts, each limb represents one of these projects. The staff of the project includes several core researchers, academics, or practitioners and staff funded by the grant or contract. When the project is over, project staff leave or move to another project. The core staff stay and look for new grants or contracts.

For a comparison of the different public health organizational models presented, **Table 1-2** shows the differences in the traditional hierarchy, a transitional model not specifically presented previously, the matrix model, and the starfish model. Structurally, we have looked at these models from centralized to decentralized. More centralized organizations tend to be focused operationally in more of a linear way than a systems way. The more decentralized an organization, the more systems based or complexity oriented it is. Hierarchical organizations tend to be more authoritarian and tend to move toward being more democratic as the organization begins to move toward fewer organizational levels in a transition from hierarchy to matrix. The management focus tends to be on the organization and less on the people. People management becomes more important in the transition model and the other decentralized models.

THE MANAGEMENT AND LEADERSHIP CONTINUUM

This chapter argues that there is an association between management and leadership. This relationship becomes even more complicated when we look at the issue of transactional leadership and transformational leadership, where the management role seems to vanish altogether. Most discussions about leadership concern vision and change. Burns has pointed out that leadership is also about reciprocity.[25]

Through the development of relationships between partners with varying perspectives on values and motivation, the partners are often in conflict and competition in relation to the overarching goals, which should bring the leaders together to realize their goals and to work together to reach these goals. Moreover, these goals are influenced by the realities of the environment or communities in which these leaders come together.

Burns defined two critical types of leadership: transactional and transformational.[26] The transactional leader engages others in the reciprocal activity of exchanging one thing for another. Most management and leadership activities are related to the exchange of one thing for another. Transformational leadership examines and searches for the needs and motives of others while seeking a higher agenda of needs. Transformational relationships are intense and raise the participants to a higher level of mutuality and morality so that the interaction between leaders or between leaders and followers changes both parties. From these definitions, it can be argued that both transactional and transformational skills are important for leaders. They are complementary types of skill. Transformational leadership demands higher level negotiation activities and leads to change at both the organization and systems levels.

The attempt to put the concept of transactional leadership into action has led to a reinterpretation of this type of leadership as a reconceptualization of management. The exchange of work for various types of rewards seems tied to the organization where there is an attempt to maintain the

TABLE 1-2 Comparison of Several Organizational Issues in Public Health

	Hierarchy	Transition	Matrix	Starfish
Leadership style	Authoritarian	Democratic	Democratic	Shared
Leadership practice	Focus on the organization	Focus on the organization	Internal and external focus	External focus
Leadership thinking preference	Linear	Linear	Systems	Complexity
Primary administrative organization	Management focus	Management focus	Partial management and partial leadership focus	Shared leadership
Structure	Centralized	Partially centralized	Partially decentralized	Decentralize

stability of the organization. Transformational leadership seems to be more about change. **Table 1-3** demonstrates how these two leadership concepts are viewed today and also puts managers in the leadership camp.[27] In recognizing that public health leaders need to transform the public health system in which they work and also change the understanding and commitment to the work of public health with their internal and external partners, the National Public Health Leadership Development Network had to define the characteristics and competencies of a transformational leader.[28] The three major activities of the public health transformational leader involve the skills necessary to engage in the development of mission and vision as well as the development of skills related to monitoring and facilitating the process of change.

In order to begin to clarify distinctions between management and leadership, it is possible to begin this dialogue by creating a continuum from management to leadership.

Figure 1-4 does this by putting management at the left side of the continuum and covering traditional management processes. Transactional leadership is at the center of the continuum and blends traditional management with the reciprocity concerns discussed by the Gallup organization in its look at great managers. It is with transactional leadership that we can begin to see the interface between management and leadership. Transformational leadership and its change and vision agenda are on the extreme right side of the continuum. Most leaders need to have both transactional and transformational talents and skills.

In order to put this leadership continuum in a clearer perspective, the continuum can be viewed as a leadership change triangle in which change affects the way a leader will function. Two other forms of leadership practice need to be added to the continuum. Managerial leadership is a transitional phase in which the public health professional

TABLE 1-3   Transactional vs. Transformational Leadership: Differences between Managing and Leading

	Transactional Leadership or Management Skills	**Transformational Leadership or Leadership Skills**
Performance:	Considered by leadership writers to produce ordinary performance	Considered by leadership writers to produce extraordinary performance.
Goal:	To maintain the status quo by playing within the rules	To change the status quo by changing the rules
Goals arise out of:	Necessity, are reactive, and respond to ideas; they are deeply embedded in the organization's history and culture	Desires; they are active, shaping ideas; may be a departure from organization's history and culture
Emphasis:	Rationality and control, limits choices, focuses on solving problems	Innovation, creativity to develop fresh approaches to long-standing problems, and open issues to new options
Attitudes toward goals:	Impersonal, if not passive, attitude	Personal and active attitude
Incentives:	Based on exchange of needs (i.e., "tit for tat")	Based on the greater good
Locus of reward:	Maximize personal benefits	Optimize systemic benefits
Requires:	Persistence, tough-mindedness, hard work, intelligence, analytical ability, tolerance, and goodwill	Genius and heroism
View work as:	Enabling processes, ideas, and people to establish strategies and make decisions	Creative, energizing, and emerging
Tactics employed:	Negotiate and bargain, use of rewards, punishment, and other forms of coercion	Inspire followers, create shared vision, motivate
	Strive to convert win-lose into win-win situations as part of the process of reconciling differences among people and maintaining balances of power	Strive to create new situations and new directions without regard to reconciling groups or power

Reproduced from Robertson, T. D., Fernandez, C. S. P., and Porter, J. E., "Leadership in Public Health," in Novick, L. F., Morrow, C. B., and Mays, G. P. (eds.), *Public Health Administration*, 2nd ed. (Sudbury, MA: Jones & Bartlett, 2007).

FIGURE 1-4 The Leadership Change Triangle

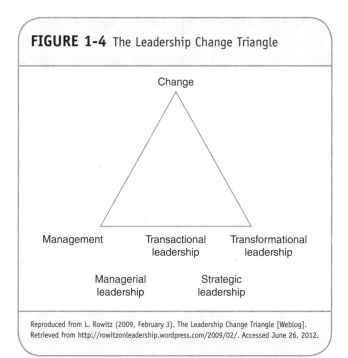

blends the skills of management with the transactional skills of people development. Strategic leadership blends the needs of making transformational change work strategically in the interface between choosing the right people to help in transformational and systems change. Leaders need to learn when to use their management skills and when to use their various leadership skills. In change, leaders need to work within their home organizations and externally with their various stakeholders. Transformational and systems change must be translated into action through transactional relationships and eventually to application at the organizational level.

THE PUBLIC HEALTH MANAGEMENT AND LEADERSHIP ROAD MAP

Now it is necessary to put the management and leadership puzzle together. By adapting the Gallup Path to the governmental sector and adding the leadership dimension as well, it is possible to develop a public health management and leadership road map such as that shown in **Figure 1-5**.[29] Because public health has strong roots in the community,

FIGURE 1-5 Management and Leadership Road Map in Public Health

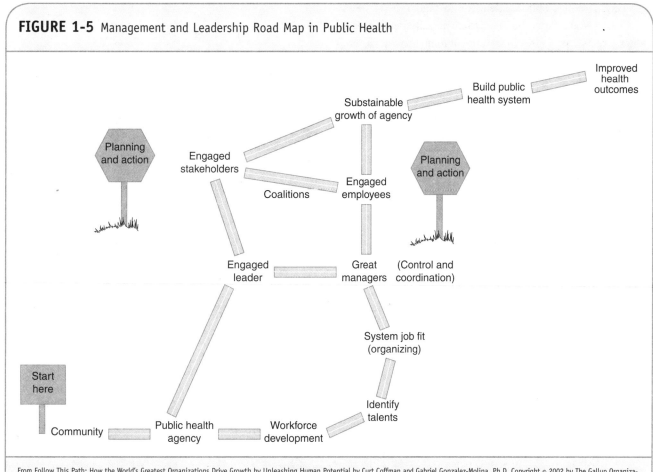

it is important to look at the context of public health as the starting point in our understanding of how the work of public health is accomplished. The public health agency becomes the coordinating organization from which to view the public health system and the specific activities of public health. The leader who is engaged is one who is able to work outside the agency with stakeholders from the political realm as well as from other sectors to improve the health of the public. This high level of planning, negotiation, and action is tied to the role of the public health administrator leader in the transformational leadership role. The public health leader is often engaged in these activities as a major part of the job of promoting the public's health. Because of the time-intensive nature of these activities, the leader often has to rely on engaged managers in the agency to carry out the day-to-day activities of the agency itself. In some instances and especially in smaller health departments, the leader may also have to carry out the activities of the manager as well.

The development of the public health workforce within the agency is often the responsibility of management. Following the work of the Gallup organization on talents, the manager has to be able to identify the talents of workers and fit those talents within the system requirements of the agency and its programs.[30] In traditional management jargon, this involves the organizing function of management. The excellent and great managers also have control and coordination responsibilities. These managers also have to engage the agency employees in the work of the agency so that they understand the vision of the agency leadership. The management staff and the engaged employee have to interact on planning and action protocols as well because this is often a team effort.

As the leader continues to work with external stakeholders, engaged employees get to work with other staff of the engaged stakeholder groups in coalitions and other groups to carry out the specific tasks necessary to help the public improve its health status. If these leadership and management tasks are carried out well, there should be sustainable growth of both the public health agency and its community partners. With this growth, the infrastructure of public health and the public health system as a whole will be strengthened. The outcome of all these activities will be improved health outcomes in the community being served.

THE LEADER'S TOOLKIT

Many public health managers and leaders have been asked by the author about the availability of tools to help them become more effective administrators and collaborators. Administrators often come to workshops and seminars looking for tools,

exercises, books, articles, drills, and tabletop simulations to add to their personal toolkits or resources to use in their agencies or with external stakeholders. This section explores tools for use by public health managers and leaders. Tools are resources that help leaders carry out the work of public health or health related endeavors. These tools can be used in multiple ways. For example, a tool can enhance the linear activities of an agency that uses tools that follow a number of steps, such as planning, conflict resolution, problem-solving, and decision-making tools. The tools of a public health leader may include the following categories:

1. Core functions and essential public health services
2. Community assessment tools
3. Assurance and program evaluation tools
4. Program development tools
5. Performance management tools
6. National Performance Standards
7. Motivation tools
8. Collaboration tools
9. Policy and law tools
10. Nominal group process and other related tools
11. Idea mapping tools
12. Strategic planning tools
13. Action planning tools
14. Quality improvement tools
15. Community and culture-building tools and methods

EXERCISE 1-2 Building a Public Health Leadership Toolkit

Purpose: to begin the process of building a public health leadership toolkit

Key Concepts: leadership tools

Procedure: Each student in the class will pick one of the 17 leadership tool categories. If there are more than 17 participants, start the selection process again. Over the next week, research your category and find five specific tools related to the category selected. Write a one-to-two page discussion of the tool, how to use it, and an example related to its use. At the next class session, present your list. List your five tools on a newsprint page related to your category. Someone can volunteer to compile the paper discussions of the tools of all students into a tool manual for all the students in the class.

16. *Creativity and idea generation tools*
17. Storytelling tools and templates

Each of these categories of tools have numerous books and articles written about them. **Exercise 1-2** involves the building of a personal leadership toolkit.

SUMMARY

This chapter has addressed the complex relationship between management and leadership. The functions of leaders and managers are clearly different even though it is necessary for leaders and managers to work together. In smaller jurisdictions, public health administrators will have to be both manager and leader. However, this marriage is not an easy one because the role of manager/leader requires multiple sets of skills. The individual may have the talent to carry out one set of skills better than the other. It is important for the individual to understand his or her personal strengths and fit his or her talents to the needs of the organization in its current state of development. The chapter also begins a discussion related to the development of a leadership toolkit.

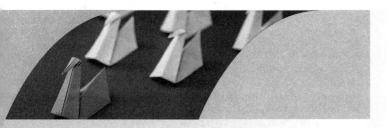

Discussion Questions

1. What are the differences between management and leadership?

2. Do you think it is possible to be a great manager and a leader at the same time?

3. What are the differences between working in the governmental and business sectors?

4. Distinguish between hierarchy, matrix, and starfish organizations.

5. What are the relationships among traditional management, transactional leadership, and transformational leadership?

6. What are organizational silos, and how can communication between these silos be improved?

7. Give examples of how the public health management and leadership road map might work.

8. How will you develop your leadership toolkit?

REFERENCES

1. M. Buckingham, *Go Put Your Strengths to Work* (New York: Free Press, 2007).
2. J. H. Fleming and J. Asplund, *Human Sigma* (New York: Gallup Press, 2007).
3. G. Browning, *Emergenetics* (New York: HarperCollins, 2006).
4. C. Cherniss and D. Goleman, *The Emotionally Intelligent Workplace* (San Francisco: Jossey-Bass, 2001).
5. M. Buckingham and D. O. Clifton, *Now, Discover Your Strengths* (New York: Free Press, 2001).
6. Browning, *Emergenetics*.
7. H. Fayol, *General and Industrial Management* (London: Pittman Publishing, 1949).
8. S. P. Robbins and M. Coulter, *Management*, 11th ed. (Upper Saddle River, NJ: Prentice-Hall, 2011).
9. R. Wagner and J. K. Harter, *12: The Elements of Great Managing* (New York: Gallup Press, 2006).
10. P. F. Drucker, *The Essential Drucker* (New York: Harper Business, 2001).
11. Fayol, *General and Industrial Management*.
12. Robbins and Coulter, *Management*, 11th ed.
13. P. H. Daly and M. Watkins, *The First 90 Days in Government* (Cambridge, MA: Harvard Business School Publishing, 2006).
14. M. H. Moore, *Creating Public Value* (Cambridge, MA: Harvard University Press, 1995).
15. Daly and Watkins, *The First 90 Days in Government*.
16. M. D. Watkins, "Picking the Right Transition Strategy," *Harvard Business Review 87*, no. 1(2009): 49–53.
17. B. J. Turnock and L. Rowitz, *NACCHO New Local Health Official Orientation Curriculum: Final Design* (Washington, DC: National Association of County and City Health Officials, 2007).
18. Turnock and Rowitz, *NACCHO New Local Health Official Orientation Curriculum*.
19. S. Goldsmith and W. D. Eggers, *Governing by Network* (Washington, DC: Brookings Institution Press, 2004).
20. T. L. Friedman, *The World Is Flat* (New York: Farrar, Straus, and Giroux, 2006).
21. Robbins and Coulter, *Management*, 11th ed.
22. P. Martin, *Quick Guide: The New Matrix Management* (Carmel, NY: Martin Training Associates, 2005).
23. P. Lencioni, *Silos, Politics, and Turf Wars* (San Francisco: Jossey-Bass, 2006).
24. Martin, *Quick Guide: The New Matrix Management*.
25. O. Brafman and R. A. Beckstrom. *The Starfish and the Spider* (New York: Portfolio Books, 2007).
26. J. MacGregor Burns, *Leadership* (New York: Harper and Row, 1978).
27. Burns, *Leadership*.
28. T. D. Robertson, C. S. P. Fernandez, and J. E. Porter, "Leadership in Public Health," in L. E. Novick, C. B. Morrow, and G. P. Mays (eds.), *Public Health Administration*, 2nd ed. (Sudbery, MA: Jones & Bartlett, 2007).
29. C. Coffman and G. Gonzalez-Molina, *Follow This Path* (New York: Warner Business Books, 2002).
30. Buckingham and Clifton, *Now, Discover Your Strengths*

CHAPTER **2**

Public Health and Adaptive Leadership

Many of the leadership books I have read over the past 25 years have taken unrealistic views of the world in which leaders live. Not all leadership activities lead to successful outcomes. The culture of organizations differs. A leader may use his or her skills more effectively in some organizations than in others. Agencies may or may not be responsive to the needs of the communities that they serve. State agencies look for uniform rules and regulations for all counties and local areas in their state rather than recognize the diversity of specific communities and their demographics. For example, a county's population may consist of 60 percent or more of people over 65 years of age. The state may require extensive development of programs for mothers and children and no priority or funding for programs for seniors. County or local health departments may be seen as successful locally but not successful according to the rules and regulations at the state level. In addition, as can be seen in the next story, politics often creates complications related to the outbreak of a public health problem. **Public Health Heroes and Villains 2-1** involves a milk contamination case with both heroes and villains (names are changed in story).

There are lessons to be learned in this case scenario. Pfeffer[3] noted that the results of many community problem-solving efforts are not positive. A leader's efforts to address an organization might not lead to a positive outcome. Much is dependent on the culture of the organization, the perceptions and reactions to the leader by employees of the organization, competition for status within the organization, and the ability of the organization and the leadership to gain trust and acceptance from the community that the organization serves. Leaders need to be realistic about their organizational and community impact. Although context is important, the presentation of public health information to our constituencies is also a critical variable.[4] One negative aspect in the milk contamination case was the delay in relaying important public health information to the population of Midwest state.

In order to increase our chances for public health victories, it is necessary to be aware of principles that we have learned from a realistic view of public health. Here is a list of some of these principles:

1. Learn from the experiences of other leaders.
2. Not all team members do the work.
3. It is managers who make leadership work.
4. Most people do not change. The weaknesses remain. Play to workers' strengths.
5. Lists and steps don't solve but can guide actions that are process based.
6. There are always unanticipated consequences to any public health outbreak event.
7. Talent and competency guide action. Talent can be enhanced but not taught.

PUBLIC HEALTH HEROES AND VILLAINS 2-1   Politics and Salmonella[1,2]

In the late 1980s, a number of salmonella cases were reported to a local health department in Midwest state. A communicable disease investigator in Maple Tree County reported four cases of salmonella infections that were seen at Maple Memorial Hospital. Several more cases were reported over the next several days in other counties. No major investigations were done over the next 4 months because a scattering of salmonella cases was not unusual. Then, 70 new cases were reported from the same counties. The largest city in the area with a local health department began an epidemiological investigation. A number of the people with the infection seemed to have shopped at the same supermarket in the area. The supermarket was inspected by food and dairy inspectors from the Midwest Department of Public Health. No new information was forthcoming and the state investigation was closed.

Several months later, cluster reports were received by the Midwest Department of Public Health Regional Center. These cases were linked to contaminated milk from Lakewood Dairy. The dairy was contacted by the state health department's food and dairy program. The state laboratory began to receive unopened milk cartons from local supermarkets. Cases were increasing over the next couple of months. The state laboratory confirmed that the milk was contaminated. The Food and Drug Administration (FDA) worked with the state to confirm the results of the investigation. Eventually, the dairy closed the plant. Over 200,000 cases were confirmed from the various outbreaks in Midwest state and around the nation.

This salmonella crisis was clearly a major one that lasted several months. Many public health professionals played critical roles during the process of dealing with the crisis and not only did these public health professionals act as leaders, they also fit our classification of public health heroes. The FDA, Centers for Disease Control and Prevention, Midwest state, and social public health people worked together to find the cause of the crisis. However, partisan politics complicated the process. Legislative hearings were held. The three-term Republican governor (Governor McNally) was blamed by the Democrats for the poor handling of the investigation. It was after all an election year and the governor was planning to run for an unprecedented fourth term. It did not help that the director of the Midwest Department of Public Health was on vacation in Mexico during the height of the investigation. Another factor was that Director Gohon Tripp was not a physician (our villain). The governor fired Director Tripp and told Tripp that he should have been home monitoring the outbreak. Both the governor and the director were seen as the villains in the case. The governor tried to defuse the political problems that ensued from the outbreak by naming an excellent public health physician well known both in Midwest state and the nation as the new director. Dr. Brian Turnkey, a Democrat and our hero, was well received by both political parties. Dr. Turnkey criticized the legislature for not providing enough funds to monitor outbreak events. The legislature provided the necessary funds for the state health department to be able to communicate disease information to local health departments. A report was issued by the state legislative committee argued that the state health department under Director Tripp had mishandled the outbreak.

What could or should have been done differently? What were the leadership issues?

B. J. Turnock, *Public Health: What It Is and How It Works*, 6th ed. (Burlington, MA: Jones & Bartlett Learning, 2015); and personal communication, Tom Shaffer.

8. Politics will inevitably affect public health events.
9. Not all leaders look or act the same.
10. No matter how good a job we do we can still lose our jobs.
11. Training does not give you all the answers or the ability to solve real-world problems.
12. Don't expect politicians, elected or appointed officials, or the public to value what public health leaders do.
13. Resilience is the secret weapon of successful leaders.
14. Public health workers do not want change and they use budget shortfalls and time constraints to justify their resistance.
15. Increasing age is not a good reason to dump professionals and other good workers on the trash heap.

Many leaders have found that reading biographies and autobiographies of leaders has helped them see leadership in action in a number of different career tracks. For example, an excellent biography of President Thomas Jefferson shows that he was an excellent leader in multiple roles: as writer of the Declaration of Independence, Governor of Virginia, Secretary of State in the Washington Administration, third President of the United States, and in retirement as one of the founders of the University of Virginia.[5] In spite of all these accomplishments, Jefferson was not always successful. He kept slaves and he had a slave mistress for many years with whom he had a number of offspring.

Another excellent tool or strategy for seeing the real face of leadership falls in the family of coaching or mentoring technique. Shadowing involves following a leader for a period of time to explore how a leader practices leadership on a daily basis. The shadow needs to see leadership in action. It is important to shadow leaders in public health as well as leaders in other fields. The leader must agree to be followed because the shadow may be seen to interfere with the actions going on or stifle the way the leader and his or her direct reports respond to key activities and processes. The leader should communicate with staff about why the shadow is present. The shadow needs to be introduced and to tell the staff about himself or herself and possible personal goals for the future. During the postshadowing conference the leader becomes a coach to better help the shadow understand why certain decisions were made and what are the leadership lessons to be learned.

The leader should be careful not to let the shadow affect the way events happen or change leadership techniques as a result of being followed. The leader needs to allow the shadow to talk to direct reports to gain a wider perspective on how leadership works in the organization. A 360-degree perspective as is used in a number of leadership inventories is also useful in shadowing. A 360-degree inventory involves a prospective leader filling out a leadership profile and other individuals evaluating the leader using the same instrument. Examples of questions that a shadow might use in a postshadowing conference include the following:

1. What are the five events today that you think might provide the best leadership lessons?
2. Would you also tell us about the following actions today and why they occurred and the leadership lessons to be learned?
3. Were there any failures in action today?
4. What is your primary leadership style and when does it work best and when the least?
5. What do you do to improve your own leadership skills?
6. (For direct reports) How do you perceive the way your boss responded to particular events today?

Exercise 2-1 gives you the chance to shadow a leader.

EXERCISE 2-1   Follow the Leader

Purpose: to learn about how public health leaders works in the real world

Key Concepts: shadowing, leadership, direct reports, tools and strategies, health department

Procedure: Select a public health professional in a leadership position to shadow for a day. Meet with the leader and his direct reports to discuss why you are there. Follow your chosen leader for a day. At the end of the day, meet with your leader and his or her direct reports and discuss some of the questions in the shadowing discussion in this chapter. At your next class meeting, discuss your experiences with your leader. Finally, write a two-page summary of your shadowing experience and what you learned about leadership.

ECOLOGICAL LEADERSHIP

Ecological leaders are committed to the development of their leadership skills and competencies throughout their professional careers while at the same time being committed to the appropriate applications of these skills within their organizations and communities. These leaders practice within the context of adapting to changing environments. Ecology involves an integration of biology and sociology. The ecological view is a systems view that has become extremely complex over the centuries. Diamond[6] has studied the development of human beings and our relationship to our environment over the last 30,000 years. Our development has evolved from hunting and gathering in small groups and then discovering and developing into bigger and bigger groups with the development of cities. As human groupings become larger and larger, germs lead to diseases that often spread quickly in large populations.

The complexity of life thus creates an interrelationship between humans, other animals, plants, and germs. As life becomes more complex and systemic, leadership grows more complex. Allen and her collaborators have pointed out that leadership needs to be seen in many different social and biological systems that are interdependent and also mutually influence each other.[7] With complexity, social structure also gets complicated. Agencies and organizations become more specialized. With this increasing complexity, leaders must understand not only these complex relationships but also their interconnections and environmental context. Constant change is also part of the process. Allen and her colleagues pointed out that there are four principles of ecological leadership.[8] First, interdependence emerges from systemic processes. The second principle involves the open system in which we work and how information gets back to the leader. Communication skills are clearly important for leaders. Third, agencies and other public health organizations require leadership processes that build the capacity of both individuals and groups. The fourth principle is that leaders use techniques and

strategies that will influence the system rather than controlling the system. Our goal is the development of health communities that promote a culture of health. **Figure 2-1** takes the next step in looking at ecological leadership. An ecological conceptual model looks at the impact on leadership for five system components: Living with Environmental Limits, Developing the Wisdom and Ethics to Respond to Scientific Discoveries, Transforming Information into Knowledge and Wisdom (Implementation), Developing the Capacity to Adapt to Changes in Social Ecology, and Globalization of Perspective.

FIGURE 2-1 Conceptual Model of the Adaptive Challenges and Their Implications for Leadership Processes

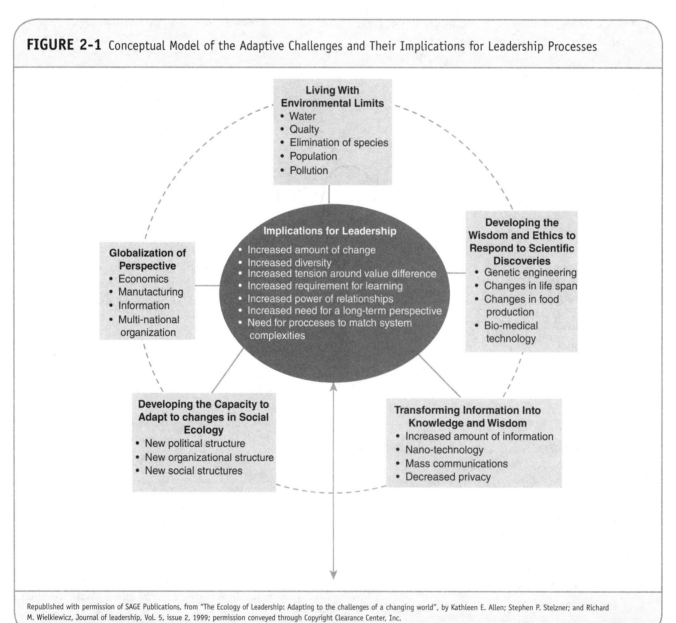

Six premises undergird an ecological approach to leadership.[9] First, leadership needs to be seen as an emergent process that comes from the interactions and adaptive actions of leaders within an agency or community context. Second, there is a necessary balance between the public health core function and essential public health services perspective and the ecological perspective if adaptation is to occur. Third, a culture of health process occurs with leaders engaged in a complex set of interdependent social and biological open systems. Adaptive challenges are affected significantly by the ecological system. Fourth, leaders require as much up-to-date health information as possible if adaptive change is to occur. Leaders also need feedback to influence community health-related issues. This premise also argues that empowering public health employees will help to increase organizational effectiveness. Conflicting feedback loops associated with public health core functions and essential services can interfere with adaptation. The fifth premise deals with diversity and the organization's need to reconcile the potential tension that can occur between the need for human and social diversity and the ability to address a common set of goals and objectives relative to all. Public health workers must believe that they are supported by the organization if they are to show loyalty and commitment to effective performance. The final premise is that leadership processes should be evaluated relative to response on long-term challenges.

Many leadership theories have an ecological component. For this text, ecological leadership is the mindset that guides our adaptive leadership practice. Using this model, we can view a number of leadership approaches as subsets of an ecological approach to leadership. Ecological leaders are committed to the development of their personal talents, leadership skills, and competencies throughout their professional careers while at the same time being committed to the appropriate application of these skills in the changing public healthcare needs of their communities. **Table 2-1** is a beginning of an exploration of the leadership subsets that we will need to address as we deal with emerging public health issues now and in the future. The leader of the future will integrate and work from a number of different skill orientations to effectively address the unexpected events that will guide our public health and other human service priorities. Skill development is cumulative and interactive.

LEADERSHIP IN PRACTICE

The ecological approach to leadership is the foundation for the following discussion. Theory gives us an approach to give our practice activities meaning. In 2007, I was a representative of the Public Health Practice Council, which was a council of the Association of Schools of Public Health. This council was composed of practice faculty of all schools of public health. One of the activities of the council was to define public health practice. Public health practice was defined as the application of public health science to the delivery of services at the community level. Public health practitioners use the paradigm of core functions and essential public health services to guide their practice activities. The performance of the functions and services will lead to improvements in the health of the public. The interventions that are used need to be evidence based. Our overall vision is to create a culture of health in all our communities. The realization of this vision will involve many technical and adaptive challenges that will require leadership to bring this vision into reality at the technical and adaptive challenge level. Thus, ecological leadership is our theory of action and adaptive leadership activities.

Adaptive leaders are individuals who motivate and mobilize others to confront tough challenges and overcome them.[10] Public health involves an ever-changing landscape in which there is constant change. The Boston Consulting Group[11] defines the four dimensions of adaptive leadership. First, the leader needs to manage the environment(agency) in which his or her collaborators interact. This is very important because of uncertainty or changing health conditions. Many different techniques will be needed if traditional approaches do not work. Shared leadership will often need to be used because of the complexity of the adaptive challenges. Leaders will need to constantly raise questions because adaptive leaders look outside the organization to realign their agencies in light of the changes in the community and elsewhere.

Second, the adaptive leader is an influencer. In order to be a successful influencer, the leader requires empathy. The adaptive leader should instill a sense of purpose in others. In public health, others need to believe that improving the health of the public is possible and that a culture of health can be created. Third, the adaptive leader realizes that experimentation will be required if solutions are to be found for adaptive challenges. This experimentation will be necessary for both individuals and teams. Failures may occur and these failures need to be learning experiences and not punishable. Organizations must become agile and able to change quickly. Agile organizations are more likely to be organized in a matrix model rather than a hierarchical one. The final

TABLE 2-1   Ecological Leadership Subsets and Leadership Skill Areas[12]

Leadership Subsets	Skill Areas	Leadership Subsets	Skill Areas
Managerial Leadership	Hierarchical Structures	Crisis Leadership	Risk and Crisis Communication
	Matrix Structures		Tipping Point Awareness
	Portfolio Management		Forensic Epidemiology
	Coaching, Mentoring		Pandemic Influenza Planning
	Developing Others		Consequence Management
	Team Building		After Action Planning
	Mission/Vision		Change Strategies
	Problem Solving		Community Rebuilding
	Decision Making		Connectivity
	Reengineering/Reinvention	Cross-Sector Leadership	Leading Across Silos
	Collaboration		Transdisciplinary Skills
	Coalition/Partnership Development		Values Integration
	Communication Skills		Goal Alignment
	Assessing the Environment		Boundary Spanning
Transactional Leadership	Creating Clarity		Multidimensional Problem Solving
	Sharing Power and Influence		Conflict Management
	Building Trust		Strategic Planning
	Developing People for Teamwork		Stakeholder Analysis
	Self-Reflection	Synergistic Leadership	
	Systems Thinking		Policy Analysis
	Analyzing Archetypes	Strategic Leadership	Futures Orientation
	Adaptive Change		Analytic Skills
	Quality Improvement		Social Network Analysis
Systems Leadership	Complexity Analysis		Partner Diversification
	Learning Organization		Web 2.0
	Scenario-Building		Systems Transformation
	Theory U		Adaptive Leadership
	Presencing	Synergistic Leadership	Sector Integration to Increase Value
Emergency Preparedness and Response	Types of Crises		Collaborative Learning
			Culture Change Agent
	Community Readiness		Thinking Skills
	Family Safety		Paradigm Busting
	Resilience	Transformational Leadership	Resistance to Status Quo
	Emergency Recovery Strategies		Strong Communication Skills
	Mitigation		Varied Change Models
	Social Change		Collaboration for Policy Change
	Public Health Law/Ethics	Global Health Leadership	Communication Across Cultures
			Understand International Health Law Regulations

dimension involves success for leaders and their partners. Adaptive leaders try to extend their influence outside their agency to the whole community. Not only do adaptive leaders want to extend their impact to the ecosystem that they serve, but they also want to create social and cultural change (social ecology) that will lead to a culture of health model for their communities.

If adaptive leadership creates change in our communities, it is necessary to put together a series of adaptive leadership tools to help in these activities. The adaptive leadership toolkit recognizes that adaptive leaders need to consider many different levels in the change process. Some of these considerations include:[13]

1. Personal understanding of the leader's role in different phases of the adaptive leadership process
2. Understanding of individual activities and leadership team activities within the agency
3. The culture of the agency in addressing change
4. The way the agency works and its outcome at the tactical and the adaptive level
5. The extent to which staff are engaged

The tools and tactics of adaptive leadership need to be built upon a systems view of change.[14] The adaptive leadership categories include a journey through the diagnosis of the system, system mobilization, the leadership system perspective, and the necessity of a leader integrating himself or herself in the adaptive challenge activities. The adaptive leadership process then involves observation of events, interpretation of those events, and finally problem solving to determine the interventions needed. Heifetz, Grashow, and Linsky present two techniques to address the adaptive leadership stages.[15] The first tool is named *On the Practice Field*. This tool needs to be with reality-based challenges as observed by others and the provision of feedback related to how the challenge was handled. The second tool is *On the Balcony*, which involves reflective thought about how challenges and their solutions are seen at the systems level. Here there tends to be reflective thinking and discussion on how the challenges were adaptively addressed from an adaptive leadership methodology.

When you attend a class or a workshop, it is beneficial to change your seat after each break or each session. Changing your seat tends to energize you and to give you a fresh perspective on the content being presented. Similarly, leadership decisions are made from different thinking perspectives and different leadership style. Leaders who are very structured and organized will view an adaptive challenge differently from a conceptual or innovative leader. Authoritarian leaders will view the same situation differently from a more democratic leader. Heifetz and Linsky[16] said we view things differently when we are on the dance floor than when we are on the balcony looking down on the dance floor (a systems view). It is possible that there is a second balcony on which complexity issues are addressed. Adaptive leaders must view challenges from multiple perspectives and synthesize the information obtained from these different perspectives into a comprehensive view of their leadership orientation.

Dance floor thinking is more a linear perspective than a systems or complexity approach. When you are acting on the dance floor, you are concerned with detail and the individuals with whom you are interacting. You are concerned with keeping the agency or community in balance and as organized as possible. You are a participant in the action on the dance floor. You concentrate on getting certain technical or adaptive solutions to your leadership challenges. You have key roles to play. You generally are working in a hierarchical agency or other organization. This type of organization, which often has a status quo mindset, feels safe for its employees who resist change even when it is necessary. Working in a programmatic silo also feels safe. You know the rules and generally what is expected of you. If you are promoted to a supervisory position or a higher level leadership position, your perspective and your challenges begin to change. You seem to be leaving the dance floor on a regular basis by going up a few steps to the first balcony. You are still a key player but your job responsibilities undergo a key shift in perspective. You find that being a manager and then a leader requires more of a systems perspective than being on the dance floor.

For the leader on the dance floor, micro knowledge is important.[17] Adaptive leaders need data and other information in order to make dance floor decisions. Micro knowledge does not mean that the leader will have to micromanage the agency. Leaders need to intensively study all the facts related to an adaptive challenge. Once the leader makes a decision, the leader backs off and assigns responsibility for implementing the solution to others. It is in this way that leadership is shared. The adaptive leader requires regular reports on the progress of implementation so that performance measurement becomes possible. With the move toward shared leadership, accountability becomes more critical.

Eventually, it becomes the task of the leader to observe the functioning of activities in several of the programs in the leader's agency. When the leader moves to the first balcony, it becomes necessary to understand how the agency functions systemically, that is, as part of the community. Systems thinking and the big picture now become the modus operandi. A move from a more traditional management orientation to a leadership orientation becomes a requirement for systems thinking and working from the first balcony. Leaders begin to notice the structure of things and how the various units interact. Leaders can look at the dance floor and see how tasks are performed and how implementation of adaptive solutions is progressing or how potential problems disrupt the activities on the dance floor. The leader uses the tools of systems thinkers to analyze events. The systems archetypes discussed by Senge[18] can guide the leader's action. Adaptive leaders will observe events off the dance floor in the hallway and outside the agency. Leaders will then begin to collaborate with outside partners.

There is a second set of steps up to the second balcony. Adaptive solutions and other events and activities appear less structured as the leader moves to the complexity level. The adaptive leadership approach allows the leader to see the mess beyond the structure. The leader needs to work external to the agency. This expansion of relationships will complicate the leader's activities, which will become less predictable. Structures become less permanent and seem to grow out of the newly cultivated relationships. Social networks expand and contract due to increasing social network relationships. Organizations grow and coevolve out of complex agencies and our community as our societies grow more complex. The second balcony can clearly be an exciting place that increases our understanding of the activities on the dance floor and on the first balcony. **Exercise 2-2** allows you the opportunity to experiment with this model to address an adaptive challenge using the balcony tool.

SUMMARY

Too many books, case studies, and reports give us the impression that most leadership practices lead to positive results. This is far from the truth. Leaders will need to learn new skills throughout their professional careers. A number of authors are beginning to write about the realities of leadership. The reality is that we hope to succeed more times than we fail. Failure is not necessarily a negative. We learn from all the processes and outcomes of our work. It is important

---

EXERCISE 2-2 On the Balcony

Purpose: to use adaptive leadership methods to address a public health challenge

Key Concepts: adaptive leadership, adaptive challenge, balcony exercise, systems thinking, complexity thinking

Scenario: In the spring of 2016, three pregnant women entered the emergency room at their local hospital complaining of flulike symptoms. They all had fevers. After an examination with a blood test, they were finally diagnosed with Zika virus. Hospital staff immediately informed the local health department.

Procedure: Shared leadership teams of five to seven people will be put together. They will be given instructions by Dr. Ridgeway (the class or workshop instructor) to meet at the hospital with Director Holmes (a member of the class). The teams are to address the problem of Zika virus in the hospital from three vantage points—the dance floor, the first balcony (system perspective), and the second balcony (complexity perspective). With this information, prepare a verbal plan on what needs to be done to address the Zika challenge. Each team will present its plans to Dr. Ridgeway. What was learned from the exercise?

---

for all young leaders to see how leaders work. The shadowing exercise in this chapter will help you to do that. The milk contamination case demonstrates that there are often heroes and villains in most events. On the theoretical side, the ecological model demonstrates the importance of context for a leader. Public health leadership takes place in an agency and a community, a county, a state, nationally, and internationally. What dance floor you are on will guide your activities. Adaptive leadership is the practice component for the ecological approach to a leadership mindset.

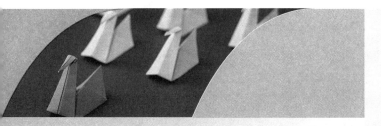

Discussion Questions

1. What are some of the principles that guide a realistic view of public health leaders?

2. In 2016 Vermont has struggled with a major drug problem. How would local public health leaders and the national Drug Enforcement Administration work together to address this adaptive challenge?

3. What is the difference between ecological leadership and adaptive leadership?

4. What are the pros and cons of having a mentor or coach?

5. What are five contemporary public health challenges that might require adaptive leadership?

REFERENCES

1. B. J. Turnock, *Public Health: What It Is and How It Works*, 6th ed. (Burlington, MA: Jones & Bartlett Learning, 2015).
2. Personal communication, Tom Shaffer.
3. J. Pfeffer, *Leadership BS* (New York, NY: Harper Business, 2015).
4. C. Klosterman, *I Wear the Black Hat* (New York, NY: Scribners, 2014).
5. J. Meacham, *Thomas Jefferson: The Art of Power* (New York, NY: Random House, 2012).
6. J. Diamond, *Guns, Germs, and Steel* (New York, NY: W.W, Norton, 1999).
7. K. E. Allen, S. P. Stelzner, and R. M. Wielkiewicz, "The Ecology of Leadership: Adapting to the Challenges of a Changing World," *Journal of Leadership Studies* 5 (1999): 62–68.
8. K. E. Allen, S. P. Stelzner, and R. M. Wielkiewicz, "The Ecology of Leadership: Adapting to the Challenges of a Changing World," *Journal of Leadership Studies* 5 (1999).
9. R. M. Wielkiewicz and S. P. Stelzner, "An Ecological Perspective on Leadership Theory, Research, and Practice," *Review of General Psychology* 9 (2005): 326–334.
10. R. Heifetz, A. Grashow, and M. Linsky, *The Practice of Adaptive Leadership* (Boston, MA: Harvard Business Press, 2009).
11. Boston Consulting Group, "Adaptive leadership," *Perspectives*, 7 (2010). http://www.bcg.com/documents/file67908.pdf. Accessed March 2, 2016.
12. L. Rowitz, *Public Health Leadership: Putting Principles into Practice*, 3rd ed., (Burlington, MA: Jones & Bartlett Learning, 2014).
13. American Public Human Services Association, *Adaptive Leadership Toolkit*, 2015. http://www.slideshare.net/karimmosa927/adaptive-leadership. Accessed March 4, 2016.
14. Heifetz et al., *The Practice of Adaptive Leadership*.
15. Heifetz et al., *The Practice of Adaptive Leadership*.
16. R. A. Heifetz and M. Linsky, *Leadership on the Line* (Boston, MA: Harvard Business School Press).
17. R. M. Gates, *A Passion for Leadership* (New York, NY: Alfred A. Knopf, 2016).
18. P. A. Senge, *The Fifth Discipline* (New York, NY: Doubleday, 2006).

CHAPTER **3**

The Six Levels of Leadership

LEARNING OBJECTIVES

- Describe the six levels of leadership.
- Learn strategies that enhance personal leadership.
- Understand the AIM Leadership Model.
- Determine the reasons and benefits for creating teams.
- Describe the importance of knowledge management.
- Discover how public health leaders work at the community level.
- Understand the factors that help in community building where collaboration exists.
- Master the eight steps in building a coalition.
- Describe how leaders can make a mark on the public health profession.

A leader is a person who inspires others to action and guides their undertakings. These others can be members of a team, employees of an agency, or heads of groups that have formed a coalition, an alliance, or a partnership, for example. In other words, leaders in public health, as in other arenas, operate on different levels. The major difficulty in conceptualizing what leadership is relates to the fact that we live in an ever-changing world that demands that leaders adapt to these changes in a continuous way. Each day leaders face new technical challenges for which solutions must be found. These challenges require more than the usual solutions tied to an authoritative position or to the standard operating procedures of an organization or community. The events of September 11, 2001, show us that the world has changed. Heifetz and Linsky pointed out that these adaptive challenges require solutions that are innovative, perhaps experimental,

and create new forms of adjustment.[1] Adaptive change may require a change in attitude, values, and behavior or a new interpretation of events.

It is also important to understand what entices people into leadership roles. Over the past 25 years, there has been a strong belief that leadership can be taught. Many public health leadership programs have come into being with the goal of training public health professionals to be better leaders with the belief that leadership is one of the key dimensions in building a stronger public health system. Parks has stated that there are important explanations of why people want to be leaders.[2] She calls these explanations "hungers" and discusses five of them as follows:

1. Hunger to contribute and make society better
2. Hunger to be in an authority position
3. Hunger to implement and explore systems issues
4. Hunger to show others how to adapt to change
5. Hunger to demonstrate moral courage on behalf of the "common good"

This chapter first discusses the abilities that public health leaders need at any level, including the personal level (i.e., when dealing with another individual one on one), then goes on to consider the particular abilities and strategies they put to use in heading a team, heading an agency, working on a community collaboration activity, shifting our perspective to the global level, or guiding their profession toward improvement. As we proceed, it is important to remember that each of the six levels of leadership provides a foundation

PUBLIC HEALTH HEROES AND VILLAINS 3-1 Dr. C. Everett Koop, a Public Health Hero

Dr. C. Everett Koop is one of the most well known surgeon generals in U.S. history and also one of the most controversial. In 1982, President Reagan nominated Dr. Koop for the position of surgeon general. It was believed by the administration that the conservative evangelicals who supported Reagan would be happy with the Koop nomination. His conservative prolife credentials upset many in Congress. Many liberal women's groups, medical groups, and public health groups called on Congress not to approve the nomination. Although critics did admit that Dr. Koop was an excellent surgeon, they argued that he did not have appropriate public health credentials or experience.

Once confirmed, Dr. Koop surprised many of his advocates as well as critics. During his tenure, which lasted until 1989, he did not let politics interfere with his work on many public health issues. He showed his leadership abilities in many different areas as he went from one health problem area to another. Tobacco issues ranked high on Koop's public health agenda. He took on the tobacco industry in a fight to have warning labels put on tobacco products. He won. He worked to have smoking prohibited in public buildings and related places. In 1984, he

was able to convince Congress to pass a bill requiring cigarette ads to include the health warning labels. His office issued a report in 1988 pointing to scientific evidence that nicotine was addictive. As of 2016, the impact of Koop's work still continues in the area of prevention of tobacco use.

The Reagan administration was slow to recognize the critical nature of the growing AIDS (acquired immune deficiency syndrome) epidemic. Once he was able, Koop wrote the official policy on AIDS and by the end of 1988, his office sent AIDS information to every household in America. Even though Koop thought the AIDS crisis was an important public health concern, he was criticized by gay activists for the way he targeted gay sex in his comments. Koop did say that the use of condoms was a preventive measure. He did pursue his comments on the crisis in spite of any criticism he might get. This is a clear leadership stance.

Koop also addressed abortion. Although he was antiabortion, he was not willing to say that abortions performed by qualified physicians were a health risk to women who chose to terminate their pregnancies. He supported the rights of newborns and children with disabilities.

for the next level. It is almost like going up a flight of stairs; we need to go up the first stair before going to the second stair. Skipping a stair might trip us up. A very good example of an individual who was able to move between the various leadership levels with very few obvious problems was our next public health hero—the former Surgeon General of the United States, C. Everett Koop.

LEADERSHIP AT THE PERSONAL LEVEL

This section considers some of the prerequisites for being an effective public health leader at any level. These prerequisites include a commitment to social justice, an understanding of democracy, an understanding of the political process, communication skills, mentoring skills, decision-making skills, and the ability to balance work and life outside work. There are at least nine learning strategies that will enhance personal leadership development activities:

1. Lifelong multidisciplinary learning
2. Systems thinking and complexity
3. Reading
4. Exploring the arts
5. Creativity
6. Family–work balance
7. Retreats and reflection
8. Experiential learning
9. Promoting a culture of health for our communities

Values

Public health leaders, to be fully effective, must be committed to the values that characterize public health, especially social justice. However, they should be careful not to let the social justice agenda prevent them from doing the tasks that need to be done. Furthermore, social justice is a broad concept and encompasses a range of different issues. The predominant social justice issue of concern to almost all public health leaders is equity in access to care. However, no consensus exists that, for instance, there should be a radical redistribution of wealth in the society at large.

A commitment to a value such as equity in access to care entails a willingness to challenge the political status quo and act as an advocate for the public health agenda. Leaders are supporters of organizational and community values and should be on the front lines in attempts to make public health practices and policies conform to these values. Leaders also must be at the front line if values need to be changed, modified, or reinterpreted.

Politics and Governance

Public health leaders need to understand the political system of the location in which their activities take place. In this country, they must understand how the American version of democracy works at the local, state, and national levels and how to influence the political process. As an example, the author, on a visit to the office of a public health professional in a state health department, noticed *The Federalist Papers* and de Tocqueville's *Democracy in America* on the shelf. The public health leader said that he often referred to these books for guidance in making decisions.

One question that arises is whether there is a difference between government (or governance, the activity of governing) and politics. Governance, in large part, consists of administering programs and adjusting them to fit policies developed as part of the political process.[3] Unfortunately, these policies are sometimes not founded on the best available evidence but instead reflect the personal concerns (including the desire to get reelected) of the politicians who vote them into existence. Several years ago, I talked to a state legislator about having a school of public health supply data on specific health issues and social determinants of health of interest to the legislator. He refused the offer, because, according to him, he did not need data to make his decisions. (As someone has pointed out, politicians have "spin doctors," whereas government agencies have "spokespeople."[4] That says something about the difference between politics and government.)

Public health agencies are government agencies, and public health leaders are implementers of policies set by politicians. This creates interesting possibilities for a partnership between the political and governmental sectors. Leadership theories often focus exclusively on organizational tasks, such as setting organizational policies and motivating the workforce, but public health leaders should develop the skills necessary for working with elected officials. Their role is to use the values, mission, vision, and goals and objectives of their agency to clarify public health issues and ensure that the policies created to deal with these issues will have a good chance of being effective.

Communication and Empowerment

The AIM Leadership Model is based on the idea that leaders have to learn to take action, learn how to influence the field, and be motivated by the process.[5] According to the model, the five building blocks of effective personal leadership are communication, the empowerment of followers, a focus on key issues, linkage to others, and life balance. Each of these building blocks is affected by leadership style and practices as well as the systems approach to organizational change.

Good communication skills are critical. Effective communication has several aspects, including slowing the thought processes, increasing understanding, testing conclusions, listening constructively, getting to the essence of things, and exploring areas of disagreement.[6] In addition, gender differences, racial or ethnic differences, and age differences can affect whether messages are received as intended.[7] Leaders need to understand all the factors that influence communication so they can synthesize public health information into effective messages.

Leaders, in trying to empower work and community associates, often act as their mentors. Interaction between leaders and constituents is critical,[8] and leaders need to empower "followers" in ways that give them the chance to be more effective as well as to develop their own leadership skills. Followers are themselves people with exceptional talents, and according to one study, 80 percent of the effectiveness of a project is due to the followers and only 20 percent to the leadership (80/20 rule).[9]

Leading and Following

Followers in one situation become leaders in another, and many public health practitioners see themselves in both leadership and follower roles. Public health practitioners who work for public health agencies see themselves as professionals first and even leaders in their profession, but those who are part of a traditional public bureaucracy are frequently expected to be less leaders than followers, which can create a contentious work environment.

Members of a board of health often see themselves as powerful individuals and therefore as natural leaders. Health administrators also see themselves as leaders rather than followers. This may lead to conflict. For example, a health administrator addressing a group of public health professionals in a leadership program said that it was his job to protect board members from gossip and controversies. A local board of health president who was in the training program said that if the health administrator kept information hidden from board members, someone in the community would give them the information instead. Board members need information and lose trust in health administrators who hold back information.

Another board of health president pointed out that the administrator of the health department was his employee, because he could fire the administrator and recommend cutting the local health department budget. This shows how important it is for the board of health members and the public health administrator to develop an understanding that they are partners. In this regard, governance has an important role to play.[10] A governance public health framework should include mechanisms for organizing values, carrying out the public health mission, formulating goals and objectives, developing realistic action plans, resolving conflicting agendas, determining the need for structural change, improving the relationship between the board and the health department, and developing mechanisms to share governance with the appropriate governmental body. As one public health leader stated:

> To create effective governing boards, we must examine our values and determine why our boards need to exist. Once we discover our common purpose, we can develop skills and processes to improve our effectiveness. Boards and administrators need a shared vision, commitment, and leadership to make goals a reality. As public health leaders, it is our job to develop boards that are a part of our leadership teams and join us in creating healthy communities.[11(p.11)]

Agenda Setting

Public health leaders should learn about and use the systems approach to organizational change and the public health core functions model to ensure that their agencies' agendas are tied to the core functions of public health. In addition, they must master the art and science of public health. Leaders are the grand integrators of science and practice, and part of their job is to explain public health issues to health professional associates and community partners.

Leaders should acquire agenda-setting skills. An organization needs to prioritize the problems that it is facing and create action plans that deal with the largest problems first.[12] Rogers and Dearing[13] developed a model for agenda setting that included the creation of a media agenda, a public agenda, and a policy agenda. The fact that public health leadership practice takes place in a government setting means that community and political realities affect the agenda-setting process. Also influencing the process are gatekeepers, the media, and spectacular news stories (e.g., a story about children becoming ill after eating in a fast-food restaurant).

Barriers to Effectiveness

In 1988, the Institute of Medicine issued a report stating that the public health system in the United States was in disarray.[14] The report listed a number of barriers that reduce the ability of public health leaders to be effective, including the following:

- A lack of a consensus on the content of the public health mission
- Inadequate capacity to carry out the essential public health functions of assessment, policy development, and assurance of services
- Disjointed decision making uninformed by the necessary data and knowledge
- Inequities in the distribution of services and the benefits of public health
- Disharmony between the technical and political aspects of decisions
- Rapid turnover of leaders
- An inadequate relationship between public health and the medical profession
- Organizational fragmentation
- Problems in relationships between layers of government
- An inadequate development of necessary knowledge across the full array of public health needs
- A poor public image of public health, inhibiting necessary support
- Special problems that unduly limit the financial resources available to public health

Without question, the public health system in the United States needs to become more effective, and public health leaders will be at the forefront of attempts at reform.[15] One problem is that public health agencies are dealing with more complex problems today, and the complexity of problems in the areas of infectious diseases and chronic diseases will probably continue to increase. Therefore, organizational stability may not be possible to achieve. In addition, public health professionals come from different disciplines with different approaches to problem solving, which leads to professional disagreements.[16] Only through collaboration will effective problem solving and decision making occur.

In a speech before the Illinois Public Health Leadership Institute in 1992, George Pickett said that public health leaders need to increase their skills transorganizationally;

that is, they need to be able to understand and communicate with others in community sectors with values and priorities different from theirs. Public health leaders are often deficient in collaboration skills,[17] and consequently they are sometimes prevented from cooperating effectively with leaders from important sectors, such as the business community and the religious community. Fortunately, obstacles to cooperation are becoming less frequent.

It should be noted that, in general, leaders who are extremely effective tend to be key players in rather than reactors to the change going on around them.[18] Effective leaders, when confronted with a problem, typically consider a wide range of options and seem to know how to select the important factors first. They also think in terms of win–win and try to arrange it so all parties are winners in a dispute. They are good listeners who try to understand others and their perspectives before trying to make themselves understood. They are excellent synthesizers who try to foster cooperation and collaboration. Finally, they constantly renew themselves through training, education, exercise, values clarification, and so on.

Leadership Style

Public health leaders need to develop an appropriate leadership style. Autocratic and directive styles work best when the leader structures the tasks and the workers are willing to do what the leader asks. In public health, the democratic style seems to work better.[19] Participative forms of leadership, in which staff members are involved in the problem-solving process, facilitate the building of a consensus and the acceptance by the staff of the decisions reached. Collaboration should be viewed as a creative process the goal of which is to discover new approaches and new solutions for old problems.[20]

Dealing with Diversity

Professional diversity in public health brings its own set of problems.[21] Practitioners from different professions view public health differently. Public health leaders need to look at public health in its totality and develop strategies for integrating the different approaches. Public health leaders need to confront not only professional diversity but gender, race, ethnic, and age diversity. For example, the so-called glass ceiling for women still exists,[22] and therefore public health leaders must conscientiously promote gender equality. The first step is to gather the data necessary to determine whether gender inequalities exist and, if so, where they exist. The next step is to hire a consultant to evaluate the agency's environment and

its receptiveness to gender equality. The third step is to use a benchmarking process (comparing the agency with the best agencies, not the average ones) to identify best practices for achieving gender equality and taking full advantage of the skills that women bring into the workplace. The final step, so to speak, is to prepare oneself for a backlash.

Diversity encompasses gender, age, race, ethnicity, sexual orientation, work and family issues, education, work experiences, tenure within the agency or organization, personality, risk tolerance, geographic region, and religion.[23] A unified diversity enhancement program for public health professionals and clients may be difficult to construct because of the different issues that are prominent in each diversity category.

One way for public health leaders to deal with diversity issues is to empower staff so that they become advocates for themselves. It is important to understand how human beings in our society act and what needs they have. In his classic work *Motivation and Personality*, Maslow defined a hierarchy of needs.[24] At the most basic level, individuals want their physiological needs met. Second in order of importance are their safety needs. In other words, issues of job security and amount of income are critical for most people. Next come social needs, including the need for recognition by colleagues. One level up, people want to experience a sense of self-esteem. They want to take pride in their work and hence want to be empowered to do a good job. A professional who works well and without the need of much direction will usually be allowed the freedom to design his or her own activities, an almost sure way of increasing self-esteem. Finally, people have a need for self-actualization—the ability to make personal dreams become reality.

Balancing Work and Play

Work has a tendency to take up most of a leader's waking hours, and family life can suffer as a result. O'Neil called this dilemma the paradox of success.[25] In his view, the myth of success is that success offers complete fulfillment, is tied to how much money is made, and increases freedom. In fact, success causes a constant craving for more success and hence can lead to a kind of bondage. Factors that can help a leader keep a balance between work life and private life include self-knowledge, managing conflicting pressures, and maintaining a concern for how others feel.[26]

Women seem to be proficient at balancing personal and professional interests. For working women with a family, work and home are full-time jobs that they typically seem to handle equally well. At work, women, by redesigning their positions and demanding employee training and development, are helping to break traditional organizational molds.[27]

They are also helping to break down the barriers between home and work by pushing for flextime, child care, and family leave.

This section raised and discussed many issues related to personal leadership development. Following is a list of leadership strategies that can be used to increase one's leadership skills and abilities:

- Be a value role model. Live the values that the community espouses.
- Understand the democratic process and how it affects the public health system.
- Translate political policy into action.
- Improve communication skills.
- Be a mentor to others.
- Learn to follow when appropriate.
- Be partners with the agency's governing board.
- Learn agenda-setting skills.
- Address barriers to effective public health practice.
- Explore community partnerships.
- Be creative in finding new funding sources.
- Balance work and family.
- Increase leadership opportunities for others.

At the personal level, leaders struggle with the issue of how they spend their time and on what. **Exercise 3-1** is a quick exercise on how you use your time, including how much of your work time is spent on management activities and how much on leadership activities.

EXERCISE 3-1 Only 100 Percent

Purpose: to define how much time is spent on management activities in contrast to leadership activities

Key Concepts: management, leadership, time, organizational needs

Procedure: Pick an organization for which you have a leadership role. Using 100 percentage points, how many points would you give to your management activities for the organization and how many points for your leadership activities. If you are spending more time on management activities than you are spending on leadership activities, how would you reduce your management activities and increase your leadership activities? Discuss these strategies with the class or workshop as a whole.

LEADERSHIP AT THE TEAM LEVEL

Public health leaders do not work alone. Public health practice is a group activity. Therefore, among the most important skills a leader can possess are those that are necessary for building and maintaining teams and increasing their effectiveness. It seems that somebody always wants to take charge when even two people are in a room. A team is a group of people who come together to pursue a common purpose.[28] The results of the team's activities are often greater than the sum of the results that would have occurred had each team member been acting alone.

Each team member should be viewed as leader although one person will generally become the official leader. The team leader will share information in an equitable manner with other team members.[29] The leader will build trust in the team process and share authority and power with other members. The leader will also intervene when necessary to move the team forward. The expectation is that all members will be involved in the performance of the team tasks.

Team members who are also members of the public health agency may need to act as a link between the team and the agency and community constituents. These team members, in particular, will need to learn the skills of conflict resolution and negotiation. When a skilled leader guides the team process, creativity and innovation are the result.

Reasons for Creating Teams

The reasons for creating teams include the following: First, a team allows an organization to use the leadership skills and talents and the multidisciplinary and multicultural backgrounds of its staff. For example, a multidisciplinary team that includes nurses, social workers, and environmental health specialists, among others, might be assembled to address the low level of prenatal care in the community. If we add multicultural team members, potential conflicts may arise due to different cultural orientations related to prenatal care. Second, creating a team allows the members time to get to know one another and to develop a sense of togetherness in the context of shared leadership. In general, team members find they can communicate with each other better even after they have left the team or the team has been disbanded. In addition, they learn how to cooperate and collaborate, and cooperation and collaboration increase productivity.[30] Finally, team decision making produces decisions that are supported by the majority of the team's members.

Teams that are created to lighten a supervisor's workload are often doomed to failure.[31] Teams are not a replacement for training and not a way for leaders to observe the opinions and working style of the staff. Teams do not necessarily increase the personal productivity of their members. They need leaders to clarify issues and set the parameters of their activities.[32] One of the strengths of teams is that they are flexible and can reorient themselves as roadblocks occur. Yet the freedom teams are given can be a weakness as well. Teams sometimes fail because they lack discipline and a sense of responsibility for achieving the desired outcomes. When team members realize they will be completely in charge of their activities and will have the power to make decisions, they sometimes abuse this power, with negative results for the agency. This risk can be reduced if the agency leaders make clear to each team how they expect it to proceed and what results they expect it to achieve.

Leadership teams work differently than management teams. Management teams carry out the instructions of a supervisor. Their tasks are circumscribed, and there is very little room for creativity or innovation. Leadership teams share leadership with the public health administrator, who openly delegates decision-making power to them. In some leadership teams, the health administrator becomes a team member. If given the trust of the agency administrator, leadership team members become committed to the agency and lose their fear of reprisal. They feel that recommendations will be seriously considered.

Facts about Teams

Katzenbach and Smith studied teams in 30 organizations, including businesses, schools, and social agencies.[33] They found that teams were critical for building high-quality organizations and improving customer service. The authors came up with 10 findings about teams in general. The first finding is that teams are created to address a performance challenge, and indeed a leadership team must have a purpose (mission) if it is to succeed. The second finding is that the team's composition and its purpose need to be thought through. Not every leadership team should be of the same size or professional composition. Third, leaders need to promote team performance opportunities. As the leaders view the organization, they will find these opportunities exist throughout. Fourth, many teams composed primarily of people at the top fail because of the other demands made on these individuals' time and energy. Fifth, organizations and their leaders find it easier to work with individuals than with teams. Everything, including the hiring of people, the determination of salary, the construction of career paths, and the monitoring of performance, is oriented toward the individual. Teamwork seems to go against the structure of individual responsibility.

The sixth finding is that organizations committed to high performance standards are more likely to use teams than organizations with lower performance standards. Seventh, very few high-performance teams exist. High-performance teams can be either leadership or management teams. However, leadership teams are generally clearer on the purpose for which they were created. They take control of their activities and promote the development of relationships between their members. They build team activities on good communication. The leaders maintain their flexibility, work productively together, and recognize the accomplishments of their leader colleagues. Leadership teams also seem to have high morale. (High-performance teams can be created using the PERFORM model, propounded by Blanchard and colleagues.[34] The acronym stands for Purpose, Empowerment, Relationships and communication, Flexibility, Optimal productivity, Recognition and appreciation, and Morale.)

The eighth finding is that teams do not replace organizational hierarchies. Instead, teams enhance these hierarchies, partly because they are able to cross over structural boundaries. Because of the strong community orientation of public health agencies, leadership teams can be used to address community concerns. These teams may include community partners among their membership.

The ninth finding is that teams are small learning organizations that integrate performance and learning. Typically, a team will do research on a subject related to its purpose. Team members also learn team-building and leadership skills. They often learn that each member is a leader or potential leader. The conjoining of performance and learning in teams is generally a plus, because their conjunction throughout an organization is often a prerequisite for the organization to increase its effectiveness. This applies to public health agencies as well.

The final finding is that teams are effective in addressing new issues as well as old issues. In the case of old issues or problems, they often discover new solutions. One reason teams are good at discovering solutions to problems is that they view the problems from a systems perspective rather than using the traditional cause-and-effect approach.[35] They are also experts at sharing information and coordinating actions, and members of one team frequently tie their activities to the activities of other teams working on different though related issues.

The important question is why so many teams fail when their importance to the work of public health is so important. Lencioni pointed to five major dysfunctions that affect the success of team-based activities.[36] First, teams fail when there is a lack of trust either in their organization or in their leadership. This includes the implicit leadership of the team as well. Second, team members fear conflict and contesting the decisions of other team members. Conflict is not necessarily a personal issue but rather is often an issue related to the challenge that the group must address. The third dysfunction relates to the level or lack of commitment of team members to the process. If there is a lack of commitment, then the fourth dysfunction occurs. The lack of accountability will often affect the effectiveness of team activities. The fifth dysfunction relates to the problem of ignoring the results of the teamwork regardless of the reasons. If the boss had the team do busywork or did not allow the team any involvement in the decision-making process, all the dysfunctions come into play. There will be no trust, no conflict on the surface, no commitment to the process, no accountability, and obviously no attention to the results.

Teams build social capital, which brings people together in a way that individuals alone cannot do. Building social capital helps to develop trust, allows for shared leadership and creativity, expands social networks for the team members, develops shared purpose in team activities, levels the playing field for the members in terms of equity, increases collaboration and commitment, enhances knowledge sharing, and fits different talents of individuals into a comprehensive whole.[37] Teamwork provides many benefits to the individual as well and creates satisfaction and sometimes personal rewards in the accomplishments of the team.

Team Classification

Many writers have attempted to classify teams. One helpful classification is as follows:[38] Natural work teams are made up primarily of individuals who work together as part of their regular activities. These teams, which can be either management or leadership teams, are usually given a set of designated activities to perform. Cross-functional teams, the second type, include members who have different functions within the organization. They are primarily leadership teams. Corrective action teams are management teams assigned to work on the solutions to problems that are already determined. Finally, hybrid teams address issues not addressed elsewhere in the organization. They may be either management or leadership teams, and they use the techniques associated with all the other types. Local public health departments use all four types of teams.

The Importance of Empowerment

Teams and their members need to be empowered by administrators to take active decision-making roles.[39] Empowerment, which gives team members the freedom to use their knowledge, experience, and skills to address important issues,[40] tends to increase their commitment to the agency and the level of their performance as well. Empowerment must come from the agency leader, and there appears to be a direct relationship between the amount of responsibility staff are given and the degree of their empowerment.[41]

The transfer of power to a team must be real and not merely nominal. A public health leadership team from a state public health leadership institute worked with a local health department to develop a lead-screening program for children. The administrator allowed the team to work on the creation of this new program because she had been told by the state to develop the program. However, the administrator viewed the team members as outsiders, and though she told them that she had respect for them and would seriously review any recommendations they made, she used the team merely to show the state that she was complying with its request and in reality had no intention of implementing the team's recommendations. This is an example of team activity subverted by a hidden agenda. The power to have an effect on the development of a program through recommendations was implied but was in fact an illusion.

Empowerment is related to organizational values, leadership activities, human resource systems, and the structure and activities of the organization.[42] Empowerment is often used as a tool for the improvement of programs and services. With empowerment, teams can improve their performance and customer service.

Teams and Leadership Style

The situational leadership model identifies four leadership styles: directing, coaching, supporting, and delegating. This same classification can be applied to team-based activities.[43] When a team is first created, the leader is involved in formulating the team's purpose and determining the activities to be performed. The leader, in other words, is using a directive style. During the next phase, the leader, acting as a coach, clarifies the team's activities. The leader then begins to involve team members in decision making, a process that falls into the category of providing support. In the final phase, the leader empowers the team members, and empowerment, as pointed out, is closely related to the delegation of responsibility.

It is also important to concentrate on the leadership activities associated with working on teams. LaFasto and Larson discussed the six tasks of team leadership.[44] First, leaders clearly need to pay attention to the goals of the project that will occur during the teamwork. Second, the critical nature of collaboration within the team to get the work done is an important leadership activity. Third, team members like to think and feel that the team process builds their confidence in the way the work is progressing. Team members want to see short- and long-term results in the work. Team leaders need to help build this confidence and be willing to keep team members knowledgeable about external events that affect the work of the team. Secrets defeat teamwork. The fourth leadership activity involves leaders demonstrating technical knowledge and abilities. This activity also means the leader will ask for help or technical assistance when necessary. The fifth leadership activity involves keeping the team on track by setting priorities. It is important to keep the team on task and prevent distractions if possible. When priorities change, leaders must inform the team. The sixth and final task relates to the necessity of managing performance, giving feedback through the group process, and rewarding results.

Of course, teams are at different places in their involvement in and commitment to the tasks they have been assigned, and leaders need to monitor team readiness, which ranges from unable and unwilling to carry out the team assignment to able, willing, and confident. In some cases, leaders may have to use planning strategies for key team members as well as for the team as a whole.

One useful team technique, based on the so-called skunkworks model, is to send a team to a neutral place away from the organization to work on issues related to the team's activities.[45] The "skunkworks" is a subteam composed of experts on the topic that is the focus of the team activities. These team members tend to be transformational leaders who will move the organization forward.

Team Members

Mallory studied the characteristics of various types of team members.[46] Some members tried to take control of the activities of the team, and these he labeled dominant members. These individuals do well in structured situations with a well-defined purpose. The influencers tend to be creative and extremely talented in interpersonal relationships. They also tend to be optimistic and try to keep the team together. The balancers look at the big picture in an objective manner and try to reconcile the differences among the team members. The loyalists are committed to the status quo. Each actual team member, although mainly of one type, has at least a little of every personality characteristic associated with any of the four types.

Team members benefit in several ways from working on a team. First, they gain experience in working together with colleagues on a project.[47] They also learn problem-solving skills, interpersonal relationship skills, and new technological information. In addition, they learn about accountability from a personal perspective as well as a team perspective and become more committed to the team's goals and objectives.

The Life Cycle of Teams

Teams have a life cycle that is similar to the life cycle of human beings.[48] A team starts out as an infant and disbands as it ages and finishes its tasks. Organizational leaders must develop the ability to function as team leaders at each stage of the team life cycle. This is especially true in the public health field, where so many leadership activities occur in a team setting.

Following are guidelines that organizational leaders should use when creating and working with teams:

- Develop teams to address agency or community public health problems.
- Choose multidisciplinary team members for their expertise and leadership qualities.
- Allow teams to make decisions and recommendations for change. Share power and control.
- Share information.
- Intervene in the team process when necessary.
- Do not create teams to alleviate your workload.
- Use the skunkworks technique for dealing with team issues.
- Tie team development to performance standards.
- Put a time limit on the activities of the team.

LEADERSHIP AT THE ORGANIZATION LEVEL

In a 2011 book on management in the health field, the authors claimed that managers nowadays have to integrate clinical practice skills and management skills.[49] The view propounded here is that public health leaders have to integrate public health practitioner skills, management, and leadership skills.

Currently, public health agencies typically have a management orientation. In the 21st century, they will need to become consumer and community driven.[50] The leadership expertise of agency staff must be increased if the agencies are to keep up with the speed of change. **Figure 3-1** shows the relationships among management theories, the healthcare environment, clinical expertise, and consumer healthcare expectations. Most of the items listed are relevant to public health as well as medical care. Two missing items that pertain particularly to public health are building community coalitions and health promotion and disease prevention.

Public health agencies, along with other types of organizations, are undergoing many reforms but need to change

FIGURE 3-1 Characteristics of the Healthcare Management Role

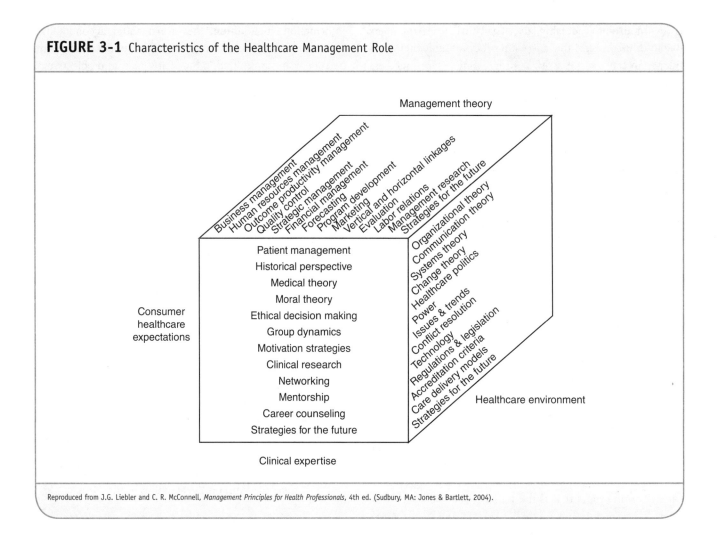

Reproduced from J.G. Liebler and C. R. McConnell, *Management Principles for Health Professionals*, 4th ed. (Sudbury, MA: Jones & Bartlett, 2004).

further. For one thing, they have not fully incorporated the lessons of business. They are still run as traditional bureaucracies, although community groups are trying to take a role in the making of decisions about public health issues.

In a bureaucracy, the managers and leaders are often far removed from the daily activities of the staff,[51] yet they feel the need to control these activities. Perhaps this is one reason that Peters and Austin urged the importance of "managing by wandering around."[52] Of course, it is true that leaders need to monitor operations, but they also need to delegate authority to managers and staff members.[53] By doing this, they can help make the professionals in their organization excited about coming to work in the morning. Leaders need to remember that associates are customers too.

In the late 1950s, Drucker noted that traditional bureaucratic organizations were gradually becoming knowledge-based organizations.[54] Public health agencies have always been knowledge based, and in fact business communities can learn much from public health leaders about knowledge-based organizations and how they work. However, the models for knowledge management are more developed on the business side. For example, Tiwana has examined the four phases of knowledge management strategies for knowledge-based organizations.[55] First, it is necessary to evaluate the current structure for dealing with knowledge in an agency (an infrastructure issue). Second, it is important to develop the system related to knowledge in terms of the analysis dimension, the design of the system, and how it is developed. Third is the issue of deployment and how to use the results of the performance evaluation of the system and to make refinements as necessary. Public health leaders have an important role in knowledge management. It will be important for leaders to apply these phases to public health and to modify the models to better reflect the knowledge management aspects of public health practice.

Public health leaders, in order to thrive in the ever-changing environment, need to make a commitment to change and to focus on increasing customer satisfaction, fostering innovation, empowering staff, and instituting appropriate structural reforms.[56] Leadership is not just a matter of charisma; it is hard work.[57]

Nanus identified four main leadership roles.[58] First, public health leaders (to keep to the focus of this discussion) are spokespeople who present the contemporary public health issues to the community. Second, they are "direction setters" and involve community leaders in prevention activities and in the search for ways to increase the level of health in the community. Third, they act as coaches or mentors for agency associates as a means of improving the agency's effectiveness. Finally, they act as organizational change agents.

Public Health Functions

From the 1840s to the 1940s, six basic local health agency functions evolved: the collection and interpretation of vital statistics, sanitation, communicable disease control, the provision of maternal and child health programs, health education, and the provision of laboratory services.[59] Between 1940 and 1980, other functions were added, including the provision of environmental health services, the development and provision of personal health services, the coordination of community health services, the operation of medical care and public health facilities, areawide planning, and the assessment of the adequacy of health services. The year 1988 saw the release of the Institute of Medicine report on public health. This report promoted the use of core functions to organize the activities of public health at the community level.[60]

Public health leaders have changed as public health has changed. They have adapted to new developments and devised innovative approaches to performing the standard public health functions. Since 1995, local health departments have continued to change. Many direct service activities have been outsourced. Local health departments have reoriented some of their activities to emergency preparedness and response activities.[61] Different organizations, performance management committees, and public health professional writers will often come up with different lists of required services and performance measures. Thus, it is important to determine the credibility of the source.

Not all states have local public health agencies. In states that do not, the state health department operates like a local agency. In states with local agencies, the activities of the state health department leaders are separate from the activities of the agency leaders. For example, state health departments have tended to stay away from the provision of direct services, especially in the case of services being provided by local public health agencies.[62] A state health department may provide special services that the local agencies do not offer. It is also likely to be engaged in overseeing and coordinating public health activities in the state.

State health department functions include communicable disease control, tuberculosis control, venereal disease control, acquired immune deficiency syndrome monitoring, sanitation, industrial hygiene, dental health, laboratory services provision, public health nursing, case management, maternal and child health program provision, public health education, technical assistance, public health workforce training, development of new local health departments, epidemiologic surveillance, regulation of healthcare facilities, licensure, inspection, cancer screening, and many more. The state health department also serves as the repository for state health data. Since 2001, the activities related to emergency preparedness and response have been added to the list. There clearly is still a need for inclusion of emergency mitigation and recovery dimensions for public health work as well.

State health department leaders are responsible for organizing the state public health system to reflect its mission, vision, and goals and objectives. They need courage to carry out their action plans in the face of community opposition and must know how to reform the state public health system without overstepping the boundaries of the state political system because, among other reasons, the state is the conduit of funding for local public health agency programs.

In order to see where our performance measurement thinking is today, a recent list of measures was determined by the U.S. Department of Health and Human Services (HHS) in 2011.[63] There are five major goals for public health and a number of objectives tied to each goal. The five major goals are:

1. Strengthen Health Care.
2. Advance Scientific Knowledge and Innovation.
3. Advance the Health, Safety, and Well-Being of the American People.
4. Increase Efficiency, Transparency, and Accountability of HHS Programs.
5. Strengthen the National HHS Infrastructure and Workforce.

The goals provide a framework for state and local agencies and their leaders to guide public health programs going forward.

Responsibilities of Public Health Leaders

Leaders of local public health agencies have the responsibility to promote their agencies. They make sure the agencies are viewed as repositories of public health information as well as providers of high-quality programs and services. They develop relationships with the leaders of public health agencies throughout their state and also develop partnerships with community health providers.

Funding, of course, is critical for strengthening the public health system, and there is currently intense competition in the entire health industry for additional money.[64] Public health leaders must be involved both in the allocation of public health funds and in the funding for related health service programs. They will need to make strong arguments for public revenues. Public health leaders have become more entrepreneurial since the 1990s. They received grants from and developed contracts with public and private funding organizations to supplement their base budgets. Fund-raising should be tied to the mission and vision of the public health agency.

Public health leaders are concerned with excellence in public health. They act as role models for emerging public health leaders. They develop benchmarks for best practices. In their oversight role, they motivate community providers to improve their performance. They work with the leaders of other organizations to develop a comprehensive, integrative approach to improving public health in the community. Public health agencies do not want to duplicate programs or services adequately provided by others, although they might offer competing services if the quality of a community provider's services is open to question.

Public health agency leaders have important responsibilities toward agency staff. They must honestly monitor and evaluate job performance and job satisfaction.[65] If job evaluations are done fairly and regularly, staff will be able to learn their full job responsibilities and meet them more effectively. In addition, public health leaders must be enthusiastic about the task of protecting public health and be able to motivate their colleagues to be enthusiastic as well, by fostering collaboration and sharing power with them, for example.[66] They also should cheer colleagues and their progress. Einstein's formula $e = mc^2$ has been reinterpreted as enthusiasm equals mission times cash and congratulations. People have to be cheered, and they also have to be paid for their efforts.

As noted already, leaders need to empower agency staff. Empowerment must occur at the team level, the agency level, and the community level.[67] Leaders empower their employees by delegating work to them and trusting that they have the skills to carry out the work activities. If the employee needs special training, the leader must provide it.

In summation at the organization level, public health leaders have the responsibility to:

- understand how the agency functions
- delegate authority whenever possible
- monitor client satisfaction
- develop performance measurement metrics
- make structural changes in the agency to accommodate new or emerging public health issues
- encourage knowledge management systems development
- explore alternate futures for the agency
- apply the core functions model to agency activities
- empower the agency staff and the community residents

LEADERSHIP AT THE COMMUNITY LEVEL

Leadership at the community level requires more systems-based skills than are used at the team and agency levels. At this level, public health leaders work to increase the visibility of the public health agency. In interviews with 100 American public health leaders, the author found consistent agreement that the public lacked in-depth knowledge about public health. Thus, public health leaders have a duty to provide public health information to the business community, the medical and health industry community, social agencies, and the general public. Public health leaders need to develop skills in community building in order to work with community groups to create an environment for positive social change.

Figure 3-2 shows the dimensions of public health leadership. Public health leaders build on the core functions model, regardless of the level of leadership, while taking into account the political and social realities that affect the agency and the community. Public health agencies must take into consideration social and political issues if they are to survive. For one thing, they are mandated by funding sources to provide certain basic services and programs. (This raises the issue of the proper balance between mandated services and community-based services and programs not included in the mandated services protocol.)

The Nature of Community

Over the past couple of decades, business discovered community.[68] Business leaders now see that community involvement needs to be part of the practice of business. Public

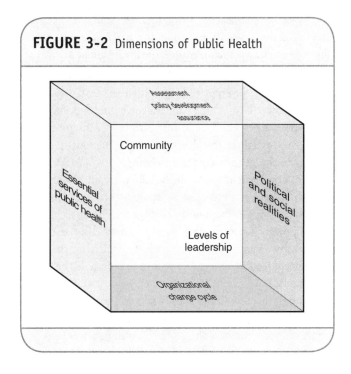

FIGURE 3-2 Dimensions of Public Health

My study of public health leaders found that their efforts at developing community coalitions have been uneven at best. Almost all of the respondents stated that public health agencies have not been successful in getting the public to understand public health.

Community is more than bricks and mortar. It is more than a place to live. It is the place in which our dreams and aspirations are or are not fulfilled. When we talk about improvement in our quality of life, community is part of the improvement process. Community is the place where values are put into action. Community is a complex system made up of individuals, families, politicians, health organizations, human services agencies, churches, schools, businesses, business organizations, and so on (**Figure 3-3**). It is a system that accepts challenges, and to develop the resources to deal with them it needs to be built on the strengths of its constituent parts, not on its weaknesses.[69]

One view currently prevalent is that we need to rediscover civility.[70] Civility requires that community leaders be open to the opinions of other people and other organizations. It also means that it is important not to degrade others. If civility training is needed, it should include a discussion of civility and its components, the relationship of civility to leadership, problem solving and decision making, conflict

health agencies, by their nature, serve communities, but serving a group of citizens who live in a specified geographic area does not mean community issues are being addressed.

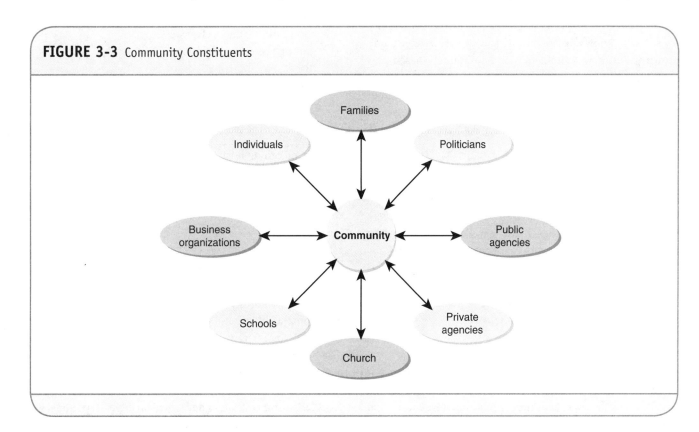

FIGURE 3-3 Community Constituents

resolution and negotiation, levels of collaboration at the vertical and horizontal levels, systems thinking, values and ethics, and the relationship of civility to trusteeship. Furthermore, public health leaders must transfer the leadership skills they use at the team and organizational levels to the community level. Leaders build communities in all their leadership activities.

Advocacy through the Media

Media advocacy is an important way to promote public health programs and services.[71] The use of social media like Facebook and Twitter is another approach. Public health leaders should learn how to use the media to create support for agency goals. For example, they should consider sending letters on a regular basis to newspapers and other sources to increase the visibility of public health.

Think of the importance of using the media in the following situation: a public health leader in a conservative, middle-class community discovers that five cases of human immunodeficiency virus infection have recently been discovered. A statistic like this can hit the nerve center of a community. It is the public health leader who will have the skills to defuse the crisis and get community constituents to become partners in dealing with the problem.

One of the most important responsibilities of public health leaders is to promote prevention at the community level.[72] Our knowledge of health and disease is constantly growing, and new technologies and community-based prevention strategies are continually being developed to address public health concerns. The public needs to be convinced of the importance of using these technologies and strategies. It is the job of public health leaders to make the case.

Linking Programs

There is a good argument that public health programs should be linked together where possible.[73] The Centers for Disease Control and Prevention created prevention research centers in a number of universities. Many, if not all, of these centers rely on community support to carry out their activities. Public health leaders, who see the future of their agencies as tied to primary prevention rather than direct services, know that linkage to academic programs will strengthen the infrastructure of public health in their communities.

Community Building

Community building is a complex process that does not occur overnight. Peck's analysis revealed four stages.[74] In the first stage, various community representatives who have formed a coalition pretend to have the community's interests at heart in order to gain acceptance for their own agendas. Peck called this the pseudocommunity stage. The second stage, which begins when the coalition realizes that community concerns are not being addressed, is one of chaos. Next comes the stage of emptiness, in which the leaders have to empty themselves of all their preconceived notions about the community and its concerns. It is extremely difficult for the leaders to leave their agendas at the door. The fourth stage is when true community comes into being.

Organizations involved in building a community need leaders.[75] These leaders must be students of the community and its culture and be able to involve individuals with different power bases in community change. Because each community resident has an agenda to which he or she is committed, leaders have to find ways to reconcile the differing agendas.

Community coalitions ideally should be learning organizations.[76] The members of a coalition need to examine their predispositions and how these predispositions affect the community-building process. In addition, the scientific perspective should be incorporated into the group's deliberations.

Community building is best achieved through the use of collaborative leadership.[77] Following are 10 factors that can contribute to the success of collaboration and community building:

1. Good timing and a clear need
2. Strong stakeholder groups
3. Broad-based involvement
4. Credibility and openness of process
5. Commitment and/or involvement of high-level leaders
6. Support or acquiescence of "established" authorities or powers
7. Overcoming mistrust and skepticism
8. Strong leadership of the process
9. Interim successes
10. A shift to broader concerns[78]

Coalition Building

Coalition building is an important part of empowering communities. Public health agencies can no longer work in isolation. Community leaders need to be involved in addressing public health issues. The major advantage of a coalition is that all voices are heard and programs can be developed that better reflect the health needs of the community. The major disadvantage is that being part of a coalition is time consuming.

Cohen and colleagues developed an eight-step model for developing community coalitions (**Table 3-1**).[79] The model

TABLE 3-1　Eight Steps to Building an Effective Coalition

Step 1: Analyze the program's objectives and determine whether to form a coalition.
Step 2: Recruit the right people.
Step 3: Devise a set of preliminary objectives and activities.
Step 4: Convene the coalition.
Step 5: Anticipate the necessary resources.
Step 6: Define elements of a successful coalition structure.
Step 7: Maintain coalition vitality.
Step 8: Make improvements through evaluation.

Reprinted with permission of Contra Costa Health Services, *Developing Effective Coalitions: An Eight Step Guide.* © 1994, Contra Costa County Health Services Department Prevention Programs.

is based on the experience of the Contra Costa County (California) Health Services Department Prevention Programs. The authors define a coalition as a group of interested parties (individuals and organizations) that want to influence the attempt to solve a critical problem. The coalition members need to develop strategies for each of the eight steps and know when to move to the next step.

A coalition can have many advantages. It can help to save resources. It can influence a large number of people in a community through its diversified membership. It can create an agenda that is more comprehensive than the agenda of any single community organization. It can create a network for the sharing of information, a network that could be used beneficially by the local public health agency for purposes of marketing and fostering change in the community. In addition, coalition members gain satisfaction when they see positive things happen, and a coalition can influence emerging grassroots organizations as they explore their roles in the community.

Building community through coalitions that are responsible and credible is an important goal of public health leaders. A report from the Centers for Disease Control and Prevention stated that public health should use a process called community engagement.[80] Community engagement involves collaboration between people who are in the same geographic area, share special interests, or are in similar situations. A mixture of social science and art, community engagement integrates the ideas of culture, community, coalition building, and collaboration. The report reviewed the literature for examples of successful engagement and presented a list of the principles of community engagement (**Table 3-2**).

Partnerships are collaborative relationships that involve more than minimal cooperation. They tend to evolve through the same steps outlined in the systems model of organizational change. Partnerships have a vision and a mission, they

TABLE 3-2　Characteristics of Successful Community Engagement

- Community engagement efforts should address multiple levels of the social environment, rather than only individual behaviors, to bring about desired changes.
- Health behaviors are influenced by culture. To ensure that engagement efforts are culturally and linguistically appropriate, they must be developed from a knowledge of and respect for the targeted community's culture.
- People participate when they feel a sense of community, see their involvement and the issues as relevant and worth their time, and view the process and organizational climate of participation as open and supportive of their right to have a voice in the process.
- Although it cannot be externally imposed on a community, a sense of empowerment—the ability to take action, influence, and make decisions on critical issues—is crucial to successful engagement efforts.
- Community mobilization and self-determination frequently need nurturing. Before individuals and organizations can gain control and influence and become players and partners in community health decision making and action, they may need additional knowledge, skills, and resources.
- Coalitions, when adequately supported, can be useful vehicles for mobilizing and using community assets for health decision making and action.
- Participation is influenced by whether community members believe that the benefits of participation outweigh the costs. Community leaders can use their understanding of perceived costs to develop appropriate incentives for participation.

Reproduced from Centers for Disease Control and Prevention (1997). Public Health Practice Program Office, *Principles of Community Engagement*, Agency for Toxic Substances and Disease Registry.

have goals and objectives, and they develop and implement action plans and evaluate their degree of success.

Each community coalition needs to be revitalized on a regular basis. A community coalition often seems to work better when a community crisis is occurring.[81] When the crisis is over, people tend to move away from the coalition back to their own personal agendas. Thus, public health leaders need to be aware of this fact and make an extra effort to keep community coalitions alive after crises are resolved.

LEADERSHIP AT THE GLOBAL LEVEL

The fifth level of leadership includes two major activities and set of tools. Today's public health leader can decide to work in a country other than the United States. The other aspect of this leadership level is the important concern of watching disease outbreaks in other parts of the world and observing whether these outbreaks will spread elsewhere. Public health issues are global in nature. Many public health professionals have pointed out that leaders need to think globally but act locally. Health and disease do not honor government or country boundaries. Epidemiologic surveillance needs to be a global as well as a local concern. Communication is critical at this level. In recent years, the Internet has helped speed up the flow of information.

National and International Communities

Thus far the discussion has been on leadership in local communities, but there are also national and international communities that offer an arena for action by public health leaders. National leaders, like local leaders, act as advocates for public health. They keep the public informed about health issues. They work on the construction of a national mission and vision as well as public health goals for the future. They collaborate with leaders at the state level on the creation of a coordinated nationwide approach to public health. They collaborate with national elected officials to address key public health concerns, including the training of the public health workforce.

On the international level, public health leaders implement public health programs in countries where public health is not a priority. These leaders need to develop skills to enhance their ability to improve the quality of life of people in these countries. Rather than reinvent public health, these leaders develop networks with public health leaders throughout the world to share model program methods for addressing specific public health problems. As already stated, public health leaders need to think globally about public

health concerns while acting locally (to protect community residents from potential health crises). Building healthy communities is partially a matter of applying knowledge gained from all parts of the world to local conditions. The importance of the 2005 International Health Regulations (IHR) cannot be overestimated. These rules and regulations were agreed upon by 193 countries. These countries believe that these international rules and procedures will help to make the world safe from potential threats to global health. The IHR were approved by the World Health Organization in the summer of 2005.[82] These rules will affect every community in the world.

Most of the strategies and techniques discussed in this chapter have universal application. Following is a list of guidelines of special pertinence for public health leaders working at the community level:

- Build trust.
- Form coalitions.
- Develop partnerships.
- Teach community groups about the core public health functions.
- Do community building with partners.
- See the community as a system.
- Encourage coalitions or partnerships to continue after a public health crisis has been resolved.
- Use the media to promote best practices in public health.
- Push a prevention agenda.
- Understand the connections between public health at a global level and public health at a local community level and their connections.

LEADERSHIP AT THE PROFESSIONAL LEVEL

Despite the multidisciplinary nature of public health, its leaders need to speak with a unified voice. Public health as a profession takes precedence over the particular educational backgrounds of the public health workforce. The following situation occurs much too often. A physician with almost no background in public health was appointed the administrator of a large county health department. He made decisions from a medical viewpoint and felt that physicians were the only ones who were qualified to do the department's work. He ran the department using a direct medical service approach and totally ignored the population-based approach to public health.

Public health practitioners tend not to travel to professional meetings or for professional development. Many local health departments have a small staff and are reluctant to let employees go to meetings. Funds for professional development are generally minimal, and paying for professional development is typically considered by taxpayers to be a waste of money. Yet public health leaders know that it is important to communicate with other public health professionals. Some of these leaders go to the annual meetings held by the various public health associations and even take a leadership role in these associations. They help to create public health policy that will trickle down to the local public health programs. Leadership development training seems to be a factor here. For example, most of the presidents over the past 22 years of the Illinois Public Health Association were either faculty members or fellows of the Mid-America Regional Public Health Leadership Institute (Illinois, Indiana, Wisconsin, and Michigan) which existed from 1992 to 2015.

Public health leaders need to become active participants of the American Public Health Association (APHA). This association represents all segments of the professional public health workforce. It is at the annual meetings of the APHA that national public health policy tends to be made. The National Association of County and City Health Officials (NACCHO) is a key national organization for local health leaders. Leaders should also consider taking key roles in the various associations for state and county public health directors. Board of health leaders can also become involved in the National Association of Local Boards of Health (NALBOH). Following is a list of guidelines for leaders who wish to make a mark in the profession of public health:

- Promote public health as a profession.
- Encourage staff to become involved in state and national public health associations.
- Be active in state and national public health associations by serving on committees or agreeing to run for an association office.

Exercise 3-2 gives you the opportunity to work with the six levels model.

SUMMARY

Leaders need to operate on six different levels. On the most basic level, they need to know how to exert their influence as leaders on other individuals at a person-to-person level. To do this, they need a whole range of skills and abilities, from communication skills to the ability to balance work and private life. Regardless of the level at which the leader works,

> **EXERCISE 3-2** The Six Levels of Leadership
>
> **Purpose:** to explore the six levels of leadership and view a public health outbreak from each of the six levels
>
> **Key Concepts:** six levels of leadership, disease outbreak
>
> **Scenario:** In August 2015, 15 cases of bubonic plague are reported in country X.
>
> **Procedure:** Put six sheets of newsprint in front of the room. Divide the class or workshop participants into six groups. Each group will take one level. The group will explore the scenario and how the group would address the problem from its leadership level (15–30 minutes). Present your findings to the whole class or workshop.

commitment and passion for the work are critical. Leaders strongly believe in what they do. Bolman and Deal believe that there is a spiritual quality to leadership that is difficult to explain or study.[83] However, it can be seen in the work and the dedication of leaders. Thus, leadership is not only about money; it is also about all the things that make us wake up in the morning with anticipation for the job we have to do today. Leadership at the personal level is about our passion in action.

Leaders also must be capable of functioning in teams, either as team leaders or as ordinary team members. Some of the leadership skills needed for teamwork are also needed on the personal level, but some are different. It is on teams that we see the mission of our work in action.[84] It is at the team level that we also see the emotional aspects of working together and creating networks of collaboration and friendship.

Public health leaders are often the heads of public health departments or agencies and thus need agency-level leadership skills as well. Their duties as agency heads include such things as mission and vision statement development, fundraising, job performance evaluation, and role modeling. At the agency level, leaders also see systems thinking in action. It is the big picture that guides our work.

Public health is obviously community oriented, and so public health leaders need to be able to play a major role in the community by acting as advocates on public health issues and building coalitions to deal with such issues. They thus need advocacy skills and coalition-building skills, among others. At the community level, we can see the passion and commitment of our partners.

At the fifth level, leaders need to address global health issues. With the ability of people to move around the world quickly, diseases can also spread quickly. It is critical that public health leaders learn to collaborate and if possible coordinate their public health initiatives.

At the sixth level, public health leaders, like other public health practitioners, have an obligation to try to improve the field of public health by becoming involved, for instance, in professional organizations such as the APHA, NACCHO, and NALBOH. Many leaders have told me that the networking that occurs at the national level is important and helps leaders to sustain their strong belief that public health can make a difference. Fighting our battles legislatively becomes easier when we work with our public health colleagues. Professional friends often become lifelong learners.

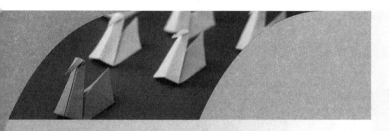

Discussion Questions

1. What is the difference between politics and governance?

2. What is the relationship between communication and empowerment?

3. What are several of the main barriers preventing public health leaders from being as effective as they could be?

4. What is one way public health leaders can deal with the increasing cultural diversity in the public health workforce?

5. What are some of the main reasons for creating and using teams?

6. What are the main agency-related responsibilities of public health leaders?

7. What are the main community-related responsibilities of public health leaders?

8. How do partnerships differ from other types of collaborative relationships?

9. How can public health leaders further the interests of the public health profession?

REFERENCES

1. R. A. Heifetz and M. Linsky, *Leadership on the Line* (Boston, MA: Harvard Business School Press, 2002).
2. S. D. Parks, *Leadership Can Be Taught* (Boston, MA: Harvard Business School Press, 2005).
3. P. M. Senge et al., *The Dance of Change* (New York, NY: Bantam, 1999).
4. A. Delaney, *Politics for Dummies* (Foster City, CA: IDG Books, 1995).
5. P. Capezio and D. Morehouse, *Secrets of Breakthrough Leadership* (Franklin Lakes, NJ: Career Press, 1997).
6. E. Tosca, *Communication Skills Profile* (San Francisco, CA: Jossey-Bass, 1997).
7. D. Tannen, *You Just Don't Understand: Women and Men in Conversation* (New York, NY: Morrow, 1990).
8. J. W. Gardner, *On Leadership* (New York, NY: Free Press, 1990).
9. R. Kelley, *The Power of Followership* (New York, NY: Doubleday, 1992).
10. J. Carver, *Boards That Make a Difference*, 3rd ed. (San Francisco, CA: Jossey-Bass, 2006).
11. V. Mamlin-Upshaw, "Creating Effective Boards," *Leadership* 2, no. 3 (1993): 1, 11.
12. J. W. Dearing and E. M. Rogers, "Agenda-Setting," *Communication Concepts* 6 (1992): 1–98.
13. E. M. Rogers and J. W. Dearing, "Agency-Setting Research: Where Has It Been? Where Is It Going?" *Communication Yearbook* 11 (1988).
14. Institute of Medicine, *The Future of Public Health* (Washington, DC: National Academy Press, 1988).
15. B. J. Turnock, *Public Health: What It Is and How It Works*, 5th ed. (Burlington, MA: Jones & Bartlett Learning, 2012).
16. Turnock, *Public Health*.
17. Turnock, *Public Health*.
18. S. R. Covey, *The Seven Habits of Highly Effective People* (New York, NY: Simon & Schuster, 1989).
19. M. M. Chemers, "Contemporary Leadership Theory," in J. T. Wren (ed.), *The Leader's Companion* (New York, NY: Free Press, 1995).
20. R. Hargrove, *Mastering the Art of Creative Collaboration* (New York, NY: McGraw-Hill Business Week Books, 1998).
21. Turnock, *Public Health*.
22. S. Wellington, "Breaking the Glass Ceiling," *Leader to Leader* 6 (1997): 37–42.
23. R. R. Thomas Jr., "Diversity and Organizations of the Future," in P. Hesselbein et al. (eds.), *The Organization of the Future* (San Francisco, CA: Jossey-Bass, 1997).
24. A. H. Maslow, *Motivation and Personality* (New York, NY: Harper & Row, 1954).
25. J. R. O'Neil, *The Paradox of Success* (New York, NY: Jeremy P. Tarcher and Putnam, 1993).
26. Capezio and Morehouse, *Secrets of Breakthrough Leadership*.
27. S. Helgesen, "Women and the New Economy," *Leader to Leader* 4 (1997): 34–39.
28. C. Mallory, *Team-Building* (Shawnee Mission, KS: National Press Publications, 1991).
29. S. P. Robbins and M. Coulter, *Management*, 11th ed. (Upper Saddle River, NJ: Prentice Hall, 2011).
30. Mallory, *Team-Building*.
31. Mallory, *Team-Building*.
32. P. F. Drucker, *Management: Tasks, Responsibilities, Practices* (New York, NY: Harper & Row, 1985).
33. J. R. Katzenbach and D. K. Smith, *The Wisdom of Teams* (Boston, MA: Harvard Business School Press, 1993).
34. K. Blanchard et al., *The One Minute Manager Builds High Performance Teams* (New York, NY: Morrow, 1990).
35. P. M. Senge, *The Fifth Discipline Fieldbook* (New York, NY: Doubleday, 1999).
36. P. Lencioni, *The Five Dysfunctions of a Team* (San Francisco, CA: Jossey-Bass, 2002).
37. D. Cohen and L. Prusek, *In Good Company: How Social Capital Makes Organizations Work* (Boston, MA: Harvard Business School Press, 2001).
38. P. Capezio, *Supreme Teams: How to Make Teams Really Work* (Shawnee Mission, KS: National Press Publications, 1996).
39. Wellins et al., *Empowered Teams* (San Francisco, CA: Jossey-Bass, 1991).
40. K. Blanchard et al., *The Three Keys to Empowerment* (San Francisco, CA: Berrett-Koehler, 1999).
41. Wellins et al., *Empowered Teams*.
42. Wellins et al., *Empowered Teams*.
43. P. Hersey, K. H. Blanchard, and D. E. Johnson, *Management of Organizational Behavior*, 9th ed. (Upper Saddle River, NJ: Prentice-Hall, 2007).
44. F. LaFasto and C. Larson, *When Teams Work Best* (Thousand Oaks, CA: Sage Publications, 2001).
45. T. Peters and N. Austin, *A Passion for Excellence* (New York, NY: Random House, 1985).
46. Mallory, *Team-Building*.
47. J. R. Katzenbach and D. K. Smith, *The Wisdom of Teams* (Boston, MA: Harvard Business School Press, 1993).
48. Capezio, *Supreme Teams*.
49. J. G. Liebler and C. R. McConnell, *Management Principles for Health Professionals*, 5th ed. (Burlington, MA: Jones & Bartlett Learning, 2011).
50. Liebler and McConnell, *Management Principles for Health Professionals*.
51. J. Q. Wilson, *Bureaucracy* (New York, NY: Basic Books, 1989).
52. Peters and Austin, *A Passion for Excellence*.
53. K. Blanchard and S. Bowles, *Gung Ho* (New York, NY: Morrow, 1998).
54. P. F. Drucker, *Landmarks of Tomorrow* (New York, NY: Harper & Row, 1957).
55. A. Tiwana, *The Knowledge Management Toolkit*, 2nd ed. (Upper Saddle River, NJ: Prentice-Hall, 2002).
56. T. Peters, *Thriving on Chaos* (New York, NY: Knopf, 1987).
57. P. F. Drucker, *Managing for the Future* (New York, NY: Truman, Talley Books, and Dutton, 1992).
58. B. Nanus, *Visionary Leadership* (San Francisco, CA: Jossey-Bass, 1992).
59. W. Shonick, *Government and Health Services* (New York, NY: Oxford University Press, 1995).
60. Institute of Medicine, *The Future of Public Health*.
61. Rowitz, *Public Health in the 21st Century*.
62. Shonick, *Government and Health Services*.
63. United States Department of Health and Human Services, Appendix B *HHS Performance Measures*, (Washington, DC, 2011). http://www.hhs.gov/secretary/about/appendixb.html. Accessed March 10, 2016.
64. Turnock, *Public Health*.
65. D. J. Breckon, *Managing Health Promotion Programs* (Gaithersburg, MD: Aspen Publishers, 1997).
66. J. M. Kouzes and B. Z. Posner, *The Leadership Challenge*, 4th ed. (San Francisco, CA: Jossey-Bass, 2007).
67. D. Tracy, *10 Steps to Empowerment* (New York, NY: Harper-Collins, 1992).
68. F. Hesselbein et al., eds., *The Community of the Future* (San Francisco, CA: Jossey-Bass, 1998).
69. J. P. Kretzman and J. L. McKnight, *Building Communities from the Inside Out* (Evanston, IL: Northwestern University Center for Urban Affairs, 1993).

70. M. S. Peck, *A World Waiting to Be Born* (New York, NY: Bantam Books, 1993).

71. L. Wallack and L. Dorfman, "Media Advocacy: A Strategy for Advancing Policy and Promoting Health," *Health Education Quarterly* 23, no. 3 (1996): 293–317.

72. R. C. Brownson and E. A. Baker, "Prevention in the Community: Taking Stock," *Journal of Public Health Management and Practice* 4, no. 2 (1998): vi–vii.

73. R. C. Brownson et al., "Demonstration Projects in Community-based Prevention," *Journal of Public Health Management and Practice* 4, no. 2 (1998): 66–77.

74. M. S. Peck, *The Different Drum* (New York, NY: Simon & Schuster, 1987).

75. R. H. Rosen, *Leading People* (New York, NY: Viking, 1996).

76. P. M. Senge, "Creating Quality Communities," in K. Gozdz (ed.), *Community-Building* (San Francisco, CA: New Leaders Press, 1995).

77. D. O. Chrislip and C. E. Larson, *Collaborative Leadership* (San Francisco, CA: Jossey-Bass, 1994).

78. Chrislip and Larson, *Collaborative Leadership*.

79. L. Cohen et al., *Developing Effective Coalitions: An Eight Step Guide* (Pleasant Hill, CA: Contra Costa County Health Services Department Prevention Programs, 1994).

80. Centers for Disease Control and Prevention, Agency for Toxic Substances and Disease Registry, *Principles of Community Engagement* (Atlanta, GA: CDC Public Health Practice Program Office, 1997).

81. Peck, *A World Waiting to Be Born*.

82. "International Health Regulations Enter Into Force," *Medical News Today*, June 16, 2007.

83. L. G. Bolman and T. E. Deal, *Leading with Soul*, 2nd ed. (San Francisco, CA: Jossey-Bass, 2001).

84. R. Wagner and J. K. Harter, *12: The Elements of Great Managing* (New York, NY: Gallup Books, 2006).

© scyther5/Shutterstock

CHAPTER **4**

Leadership at the Personal Level

LEARNING OBJECTIVES

- Discover the five essentials of successful leadership.
- Investigate how the arts can improve leadership performance.
- Show ability to write a personal leadership philosophy.
- Understand personal risks.
- Describe the dimensions of leadership presence.
- Develop a leadership learning contract.
- Begin journaling.

If we were to try to look at all the literature on leadership and distill all the literature down to the five essentials of being a successful public health leader, what might we expect these essentials to be? Here is one possible list:

1. Knowledge with the intelligence to use it. Leaders are bombarded with new information on a daily basis from new health statistics, new public health technical reports, new funding opportunities, and new demands for service based on emerging threats or the need for new programmatic directions. All the new information has to be translated into the context of public health and the governing paradigms of core functions and essential services that drive public health action and practice.

2. Empathy and motivation of others. Leaders have learned that the technological expertise that brought them into public health careers has become secondary to their relationships with colleagues and external partners. Leaders struggle to develop the social skills necessary to be effective and able to collaborate with others with ease. This set of basic skills has come to be called emotional intelligence.

3. Risk taking with action and follow-through. Leaders need not only to be visionary and creative, they need to be able to take risks and to get their ideas translated into action with well-defined projected outcomes. Every new vision or creative idea has a potential risk associated with it. Many people including colleagues are fearful of change. Risk taking is the attempt to change the status quo in spite of much resistance in order to move their agencies in new directions.

4. Ability to communicate at many different levels. Leaders have to communicate both verbally and in writing in both traditional ways or through the use of social media. Social networks may become critical to their work. They need to listen to others carefully. They may also have to communicate cross-culturally or to others who speak in another language. Most leaders are excellent at using real life events to demonstrate how their theories work. They also become skilled as storytellers.

5. Systems thinkers with an understanding of how complexity affects their work. Leaders understand that most of their work relates to the big picture of their communities. They also look at their agencies as whole organizations with interacting parts. They see their organization within the context of the whole community. They understand that most of their work is about change and upsetting the status quo. Leaders tend to support a social justice philosophy with a belief in improving the health of all people in their respective communities. They also realize that the best plans may also have unanticipated consequences.

It is clear that leadership is a complex process. The leader needs to develop himself or herself at the personal level and incorporate all types of leadership tools to guide the personal growth process. The leader also needs to develop a leadership mindset or mental model that incorporates leadership and lifelong learning into what it means to be a leader. Because leadership is interactive and also oriented to change, the personal skills related to relationship-building and change management become an important set of tools for the leader to master at the personal level. The leadership mindset involves the importance of realizing that the community context is critical in public health for addressing adaptive challenges.

As leaders or future leaders, we need to commit ourselves to lifelong learning at all six levels of leadership—personal, team, organizational, community, professional, and global. Each leadership level requires a portfolio of learning activities to enhance our leadership. This chapter addresses our personal development as leaders. A personal leadership portfolio contains all the results of various leadership instruments that a leader uses to learn more about his or her leadership strengths and skills. I would recommend that you start this process with *Strengths Finder 2.0*.[1] The portfolio also documents key leadership decisions made in different settings. Part of lifelong learning is to continue learning as much about yourself as a person as possible.

To be a successful lifelong learner, learning to be a leader should not be limited only to leadership. Leaders need to be well rounded. We need to go beyond the academic specialty in which we were originally trained. If you are a leader originally trained as a physician, now you need to learn about management, leadership, and behavioral sciences such as economics, sociology, and psychology, political science, biostatistics, epidemiology, community engagement, and so on. It is the multidisciplinary perspective that broadens our view of the context in which we work.

Most of our education involved the development of a linear thinking approach to problem solving in our agency or other unit within it. We need to develop tools that help us to organize a systems thinking perspective. Senge[2] has provided us with a number of systems tools called archetypes to help us in this endeavor. With mastery at this level, we are able to see the chaos that must be addressed in our community work. It becomes imperative that leaders develop a complexity perspective that uses tools to bring order out of the chaos that we see. The composition of the group that is doing the problem solving is clearly affected by the individuals in the room. If the group changes its composition over time, the problem solving will change with the new members. With complexity then, unanticipated happenings are common.

Leaders love to read and read widely. They read books in many fields and even learn to use fiction to help them understand the world better. I give you two books a month to add to your leadership learning in my leadership blog book club.[3] Another way to add to your knowledge is to visit a local bookstore or to explore new books and literature. There is also the excitement of visiting a good library as well as many Internet sites that give you many interesting articles to read.

Exploring the arts also enriches us at many levels. Movies, concerts, museums, opera, classical music, theater, art exhibits, sports events, travel, and new restaurants teach us much about our culture and other cultures. Not only do these events give us much to talk about, they help us view the world from many perspectives. I find that I begin to understand our country better after a trip to another country. Travel also gives me the chance to see us from a number of different perspectives. The arts also provide us with many tools that are also useful in our leadership work. Here are a few examples of how the arts can help us in our work:

1. Use of the tools of the arts will strengthen the mental models of the culture in which leaders work.
2. Theater arts allow leaders the opportunity to test leadership principles and practices in our social lives.
3. Music provides the chance to see how leaders function with music in the background and how music affects leadership performance.
4. Communication strategies and techniques can be improved by the arts.
5. The arts provide innovative approaches to conflict resolution strategies, problem solving, decision making, and team building.
6. Theater games will be useful in emergency preparedness and response practices.
7. Coaching opportunities are possible in theater arts scenarios.

It is important for leaders to explore their creativity by doing different things as well as stepping back from a conflict situation in order to experiment with innovative and nontraditional approaches to addressing adaptive challenges that have been presented. We can use new group process strategies like six thinking hats,[4] open space technology,[5] and the world café[6] that employ creative approaches to solving challenges of many kinds. Another technique I have used in workshops is the employment of theater games to experiment with different leadership strategies. In the area of conflict resolution, for example, two people are arguing about closing a window. One person wants to close the window and the other person does not. Who will win the argument?

Leaders need to know that it is important to maintain a balance between their personal lives and their work lives. Leaders sometimes let their work lives overpower their personal lives. Because we have only so many hours of awake time, the important issue is how we will use those hours each day. The choices we make can affect our lives over the long run. Because leaders are embedded in their home communities, it is important that leaders strengthen their personal connections both within our household and also within the community at work and play.

John Gardner[7] believed that leaders needed to set time apart for personal reflection. Time needs to be set aside on a regular basis for this self-renewal process. Retreats at a remote site are another mechanism for leaders to collaborate with their work colleagues or external partners to review, evaluate activities, or plan for the future. Retreat participants can use creativity exercises and strategies to develop new programmatic directions or to explore and develop their personal leadership knowledge and skills.

Leaders often learn from their action-based activities. If a leader goes out into the community to be actively involved in the health promotion activities of the community, leaders and their partners should learn new strategies from their activities. Experiential learning will also enhance leadership and give

PUBLIC HEALTH HEROES AND VILLIANS 4-1 Paul Farmer, Humanitarian and Hero[8]

Paul Farmer was born in Massachusetts in 1959. As he was growing up in Florida, his family picked citrus fruit with Haitian migrant workers. He and his family lived in a houseboat on the Gulf, bathed in a creek, and brought water in jugs from a creek. Despite these unusual family circumstances, Farmer did exceptionally well in school. He won a scholarship to Duke University where he studied medical anthropology. He spent 6 months in Paris where he attended classes of Claude Lévi-Strauss, a world-renowned anthropologist. Farmer returned to Duke speaking fluent French. He became interested in the poor farm workers, some of whom were Haitians living not far from Duke. He became interested in Haitian culture and learned Creole during this period. Farmer graduated from Duke *summa cum laude* and went to the University of Pittsburgh where he completed a postgraduate fellowship.

Farmer next went to Harvard where he completed a joint degree program in medicine and medical anthropology in 1990. He also became interested in public health. During this time, he travelled to Haiti with the intention of working in a public health clinic. He was able to secure funding from Project Bread to open a bakery in Cange, Haiti to supply bread to a community with a high percentage of people with chronic malnutrition. Next, Farmer founded Zanmi Lasante, a community-based health project. In 1985, Farmer and a colleague opened Clinique Bon Saveur in Cange. Cases of acquired immune deficiency syndrome (AIDS) were discovered.

In 1987 Farmer and his friends founded the organization Partners in Health in Boston. This organization's mission is to change the way we work to help people on a global level. Patients are to be helped in their homes and local communities. Health workers will develop partnerships with local government officials and medical and academic institutions around the world. Through these partnerships, medical and public health service capacity will be built in order to strengthen health systems. In this work, the priority will be to help the poor.

Through the 1990s, in Haiti, Farmer helped the Zanmi Lasante clinic grow into a hospital. Farmer's work was recognized by the MacArthur Foundation in 1993 and he received a MacArthur genius grant. By the end of the 1990s, Zanmi Lasante had built homes for the poor, schools, improved sanitation, and water facilities. On the disease front, outbreaks of drug-resistant typhoid decrease in the incidence of tuberculosis.

Over the last 2 decades, Farmer has written a number of books and articles. He has continued his work in Cange as well as work with the Partners in Health organization. He travels all over the world to help the poor improve their health and was named the United Nations deputy envoy to Haiti by the Special Envoy Bill Clinton in 2009. He is now the department head of global health and social medicine at Harvard Medical School. Paul Farmer is clearly a leader with passion for his work in Haiti and elsewhere. He lives his life for the improvement of the health of the poor around the world. He is one of our major public health heroes.

leaders the opportunity to apply leadership knowledge, skills, and tools in real time. Leaders become expert in applying all of these learning strategies to adaptive leadership challenges synergistically. Each leader puts all these tools and skills to work in innovative and creative ways. Paul Farmer is one such person. He is a true public health leadership hero. See hero story above.

From several decades of leadership in both the public and private sectors, Robert M. Gates, former Secretary of Defense in the administrations of both Presidents George Bush and Barack Obama has clearly learned some facts about being a successful leader.[9] Gates states that most leaders are concerned with change. Leaders also need to be careful not to let their egos interfere with the work that needs to be done. Paul Farmer was extremely careful to do this although he was clearly passionate about helping the poor. Gates believes that leaders need to be trustworthy and have integrity, within both the public and private sectors. Paul Farmer was able to work with both sectors with great success. He was seen as trustworthy by both sectors as well as the people of Haiti and other poor nations. Gates also points out that leaders need to be self-disciplined. Collaboration requires self-discipline. A leader needs to be able to listen to others and not always dominate the proceedings. This is another characteristic of Farmer. Gates also points to the need to be humble and not give the impression of being the smartest person in the room. Farmer seems to excel here as well. Gates argues that leaders need to have courage, work with others for change, know and understand that compromise is important, follow their principles, and finally realize when their work is done. Dr. Farmer excels here as well. Most of Gates' principles of successful leadership fit our heroes including Dr. Farmer. Gates also advocates the importance of humor. This characteristic is harder to ascertain for our heroes.

Heroes and leaders need to be reality based. There are at least three competencies that a leader must address.[10] Dr. Farmer also seems to have mastered these three competencies. First, leaders must be able to address heath crises. Because leaders are working in an environment of constant change, they should be prepared for any contingency. Second, leaders need to be oriented toward success. Third, leaders need to have the willingness to resolve conflict as quickly as possible.

One thing that leaders can do to improve their leadership skills is to develop a personal leadership philosophy. At this point, your philosophy statement should be no more than one page. The statement should include your approach to leadership at home and at work. It should also include your approach to lifelong learning. **Exercise 4-1** is an opportunity to develop a philosophy statement.

EXERCISE 4-1 My Leadership Philosophy

Purpose: to develop a personal leadership philosophy statement

Key Concepts: personal leadership, philosophy statement, reality based

Procedure: Write a one-page personal leadership philosophy statement for your future work in public health. You should include the issue of work and family in your statement. You should also address your approach to your lifelong learning agenda. Present your statement to your class and get recommendations for improving your statement. Revise statement and use it in your work going forward.

A BRIEF NOTE ON RISK

In a complex world such as ours, leaders find the rules of the leadership game involve change that becomes a reality in which to work. This is especially true in public health and the other health services areas. We seem to have multiple stakeholders watching whatever we do. These stakeholders are elected officials, governing boards, community residents, religious leaders, and business leaders. With all these stakeholders watching us, leaders often need to take personal risk in addressing community health-related concerns. Personal risks often become entangled with health risks of many kinds. There are several personal risks that are involved.[11]

First, we do not always have the option to select the people with whom we work. Respect between leaders and their staff is important if we are to accomplish our goals. Personal risk taking to improve these relationships may or may not be successful. Second, risk taking becomes complicated if we work for an organization where our personal values and ethics are not similar to the values and ethics built into the agency culture. Third, the leader needs to be concerned about the risk of compromise where the critical part of a solution is lost as a result of the compromise. Fourth, there is a risk of making a decision that a leader does not care about. A leader needs to be committed to the decisions that are made. Next is the related concern of a decision that goes against a leader's belief system. Finally, there is the important risk of working in a field such as public health when you really wanted to go to medical school.

Risk taking should be strategic.[12] Even at a personal leadership level, risk taking has consequences at the team, organization, and community levels. All risks need to serve the mission of our agencies. All risk-taking activities by a public health leader have the possibility of leading to failure. A failure needs to be seen as a learning experience. Before the leader takes a personal risk, he or she needs to be aware that taking the risk is a choice. The leader weighs all the factors that affect the risk-taking choice because risk taking may have financial effects as well as social and psychological costs. Risk taking may not have immediate effects. Change takes time to show results.

LEADERSHIP PRESENCE

In recent years, leaders have become concerned about how they are viewed by others.[13] If you give a talk before others, do you do any personal things to enhance your performance? How do you want to be seen by others? Presence provides added features beyond the leader's behavior. Glasshammer, which is a career consulting firm for women, provides a number of tips for helping leaders increase their presence.[14] Most of the tips would be useful to men as well:

1. A positive attitude enhances the relationship with others.
2. Listening to others is a sign of respect.
3. You need to be outgoing and friendly to others.
4. The 80/20 rule applies. You need to listen 80 percent of the time and speak only 20 percent of the time and not about yourself.
5. Empower others to solve problems.
6. Your appearance is important.
7. Try to be early to events.
8. Be as clear as possible in what you say. Avoid jargon.
9. Be open to criticism.
10. Be able to share credit with others.
11. Show empathy and give feedback where appropriate.
12. Be careful about losing your temper. Your composure is important in maintaining the balance in a given situation.
13. Have individual conversations with others and especially with coworkers and community stakeholders.
14. If conflicts arise, deal with them quickly and fairly.

Leadership presence involves the integration of public, private, and personal leadership.[15] Public and private leadership involves what leaders need to do at a behavioral level with individuals and groups. Public leadership relates to the actions and behaviors that we do with two or more people in creating a vision, empowering others, planning, agenda setting, problem solving, decision making, and implementing our decisions. Private leadership is a leader's work with one individual on purpose and individual performance on tasks and helping a direct report to build skills. At the personal leadership level, we are addressing our needs for knowledge and skills to carry out our leadership activities. We need to make sure our personal attitudes are in agreement with others both inside and outside our organizations. The complicated concerns related to psychological self-mastery are also critical here.

In summary, the integration of public leadership, private leadership, and personal leadership leads to the way our authentic self is seen by others. This affects our leadership presence. For each unique leader, Scouller[16] points out that there are seven qualities related to presence:

1. Personal power
2. High self-esteem
3. Desire to learn more
4. High service orientation and respect for others
5. Intuition
6. Living in the present
7. Inner peace of mind

LEADERSHIP LEARNING CONTRACT

Leaders need to be open to new tools and perspectives. Flexibility and resilience are important. Personal leadership development is an evolving process. Because of this, leaders should take time for personal reflection. As a leader, we need time to grow. No one approach to leadership will work in the long run although the ecological approach does have the flexibility to expand and include new techniques and tools. Adaptive challenges will always present themselves. A culture of health will also allow leaders to approach community health concerns with flexibility as new health challenges and health breakthroughs occur. In addition, the way Leader A did the leadership work in his or her agency is not the way Leader B does leadership work in his or her agency because the demands of each agency are different. One size does not fit every situation.

Leaders tend to look for ways to develop and expand their leadership skills throughout their work lives. In fact, many public health leaders tend to continue their leadership into their retirement years. The leadership learning contract is a tool that many leaders use. The contract has the leader prepare a yearly learning plan to guide his or her personal learning each year. As these plans are developed, the leader may have to decide if an executive or life coach is needed to help prepare the plan and evaluate progress in meeting the goals of the plan. The leadership learning plan needs to be seen as a contract in which the leader views the plan as a set of obligations that guide the leader in ways to become more effective.

Some of the questions that the plan needs to address are:

1. What are the key learning objectives for the year?
2. What is my reading agenda and conference agenda for the next year?
3. What are my objectives for my agency over the next year?
4. Are there new internal and external collaborations that I want to initiate over the next year?
5. Which two or three employees can I mentor next year?

It is the actual writing of the plan that is critical. The tendency to write a plan and put it in a file or in your bottom desk drawer is not the purpose of this exercise. This plan, if implemented correctly, can be merged with a leadership journal over the next year that documents your progress toward meeting your personal goals. Regular meetings with an executive coach might also be helpful. **Exercise 4-2** involves your writing a leadership learning contract.

JOURNALING

Over 25 years ago, I made my first visit to the Centers for Disease Control and Prevention (CDC) and noticed that most CDC public health professionals that I met were carrying a green book. Throughout the meeting, each CDC person opened the green book to take notes or write comments on the proceedings. These green books were journals. Since that time, I have noticed that many public health leaders and other professionals carry these journals with many multicolor covers. Today, many of these leaders carry a laptop computer, a tablet, or a phone in which they now write their commentaries. I started carrying a journal 25 years ago and entered the 21st century carrying a computer tablet on which I continue to jot down my thoughts and ideas. In the public health leadership institute that I ran for over 20 years, we gave all participants journals in recent years. This one tool has become essential for many managers and leaders.

Our lives are so busy with all sorts of activities including work, school, home, and social lives. Ideas seem to come at breakneck speed. As leaders, we need to keep our eyes and ears focused on many things and issues in the course of a working day. Our journals prevent us from losing many of these high-speed ideas. One use of our journals is going back at the end of each week with a new entry that prioritizes the ideas of last week. This priority list allows us to determine which ideas need further development. Give each idea a score from 1 to 3 with 1 being an idea to continue to develop and 3 being an idea that is interesting but not of high priority at the present time. Write a few lines on the issue ranked 1 and what might be the next steps in developing the idea. Each month, look back at the high-scoring ideas and determine the progress in addressing these ideas. You can now answer the question whether some of these ideas should be dropped because a dead end has been reached.

A few other things that you can include in your journal are:

1. Book and article summaries
2. Meeting notes and your assignments
3. Summary of presentations at meetings
4. Progress notes related to work assignments
5. People to meet with and a brief personal background of these people

A leadership journal needs to be a living document. You can share your ideas or book and article recommendations with other leaders. This will allow idea generation and sharing to be a collaborative activity. **Exercise 4-3** allows you to start your leadership journal. You can use a book or start a journal on your laptop or other electronic device. Journaling is the process of writing in your journal.

EXERCISE 4-2 My Personal Leadership Learning Contract

Purpose: to develop a personal learning contract for the next year

Key Concepts: leadership learning contract, executive or life coach, personal goals

Procedure: Using the five contract questions in this section of the chapter, prepare your plan. Are there other questions you want to add? Discuss your contract in a personal meeting with your instructor playing the role of coach.

EXERCISE 4-3 Leadership Journal

Purpose: to begin and develop a leadership journal to guide your leadership journey and to document your leadership ideas

Key Concepts: leadership journal, journaling

Procedure: You will develop a leadership journal. On the first entry, decide the topics that your journal will cover. The format of your journal might be a hardcover book or a computer-based one. It is also possible for you to develop your journal using a blog format.

EXERCISE 4-4 Development of a Checklist

Purpose: to develop a checklist

Key Concepts: public health checklist

Procedure: You have a term paper due in 3 weeks. Develop a checklist to help you meet the deadline. Share your checklists in class.

PUBLIC HEALTH CHECKLISTS

Another important personal leadership tool is the leader's checklist. A checklist includes a set of steps for carrying out a defined task or activity. The checklist can be used for many activities such as preparing for a vacation, remodeling a kitchen or bathroom, carrying out a case management strategy, responding to a crisis event, or the procedures to follow during brain surgery. Gawande has explored the checklist in detail in his book on the use of the checklist in medicine.[17]

In public health, the checklist can become an important tool for managers and leaders. It is specifically useful when multidisciplinary teams deal with a problem or adaptive challenge. The checklist allows leaders and their teams to outline the process of activities to be done in order. In addition, an entire program or activity can be defined. This is important when activity one has to be performed by an intake nurse and has to come before an activity by another health professional. A checklist may help a leader carry out activities in a learning contract. An interesting exception involves the possibility that leadership checklists may be more abstract

and involve a number of leadership events that might occur simultaneously. **Exercise 4-4** allows you to experiment with the development of a checklist.

SUMMARY

This chapter introduces us to the first of six leadership levels. Personal leadership development is critical to what happens at all other levels. Certain characteristics seem to apply to most public health leaders. These five characteristics are reviewed in this chapter. Leaders gain knowledge that helps them become more effective leaders. This life-long learning process comes not only from reality-based experience and increasing knowledge of public health information; it also comes from the arts and books from many different fields. Leaders also have to become aware of the way they are seen by others. Presence is very important for leaders. Finally, there are a number of leadership tools presented to help leaders to become more effective and efficient including the development of a personal leadership philosophy, learning contract, leadership journal, and public health checklist.

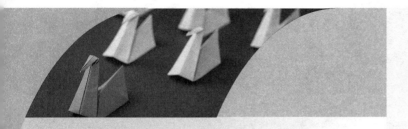

Discussion Questions

1. Why is personal leadership development important?

2. What are the five essential characteristics of a successful leader? Do you agree with the list?

3. What types of risks do leaders take? Do they have a choice?

4. How do you integrate data from the several leadership tools presented in this chapter?

5. What are five things you can do to improve your personal presence?

REFERENCES

1. T. Rath, *Strengths Finder 2.0* (New York, NY: Gallup Press, 2007).
2. P. M. Senge, *The Fifth Discipline: The Art of the Learning Organization, revised and expanded* (New York, NY: Doubleday, 2006).
3. http://rowitzonleadership.wordpress.com. Accessed February 15, 2016.
4. E. deBono, *Six Thinking Hats, Revised and Updated* (New York, NY: Back Bay Books, 1999).
5. H. Owen, *Open Space Technology: A User's Guide*, 3rd ed., revised and updated (San Francisco, CA: Berrett-Kohler, 2008).
6. J. Brown and D. Isaacs, *The World Café: Shaping Our Futures through Conversations That Matter* (San Francisco, CA: Berrett-Kohler, 2005).
7. J. W. Gardner, *Self-Renewal, revised edition* (New York, NY: W.W. Norton, 1995).
8. See http://www.achievement.org/autodoc/page/far1int-1. Accessed February 15, 2016.
9. R. M. Gates, *A Passion for Leadership* (New York, NY: Alfred A. Knopf, 2016).
10. C. Wakeman, *Reality-Based Leadership* (San Francisco, CA: Jossey-Bass, 2010).
11. R. Komisar, *The Monk and the Riddle* (Boston, MA: Harvard Business Review Press, 2001).
12. M. Zetlin, "5 things the smartest leaders know about risk-taking." http://www.inc.com/minda-zetlin/5-things-the-smartest-leaders-know-about-risk-taking.html. Accessed February 20, 2016.
13. J. Scouller, *The Three Levels of Leadership: How to Develop Your Leadership Presence, Knowhow and Skill* (London, England: Management Books 2000 Ltd., 2011).
14. J. Keyser, "14 Tips for Developing 'Leadership Presence,'" http://theglasshammer.com/2014/08/14-tips-for-developing-leadership-presence. Accessed February 20, 2016.
15. Scouller, *The Three Levels of Leadership*.
16. Scouller, *The Three Levels of Leadership*.
17. A. Gawande, *The Checklist Manifesto* (New York, NY: Picador, 2011).

CHAPTER 5

Leadership and Quality of Life

Have you noticed how successful leaders look? Most of the time, they seem positive. They seem vigorous and energetic. They appear excited with the leadership game. They love innovation and see change as a positive force. They love meeting new people and excel at building relationships. Public health leaders are excited and challenged by each new public health event. Being a leader is often a healthy endeavor. Research supports this in that traits of leaders are seen as healthy although leadership is often not mentioned as a healthy outlet for these traits.

There are many health-related research findings that affect leaders and other people. First, married people tend to be healthier than single people. Leaders who balance work and family tend to be healthier than leaders who sacrifice solid family relationships for work. Research has shown that people who are good at building relationships that they maintain and develop are healthier than those who do not build relationships. People with solid family networks also tend to eat more healthy foods than those who live alone. Second, leaders know the importance of exercise and many leaders tend to follow an exercise regimen. They find that exercise improves mood, makes them more positive, and keeps their bodies in shape. Gardner[1] argued for the importance of

reflection as a renewal process. Sharma[2] has discussed how successful leaders often meditate to reduce stress. Third, leaders are team players and stress collaboration as a positive force for change and a way to make life more meaningful. Collaboration tends to improve the mental health of the participants. Fourth, public health leaders are often believers in social justice and share themselves with those in need. Service to others results in good feelings, positivity, and helping others improve their health and quality of life. Thus, personal leadership development has the unanticipated consequence of improved health and well-being.

There are at least two sides to the issue of quality of life. From a personal leadership dimension, leaders will define quality of life from the perspective of subjective well-being. From a research perspective, quality of life will be determined relative to the general well-being within a community. The argument can be made that a culture of health perspective in a community is to promote health and improve the quality of life for all community residents as an ongoing set of activities. A standard set of indicators related to quality of life would include nutrition information, impacts of exercise, income and employment status, good sleep patterns, social integration into community life, physical and mental health status, educational level, recreation and leisure time, and the effects of retirement and aging. All of these indicators and possible others will interact and be viewed by each individual in a different way related to their individual quality of life.

At its foundation, public health is about improving health in order to improve the quality of life of all citizens in our communities, counties, and states. If our personal health initiatives improve as a result, we are moving toward change in our

PUBLIC HEALTH HEROES AND VILLIANS 5-1 Get Up & Go: An Heroic Initiative

St. Clair County in southwestern Illinois is located in the Mississippi River Valley. Sixty percent of the county land is agricultural and involved in grain production and the production of fruits and vegetables in many small gardens. In terms of population, the county is 89 percent urban and 11 percent rural. Despite these positives, access to healthy food is a concern in many poor communities and rural communities in the county. Seventeen percent of the county's population lives in poverty. The county health department is located in Belleville, Illinois. There is a second health department in the county located in the economically poor location of East St. Louis.

Our story goes back to 2005 when the county was participating in its 5-year cycle in carrying out a community health assessment. One of the findings in the 2005 cycle involved the importance of quality of life. The poorest areas of the county had the lowest quality of life scores with major concerns for safety. Other factors included lack of community support, transportation problems, lack of economic opportunities, and little access to healthy foods and health resources. It was decided that a goal of the county health department was to create a broader program of community connectedness over the years of 2006–2011. This goal led to the start of a special program eventually called "Get Up & Go."

Mark Peters is the director of community health for the St. Clair Department of Public Health and had taken a leadership role in the St. Clair community health assessment process. He had a meeting with Rita Arras-Boyd who taught public health nursing at Southern Illinois University School of Nursing. In 2007–2008, they worked on the development of a 30-day challenge program to take place in April 2008. They found community sponsors for the challenge in addition to a small grant that they received. Many community groups joined in the challenge

to improve health. This was followed in May 2008 by a health and fitness fair hosted by Belleville High School. These events led Peters and Boyd to codevelop the Get Up & Go program. The program became a nonprofit organization with a team of volunteers who became part of the original board.

A website was developed and a newsletter began to be published early in 2009. The underlying mission of the program was to help build healthier communities, neighborhoods, and families. It was strongly believed that the initiative needed to be long term if health improvements were to occur. It was also believed that community connectedness would increase the chances of success in improving the quality of life of county residents. Four priority areas were designated for the program: youth and schools, cities and neighborhoods, faith-based organizations, and worksite wellness.

In 2009 the planning proceeded for the second annual Get Up & Go 30-day health and fitness challenge. Collaborative partnerships continued and expanded. Improving the effectiveness of the program was stressed and communities were encouraged to continue the health initiatives all year long. Grants and contracts were applied for with successes as well as failures. The Get Up & Go program continues to exist, and Mark Peters and Rita Arras-Boyd are still playing leadership roles in the project. Professor Emeritus Arras-Boyd was a president of the board. Over the past several years, the program has been a cosponsor of county health policy summits. This program clearly deserves its label as a hero organization. It has benefitted St. Clair County for over 10 years. Many heroes can be found in the organization including Peters and Arras-Boyd as well as the hundreds of volunteers over the years. Get Up & Go is built on a leadership mindset that stresses service and a strong culture of health perspective.

cultural value system. This move makes a culture of health more possible. The next story involves a hero county that has been struggling with this quality of life issue for the past 10 years.

TIME MANAGEMENT

Quality of life is affected by our use of time. The use of time is largely a choice. Most of us manage our time on the computer, on our phones, or on paper. Despite using some time management process, we still manage not only to waste the time we have but not use other time we have to improve the

quality of our lives. With better time management, we can reduce stress, become more balanced, increase our productivity, and become more goal oriented.[3] There are numerous time wasters that stop us in our attempt to manage our activities at home and at work. Leadership activities increase the distractions. Some of these time wasters include:

1. Too much television watching
2. Gaming
3. Travel to and from work by car
4. Going from crisis to crisis

5. Telephone interruptions
6. Too much time with reading and responding to emails or the inbox
7. Time in socializing and gossiping at work
8. Too many meetings
9. Not learning how to say "No"
10. Too little planning
11. Too much open door policy and drop-in visitors
12. Ineffective leadership and delegation
13. Procrastination
14. Not enough staff for the work
15. Children with too many extracurricular activities
16. Poor communication skills
17. Duplication of work due to poor assignment by the boss
18. Too many home activities assigned by spouse
19. Not finishing work assignments

Each of us can probably add to these 20. The lesson of this list is that poor time management cuts down the time for those activities that improve our lives. It would be interesting if you could come up with a series of recommendations for preventing these time wasters from happening.

Time and quality of life are also affected by the society in which we live, the type of individual, and the belief system that defines us. Covey[4] has also studied the issue of what quality of life means to each of us. He pointed out that there are four endowments that define human beings. First, there is self-awareness, which allows each of us to define our life priorities. Second, we have a conscience, which helps us to determine what is important to us in matters related to how we live our lives. Third, we have independent will, which affects our ability to think through what we want our destinies to be and the way we can use our actions to achieve our desired future. In fact, our creative imagination permits us to define a mission and a vision for our lives. **Exercise 5-1** starts us on the road to defining what we want our quality of life to be.

Habits and routines are hard to change. Here are a dozen tips for managing personal change to get you started:

1. Limit the amount of time you watch television or the time you spend gaming.
2. At both home and work, prepare "to-do" lists but be realistic about the time to complete activities.
3. Consider public transportation instead of driving your car so that you can do some work-related activities while you travel.
4. Develop a time for returning phone calls and answering emails. Put the time allocation on your calendar. Turn the ringer off your phone and computer.

EXERCISE 5-1 My Personal Calendar

Purpose: to use my personal calendar to see how my schedule affects my quality of life on a daily basis

Key Concepts: personal calendar, quality of life, mission, time, leadership

Procedure: Using your personal calendar, list all the activities of your day for 3 days including when you slept, had meals, etc. Examine your 3-day calendar and identify any patterns.

1. Which activities do you find that you require and probably cannot change?
2. Which activities do you want to retain and which activities do you want to change?
3. Which activities affect your own quality of life?
4. Which activities do you want to add to enhance your quality of life? For example, do you want to lose weight, which will affect the food you eat or the amount of exercise in which you will engage?
5. How will you change the time you allocate to your family or to leisure activities?
6. Write a quality of life mission statement for yourself and put it in your leadership journal.

---

5. Limit office socializing to an hour a day when your energy is at its low ebb.
6. Limit the number of meetings if possible. Keep the meetings you have to attend to less than an hour.
7. Learn to say no if your calendar is full or learn to delegate whatever assignments you have that can be done by others.
8. Plan ahead.
9. Do not assume that you as leader are the only one with the knowledge to do the work.
10. Do not take on more assignments than you or your staff can do.
11. Procrastination has bad results.
12. Share home responsibilities. If your spouse or roommate cooks, you clean the dishes.

RULES FOR HEALTHY LIVING

Public health leaders need to be committed not only to the development and enhancement of their personal leadership skills, but they must use their public health knowledge to improve their personal health skills. In other words, public health leaders need to practice what they preach. If they do so, both their leadership abilities and their quality of life will be improved. In this section, we explore a dozen rules for healthy living. First, it is important to address nutrition. How many times a week do you eat a fast-food lunch or go out for dinner? Eating healthy food for 80 percent of your meals will help you to improve your health status. The other 20 percent allows you to have some freedom in your food choices. It is fine to have a pizza once in a while and in moderation. Second, avoid too many sweets. Diabetes cases are increasing. If you need sugar, try a piece of fruit.

Third, a leader should maintain a healthy weight appropriate to his or her height. With the high obesity problem in the United States, it is important for our leaders to be role models for normal weight. Our fourth rule helps in maintaining our weight. We should be exercising five or more times a week for 30 minutes or more. Many leaders argue that they do not have the time. Try taking a walk as part of your lunch hour and get away from your desk.

Fifth, sleep is important to our ability to function with high efficiency. Many sacrifice their sleep hours to catch up on work-related activities. Leaders generally need 7–8 hours of sleep a night. If a leader or anyone else does this for 7 days a week, a pattern will develop and you may not even need an alarm clock to wake you up in the morning. Sixth, develop stress reduction techniques to keep your productivity in high gear. A good night's sleep and ability to control stress will help both your energy level and your productivity.

Seven, stop smoking or do not smoke or use recreational drugs. I visited a local health department a few years ago where I saw health department staff smoking cigarettes in the parking lot. This is clearly something that we do not want our clients to see and it undermines our image of being advocates for the public's health. The issue of alcohol use can also be mentioned as part of this rule. If a leader drinks, it should be done in moderation.

The eighth rule involves the importance of getting an annual checkup from your physician. If the leader has diabetes or some other chronic health problem, he or she may visit a physician more than once a year. The ninth rule is another way to protect your health. Fresh air is important. Try to spend an hour a day out of doors. A leader may want to combine this with his or her lunchtime walk.

The 10th rule relates to the leader drinking clean water. Many nutritionists argue that eight glasses of water should be consumed each day. The 11th rule argues for the importance of good hygiene and frequent handwashing. The final rule relates to our mental health and doing whatever is needed to maintain our health. For some people, our adherence to our

religious faith helps us. For others, volunteerism and helping our neighbors helps our mental health.

Practicing these 12 rules for healthy living is clearly related to our quality of life. **Exercise 5-2** allows you to grade yourself from A to E on how well you practice the 12 rules of healthy living.

WELL-BEING

Well-being is another perspective on quality of life issues. Rath and Harter[5] reported on the findings of a comprehensive international study of over 150 countries on the issue of well-being. They found that there are five interdependent factors that help

---

EXERCISE 5-2 The 12 Rules of Healthy Living

Purpose: to allow leaders to develop plans for improving their adherence to the 12 rules of healthy living

Key Concepts: rules of healthy living

Procedure: Grade yourself as to how well you are following each of the 12 rules of healthy living. Develop a plan for improving your grade for each rule.

---

12 Rules of Healthy Living Report Card

Rule	Grade	Plan
1. Healthy eating		
2. Sweets in Moderation		
3. Healthy weight		
4. Exercise 5 days/week		
5. 7–8 hours of sleep/night		
6. Stress reduction techniques		
7. No smoking		
8. Annual physical		
9. Hour of fresh air/day		
10. Drink eight glasses of fresh water/day		
11. Practice good hygiene		
12. Practice faith or volunteerism		

us to determine and improve our well-being and overall quality of life. The first factor is career well-being. On the whole, many of us enjoy our work lives. Leaders can use their strengths to be more effective and efficient leaders. We can improve our work life through the use of mentors and coaches. We can search for and discover organizations for which we love to work. We also develop friendships with those at work. These friends enhance our social lives as well.

The second factor relates to social well-being. The hours that we spend with friends often increase our happiness level. We also keep stress levels low when we are enjoying our friends and our social activities. Each friend offers us unique experiences. Our friends provide us with social support and encouragement to improve ourselves. Rath and Harter encourage us to spend 6 hours a day with friends, colleagues, and family. They also encourage us to work on our physical activities with our friends.

The third factor involves the element of financial well-being. On a personal level, each of us determines how much money we need to make us happy. If the problem of never enough money is resolved, then the determination of how we spend the money we have will be more important. Vacations and outings with friends and family are well-being enhancers. A leader can take a friend or colleague to lunch, for example. Saving money is another way to enhance well-being.

The fourth factor involves physical well-being. As pointed out earlier, what we eat, how much we sleep, and how much we exercise affect our well-being. Eating too many fast-food lunches, getting too little sleep, and not exercising does not set a good example for others. Just think about the cost to society for our bad habits. Public health leaders need to practice what we preach. Thus, we need to shop better, eat healthier foods, get enough sleep, and exercise.

The final factor relates to the well-being of our communities. The air we breathe and the quality of the water we drink are important to keep our communities healthy. The safety of our streets is another important concern. Involvement in community life is also important as was seen in the Get Up & Go hero story. To help improve community well-being, determine how you can use your leadership skills to contribute to the promotion of a culture of health in your neighborhood. Find ways to relate to others. You can look to increase your social networks. Share your interests by joining community groups.

Rath and Harter[5] have developed the Well-being Finder to measure your well-being. Are you thriving, struggling, or suffering?

THE WELBE™ MODEL

In his second book on quality of life issues and personal well-being, Rath[6] discusses the impact of eating, sleeping, and moving on our lives. Choice on how to live our lives is the critical factor. We need to make choices consciously through the creation of a plan, reading widely on health-related issues, and making 30-day challenges for ourselves. It is important to be realistic. A 30-day plan is realistic. Long-term planning is not so realistic. We will find that our health improves through making small adjustments. Rath is not talking about fad diets. Inactivity is one of the culprits. Too much or too little sleep is not the answer. Personal health choices need to be made one at a time. It is important to make these healthy life changes a critical part of our everyday life.

Eating, exercise, movement, and sleep all work together to improve the quality of our lives. Leaders need to live this healthy lifestyle if our families, our friends, colleagues, and communities are to improve their health and create a culture of health. Rath has created a Welbe™ application for our phones and computers to monitor our health-making process. The application includes nutrition, exercise, and sleep as pillars for taking action for us, our friends, colleagues, and place of work. We can make our organizations models for healthy living in our communities.

FULLY CHARGED

In his third book on wellness and quality of life, Rath[7] explores three keys that are important to our overall well-being on a daily basis. When our energy level is high, we tend to be more motivated and productive. Rath associates energy with being fully charged. The first key to a full charge is associated with meaning. There are a number of ways to create meaning including small wins, meaningfulness from inside ourselves and living our values, having a mission and purpose for the work we do, addressing the needs of our communities, and wanting to shape the future of our public health work and healthy community outcomes.

The second key relates to interactions. Leaders work to make their interactions count. Emotional intelligence skills are extremely useful. Being positive most of the time is also a significant interaction skill. It is important not to overpower the people with whom we interact. It is important to listen and to make time for social interaction. Working with others creates positive experiences as well as making our experiences meaningful.

The third key specifically addresses energy. As pointed out in the last section, it is important to protect our personal health. If we maintain our activity throughout the day, our energy levels seem to remain high. Our stress levels are affected by our personal health habits. Seeing stressful situations as a challenge tends to improve our resiliency.

EMOTIONAL INTELLIGENCE

Leaders spend much time in building their relationships with others. Networking with colleagues at work, friends in the community, and family is a quality of life indicator. Although intelligence and the intelligence quotient (IQ) seemed to be the critical requirements for leadership during the previous century, leaders of the 21st century need to have emotional intelligence as well.

Today, leaders need to develop an ability and capacity to recognize their personal feelings and the feelings and emotional reactions of others.[8] In addition to developing this emotional awareness, leaders need to become motivated to manage their emotions and feelings in their relationships with others as well. In his classic book on leadership, Burns said that a critical activity for leaders is to help others become aware of their feelings, feel these needs in a strong way, understand their values and how they emotionally respond to these values, and then become involved in meaningful actions based on these emotional realities.[9] Mayer and Salovey coined the term emotional intelligence to refer to these important leadership skills.[10] Effective leadership thus occurs in the context of emotional intelligence.[11]

Emotional intelligence is critical to effective leadership.[12] In reviewing extensive research, Goleman pointed out that it may be technical and cognitive skills that get a person a leadership position, but it is emotional intelligence that helps leaders keep their jobs. It is also interesting to note that leaders have to rely on these emotional skills more and more as they move up in the organization. These leaders promote the development of technical skills for those individuals who work in the more technical positions in the organization. It is also clear that leaders will have to be proficient in emotional intelligence as they expand their activities outside the organization in collaborative groups or other community-based activities. Emotional intelligence distinguishes the outstanding leaders and is clearly an important indicator of strong and effective performance.[13] This finding was strongly supported by Mayer and Salovey to explain how two people with similar general intelligence and technical expertise can end up in entirely different parts of an organization and at different leadership levels in the organization.[14]

The relationship between technical skills, cognitive skills including IQ, and emotional intelligence needs to be evaluated further. If we were to create a recipe for successful leadership, it would be necessary to determine the percentage of these three ingredients for different types of professional work. Although it seems clear that emotional intelligence increases in importance as leaders work more with others, it also seems apparent that the relationship of the three ingredients will fluctuate over time and place.

An interesting set of issues relates to the question of whether emotional intelligence can be learned. Intelligence and emotional intelligence are separate sets of competencies.[15] Having a high intelligence quotient is not a guarantee of strong social skills or high emotional intelligence. General intelligence is less flexible than emotional intelligence.[16] People do not generally increase their general intelligence over time, but emotional intelligence does increase as people become more adept at personal relationships. Emotional intelligence is not fixed at birth by genetics.[17] It can grow over time. In making the argument that emotional intelligence can grow and be learned, there is evidence that emotional intelligence increases with age.[18] Emotional intelligence is related to neurotransmitters in the limbic system of the brain, which is tied to feelings, impulses, and drives. It will be important for training programs to orient their activities to changing behavioral patterns that are associated with the limbic system. Increasing the motivation to make these changes must be a goal of training. Learning to be empathic is a critical part of the development of emotional intelligence.

It has become clear in the past several years that emotional intelligence skills are important both for individual leaders and for their relationships with others. This is not to denigrate the importance of technical and cognitive skills. The real concern is related to balance. The leader needs to use the head as well as the heart. An interesting view of this issue is found in an inspirational writing by Rabbi Lori Forman.[19] She was responding to a religious document called the Midrash in which ancient Jewish scholars defined the wicked as those who are controlled by their hearts and the righteous as those who have their hearts under control. Rabbi Forman explained this passage in terms of balance. It is not possible to separate our rational self from our feeling self. Our thoughts guide our feelings and vice versa. It is through the combination of thoughts and feelings that humankind addresses the world. Self-control is important because feelings without control can lead to chaos. It is important for the leader to realize that the mind skills and the heart skills all need to be developed if successful leadership is to occur.

Many writers have come up with frameworks for determining the important components and competencies of emotional intelligence. Three of these frameworks, developed by Goleman, Cooper and Sawaf, and Feldman, are discussed here. All three involve the development of personal skills as well as skills involved in dealing with others. All three models also have assessment tools tied to them that the reader can access.

Goleman's Emotional Intelligence Framework

The first model relates to the structure defined by Goleman.[20–23] Goleman and his colleagues in the Consortium for Research on Emotional Intelligence in Organizations have been working with this model for a number of years. The framework now has four components, with 20 subcompetencies associated with each of the four categories. Two of the dimensions (self-awareness and self-management) involve personal competencies, and two of the dimensions (social awareness and relationship management) involve social competencies.

The self-awareness domain includes emotional self-awareness, accurate self-assessment, and self-confidence. The competencies involved here include an ability to understand and recognize moods, feelings, and drives. Specifically, emotional self-awareness includes the ability to recognize moods and emotions and how they affect personal behavior. People with this competence not only understand their moods but also understand why they are feeling as they do.[24] These people also recognize the link between thoughts and feelings. They also know that their performance is often affected by these feelings and thoughts. Competency in accurate self-assessment includes the knowledge of one's strengths and limitations. This skill clearly involves learning from experience. These people also are willing to accept feedback on their behavior. The third competency in self-awareness involves self-confidence. These people are willing to take a stand. They are often the risk takers.

The second component of the Goleman model involves self-management, which has several subcompetencies associated with it. This component includes the ability not only to understand one's feelings and moods but also to use these feelings and moods to guide oneself toward personal goals and objectives. There is a strong motivational factor here in that the leader not only is aware of personal moods and feelings but needs to stay flexible and positive in directing these moods and feelings into change.[25] The first subcomponent is emotional self-control, which means that the leaders know or learn how to control feelings and emotions. People strong in this competency have also mastered the ability to stay focused. Being trustworthy is an important part of self-management. Action in an ethical manner is a critical leadership responsibility. People strong in this competency work vigorously to build trust. They also admit their mistakes and address unethical behavior in others. It is important

to remember that trust takes time to build, and it can be destroyed in a moment. Part of trust is carrying through on promises, which is also involved in the competency of conscientiousness. Thus, these leaders keep their promises.

The next competency related to self-management involves the skills related to adaptability, involving flexibility in managing change. Leaders are always oriented toward the future and the changes necessary to get there. They look for new approaches and new methods for attaining goals. They are innovative and want to generate new ideas. Leaders are excellent multitaskers, and they can handle shifting priorities. They are flexible. The next competency of leaders having an achievement drive is closely tied to the competency of adaptability and innovation. These people are results and outcome based. They also take calculated risks to achieve the ends they seek. These people would be concerned with the tools of performance measurement. They would also want to create performance standards and then surpass them. The final competency for self-management involves initiative, which is a readiness and ability to act on opportunities whenever they present themselves. Optimism is part of this competency because leaders are positive in addressing challenges.[26] If you are to seize opportunities, a positive perspective helps. Leaders create visions and then surpass them. They will do whatever is necessary to get the job done, although they will always practice ethical standards in doing so. These people are able to inspire others to follow their lead.

The next dimension of the Goleman model addresses the issue of social awareness.[27] An important ability of leaders is to be able to recognize and read the emotions, feelings, and reactions of others.[28] The interesting challenge here is to do this when you might feel differently than other people about a situation. Three competencies are tied to this dimension of emotional intelligence. The first critical set of skills is empathy or understanding others. Empathy requires the ability to be an active listener who is able to pick up emotional cues from other people. Empathy includes sensitivity to the needs of other people. Mentors and executive coaches need to be strong in this competency. If we as leaders are to enable others to act, then we must learn to empower others. One way to do this is to show others that we understand their needs and desires. Good leaders make others feel strong and capable.[29] In doing this, those who follow often exceed their own expectations.

The second competency is service orientation. This competency is familiar to those who are proponents of continuous quality improvement methods. This competency involves the development of skills to anticipate, recognize, and meet the needs of others, whether they are the clients of a public health agency, the residents of a community, or our community partners. Leaders competent in this area are concerned about how others react to public health decisions. Public health leaders have a strong concern for others, which is tied to the belief that all people are entitled to the best that health and public health have to offer. Social justice concerns drive the public health agenda, and yet political and budgetary decision sometimes lead to health inequities.

The final competency in the social awareness cluster involves organizational awareness. This competency can be defined as an ability to increase awareness of the emotions and political realities of those with whom the leader works.[30] This competency involves the skills of networking, collaboration, influence building, and systems thinking. The leader with this competency must understand the interdependencies of groups and how feeling and emotions affect outcomes. Almost all leadership skills require this competency to be well developed.

The fourth dimension of the emotional competency model of Goleman involves the critical sets of skills related to relationship management. In fact, the skills of social awareness are closely allied to this cluster of eight competencies. Such skills as strategic planning, conflict resolution, problem solving, decision making, and other traditional leadership and management tools are subsumed under this component of emotional intelligence. The value-added piece of the current discussion relates to the effect of emotions and feelings on these traditional leadership activities. A major competency involves the development of others, which appears closely allied to the empathy competency discussed previously. Leaders need to be concerned about the future and the issue of succession planning. It is important to recognize the skills and potential of others. Leaders need to be realistic. No leadership position is forever.

The ability to be influential is another competency related to relationship management. Influence and skill in persuasion are tied together. The leader has to become skillful in getting others to buy in to his or her message. This means that complex strategies need to be developed to build consensus and support for the issues that the leader considers to be important. Successful leaders are able to put the pieces together in effective ways. They make their point and convince others of the validity of their position. It is important that the enthusiasm and positivity of the leader be contagious for others to follow.

The next competency involves the ability of the leader to listen with an open mind, monitor personal emotions and feelings, and be able to send effective messages in a number of different ways. Leaders emphasize the importance of communication in all its aspects. Communication is more than interpersonal in nature and covers many things, including written communication strategies and public discussion and dialogue. People who are strong in this competency excel at reading emotional cues in others.[31] These leaders are also effective in addressing complex issues in a straightforward manner. They are good listeners and seek to understand what is said to them at both a verbal and an emotional level. They foster communication, and they try to listen to information about good and bad events. Collaboration not only improves performance; it also creates a strong level of trust.[32]

The next competency in relationship management involves conflict management. People strong in this competency know how to handle difficult people in tense situations.[33] This ability involves the use of tact and diplomacy. These leaders know how to diffuse tension and move from conflict to collaboration. They do this by addressing conflict in an open manner and encouraging the expression of diverse views. These leaders want to create win–win situations. The leader really needs to be able to spot trouble before it explodes in a major crisis situation. The leader also needs to determine when an objective negotiator needs to be brought in to resolve conflicts because the emotions are overtaking rational decision making.

The competencies of visionary leadership and catalyzing change are clearly competencies of leaders. Leaders need to be able to create a vision with an awareness that emotional factors will guide the vision process. To attain the vision, the leader needs to convince others to go along with the steps necessary to bring about change. Leaders are catalysts for change; they need to not only recognize that change is necessary but also challenge the status quo and remove the barriers to change.[34] Leaders will have to get others to emotionally invest in the change process and be part of the vision that the leader has.

The next relationship management competency addresses the building of bonds between people. Building networks between people is important if strong relationships are to be built. One of the hidden functions of leadership development is fostering the connections and friendships that develop among the trainees. These leaders think that one of the benefits of training relates to the leadership networks that this training generates. Relationships that evolve through training or through building bonds between people in other arenas often create trust and goodwill. Strong leaders build bonds. When these bonds develop, social capital increases.

The final competency in the Goleman framework involves teamwork and collaboration. At the emotional intelligence level, this competency involves the creation of a balance between the work or task to be performed and the relationships necessary to carry out the work.[35] Collaboration has emotional components. The sharing of information and future plans or resources can lessen stress in many situations, although not in all of them. Feelings of competition have strong emotional reactions. The goal of leaders strong in collaboration is to build positive working and personal environments. These leaders want to nurture teamwork and collaboration in coalitions, alliances, and partnerships.

An important factor to note is the specific competencies that seem to predominate in the authoritarian or democratic leadership style. Which is your predominant style? If you go through the list of the 20 Goleman competencies, which competencies would you say are your strong ones, and which do you want to develop competence in for the future?

Cooper and Sawaf's Four Cornerstone Model

The second approach to emotional intelligence is built on the four cornerstone model.[36] As the following discussion shows, the four cornerstone model overlaps with the Goleman model just discussed, and yet there are some different perspectives that the authors give that can enrich the skills of the prepared public health leader. High-level executives with a strong emotional quotient (EQ) as well as a strong IQ (intelligence quotient) tend to make the best decisions and run the most dynamic and creative organizations.[37] These leaders also report that they are living very satisfying lives. The following discussion involves a look at the four cornerstone model developed by Cooper and Sawaf and the four competencies associated with each of the cornerstones.

The first cornerstone relates to emotional literacy, which is tied to the emotional center of all our activities. It is emotional literacy that affects our energy and motivation. This cornerstone has four competencies associated with it— emotional honesty, emotional energy, emotional feedback, and practical intuition. Many of our emotional reactions are tied to the first competency of honesty. Being true to yourself and others undergirds much of the preceding Goleman discussion. The way the leader is seen by others is important here. The honest leader needs to judge him- or herself in an honest manner as well. Whenever a leader is asked to evaluate personal skills on a leadership assessment tool, it is assumed that the leader will be honest in filling out the form and not answer the questions in such a way that the leader thinks the tester will evaluate so that their skills are seen in a more favorable light. One little exercise that you can try to evaluate this honesty dimension is to evaluate your energy level, openness, and level of focus on a scale from 1 to 10 for each dimension before and after a meeting that you have to attend.[38] Your

honesty in rating yourself on this scale from 3 to 30 will give you insights into your ability to address issues. If you have trouble being motivated during the meeting, evaluate the strategies that would help you become more involved.

The second competency in this first cornerstone is emotional energy. People do better when they have the energy to address tasks and develop people relationships. There are two major components to this competency. The first relates to the level of tension that the individual feels, and the second component is the level of energy itself. If the tension is high and the energy is high, the authors call this tense-energy. This pattern occurs when you push yourself to extremes and leave your personal needs at the doorstep. This pattern may lead to burnout. If you have low tension and high energy, you have calm-energy, which can lead to some very productive work. The unfortunate part is that leaders do not feel this state very often. When we feel calm-energy, it is more possible to be proactive than in the previous state, where behavior tends to be more reactive.

The third energy pattern is high tension with low energy, which can be called tense-tiredness. This is how we often feel after we get home from a busy day and a difficult freeway drive. The stress is high and the tiredness is great. In this state, individuals need to be careful not to overreact to the demands of family members or colleagues who need help in some matter. The final state is low tension with low energy, which is the state of calm-tiredness. This is the good state of just feeling content and relaxed. Leaders need to understand their energy levels and how to react to them.

The third competency involves the skills related to understanding emotional feedback. Leaders need to realize that every feeling or emotion is sending a message. Leaders who understand this will become adept at managing emotional impulsivity. This competency is similar to the competencies discussed by Goleman in the area of self-awareness and self-management. The leader needs to take responsibility for his or her actions. An interesting exercise that you can do for better understanding this competency is to ask yourself, "If you were to take responsibility for a specific feeling you have, such as anger, what would happen?"

The fourth competency relates to emotional literacy and the development of intuitive skills. Intuition is closely tied to the empathy competency in the Goleman model. The empathic individual is one who can read the feelings beneath the words that are spoken. Sometimes our gut reactions to a situation should guide our behavior rather than our rational thoughts. Trust is also important here in that relationships built on trust allow others to say and show their authentic reactions to events.

The second cornerstone in the Cooper and Sawaf model involves emotional fitness, which includes the four competencies of authenticity, trust radius, constructive discontent, and resilience and renewal. Authentic power includes the issue of personal power. Authentic presence is affected by the factors of showing attentiveness to others (another aspect of empathy and building bonds), concern for others (also a part of empathy), your agenda and motives to get people involved in your vision, and the complex issue of entitlement that is affected by your organizational position or personal relationship to the other person. Authenticity also involves convincing others that you are taking discussion and dialogues seriously. The authentic leader is also one who admits to mistakes and is willing to forgive him- or herself and others. The second competency, which also exists in the Goleman model, relates to the importance of building trust. The new wrinkle in the present model is the connection between trust and believability. In addition, there is a trust radius that answers the question of how far the leader is willing to extend his or her trust network. Trust relationships take time to build, and a leader must struggle to be sociable to strangers where the trust is not yet apparent.

The third competency related to emotional fitness is constructive discontent. As a facilitator, the leader may have to create conflict in a group and get group members to address an issue in a different way than they may have in the past. Creating discontent can have positive effects even though the stress and tension levels will increase significantly. Goleman would have included this competency under conflict management. Some of the details in this constructive discontent include the process of increasing awareness, exposing problems in the group, using empathy to explore diverse views, promoting the development of trust in a group, understanding and promoting inclusion and participation when values and goals are in conflict, collaborating for creative solutions to problems, developing learning organizations with your colleagues in order to learn in action, creating an environment that promotes the enjoyment of the process, and believing that constructive discontent leads to real problem solving and decision making.

The final competency for this cornerstone relates to resilience and renewal. The resilience factor is critical to creating change. It is important to point out that resilience is tied to adaptability and the ability to adjust to change. Resilient people have great curiosity. The issue of renewal is important as well. Leaders need to renew themselves. Renewal may involve taking a new job in a new place. It may be a walk on the beach or sitting in a favorite chair and reading a new book. Each of us will have different ways to address renewal.

The important message is that leaders need to allow time for this sabbatical experience if they are to remain effective. We spend time taking courses or going to training workshops to expand our leadership skills, and we need to spend time on expanding our emotional intelligence skills as well.

The third cornerstone involves the critical concerns related to emotional depth.[39] This cornerstone is involved with the issue of character and how individuals over their lifetimes become more and more adept at people relationships. How we practice the skills of emotional intelligence becomes a critical indicator of emotional depth. You can experiment with some of the issues involved in this cornerstone by exploring the technical and emotional aspects of the real purpose of leading by walking around. Why do leaders walk around their organizations and communities? What is the real meaning of this activity? The four competencies of this third cornerstone include unique potential and purpose, commitment, applied integrity, and influence without authority.

The competency related to unique potential relates to the individual who is adept at analyzing personal strengths and weaknesses. Leaders need to have a purpose—a personal vision. The ability to engage in some self-analysis often gives us insights into who we are. Here are some possible questions for you to consider:

1. What are my five greatest strengths?
2. Who are the five most important people in my life?
3. What are the five major accomplishments I have achieved in the past year?
4. What are the five personal things I want to do for myself in the next year?
5. What are the five work products I want to produce in the next year?
6. When I die, what are the five things I want people to say about me?

As you answer these questions, ask yourself why the five things you discuss are important. What feelings are created as a result?

Commitment is another competency involved in emotional depth. When you add purpose to your level of commitment and your need to be accountable for your actions, you also need to be aware that you may have some resistance to the changes required to carry out your vision.[40] Underlying the discussion of commitment is the need to abide by ethical standards of behavior. Accountability involves the practice of ethical behavior in a committed way. For Goleman, commitment is significantly associated with leadership.[41] The third competency of integrity is closely tied to the commitment and accountability competence. Integrity is also a part of trustworthiness. Integrity involves the recognition of the difference between right and wrong. Cooper and Sawaf called this discernment and said that discernment needs to be tied to personal actions and the way words are used to explain action.[42] Thus both the competency of commitment and the competency of integrity speak to the importance of ethical standards and how they affect thoughts and feelings. Integrity really gets to the heart of the question of what the leader represents to those who follow.

The final competency related to emotional depth is influence without authority. Influence must occur without manipulation and without authority. Influence involves perception, relationships, innovations, setting priorities, empathy, and taking account of emotional reasons for actions and not just the logical analyses. Successful leaders have influence regardless of the positions they occupy. People who are influential seem to have high energy and the ability to motivate others. They respond to the show of emotion in an understanding and nonthreatening manner. For Goleman, influence serves as the core of the relationship management component of his model.[43] One way to demonstrate this is through the use of leadership stories.[44] When you read a story of someone you consider to be a leader, look specifically for the role of the influence competency in their demonstration of leadership.

The final cornerstone in this model of emotional intelligence is emotional alchemy. Emotional intelligence is about synergy and how to use your emotions to create more value in the things you do. The four competencies tied to this final cornerstone include intuitive flow, reflective time shifting, creating the future, and opportunity sensing. In discussing the idea of flow, Csikszentmihalyi defined flow as related to the positive aspects of life and human experience.[45] Flow is demonstrated through such emotional processes as joy, creativity, total immersion in actions and all of life's experiences. Flow indicates a total concentration and involvement in what you are doing. Flow can be controlled and not left to chance. Intuitive flow is tied to strong feelings of self-worth and personal satisfaction.[46] The ability to experience intuitive flow is almost like an ability to see the real meaning of things, even when they seem obscured by rational thought. Leaders with this competency learn to use the intuition they have in more effective ways.

The next competency expands the concept of self-reflection to address the issue of shifting time. People sense time in unique ways. Some of us notice changing daylight patterns. Some of us check our watches on a regular basis. Some of us let another staff member or family member remind us of where we are supposed to be. With the skill of reflective time shifting, the emotionally competent leader can picture events in the past, the present, and the future. Shifting time also requires shifting perspectives on events. This competency allows the leader to learn to shift reactions and feeling states to a given situation at a moment's notice. Cooper and Sawaf called this feeling yourself in time.[47] This set of competencies is critical in visioning activities. The next two competencies are related to visioning as well. The first is the competency of opportunity sensing. Leaders need to sense things and to push traditional sensory limits. This can be called an extension of the opportunity horizon. Leaders work to expand their awareness and to explore the larger field of possibilities. This is sometimes referred to as thinking (and sensing things) outside the box. The final competency relates to creating the future with a vision to guide the process. Goleman subsumed these three competencies within the general competency of visionary leadership.[48]

The Feldman Framework

The third framework is somewhat different from the first two frameworks. The Feldman framework is very practical and built on words that are less technical than the categories discussed previously.[49] The Feldman model is also clearly based on the emotional intelligence competencies for leaders. This model integrates many of these competencies into five core skills:

- Knowing yourself
- Maintaining control
- Reading others
- Perceiving accurately
- Communicating with flexibility

It is necessary for a leader to learn these basic skills before he or she goes on to develop higher level skills such as learning to take responsibility, learning to generate different choices, developing and embracing a vision, having courage, and demonstrating resolve. This model is of interest because it tries to distinguish different levels of emotional intelligence. If you take the lifelong perspective on leadership, it seems obvious that different skills and competencies are needed at different points in a leader's career. If emotional intelligence skills expand over time, then it is clear that leaders should hone these skills as they go through life.

The first Feldman competency of knowing yourself is an obvious component in all emotional intelligence frameworks. It entails the recognition of personal emotional reactions, the ability to understand how emotions affect action, and also how to differentiate an emotion such as anger and how it is perceived in different social situations. My anger on a freeway shows itself in interesting ways, whereas my anger at a coworker is displayed in entirely different ways. Look at a leadership challenge you face and the emotions you display. How does your decision-making process change when you learn to control your emotional reaction to the challenge?

This first core competency affects the second competency of controlling emotions (maintaining control). The important concern for the public health leader is how the leader controls emotions during an emergency situation. Others will respond to the leader in terms of the emotions they see displayed. Others expect their leaders to appear calm during a crisis. In fact, maintaining control is all about remaining calm when chaos reigns.[50] If a leader feels that his or her emotions are getting out of control, the leader needs to briefly step back from a chaotic situation and take a deep breath. The leader in stressful situations needs to think of positive outcomes.

The third competency of reading others is in many ways similar to the empathy competency in the other two frameworks. It involves not only an awareness of the emotions of other people but also the appreciation of the emotions of others as well as excitement involved in the diversity of other perspectives. Leaders increase their effect when they better understand the reactions of others to crisis as well as noncrisis situations. This competency also requires active listening. Respect needs to be shown to others as well. The fourth competency of accurate perception is related to this third competency. Leaders need to develop skills in assessing different types of situations. They also need to be guided by a vision as pointed out in the first two framework models. Leaders as systems thinkers need to keep their view on the big picture and try to maintain their objectivity if at all possible.

The final core competency is the importance of learning to be flexible when communicating with others. Flexibility is all about bringing our verbal and nonverbal words and actions into alignment. The messages that we send need to be clear. Others will listen to our words but will also pay attention to our actions. Leaders should be aware that not everyone will react to them in the same way. There are many ramifications of our words and deeds.

In this section, three frameworks of emotional intelligence have been presented. The first two frameworks by Goleman and Cooper and Sawaf have assessment tools tied to them. The third is a more practical one, with guidelines for developing each of the competencies discussed. If you would like to experiment more with emotional intelligence models, look at the Bradberry and Greaves book, which is close to the Goleman framework, and then take the online version of the emotional intelligence assessment tool developed by the authors.[51]

Kravitz and Schubert reviewed the various models of emotional intelligence and believed that this field needs to be tied to an applied perspective that they designated people-smart strategies.[52] People need to learn how to make choices in their lives. These choices extend to all the things you say and do. People-smart strategies mean you have to not only think smart but act smart. To think smart is to understand how you function as a person, to learn self-awareness skills, to practice optimistic thinking by thinking positively, to value the work you do, to develop a support network, and to learn the skills related to caring. The three aspects of being smart involve the learning of communication skills to effectively talk to others, learning to control emotions, and developing flexibility to change. People-smart strategies are adaptive emotional intelligence that translate into the following activities:

1. Showing flexibility in communication
2. Managing personal stress
3. Helping others who express pessimism about the future
4. Showing respect for others
5. Managing work rage
6. Becoming a servant leader

SUMMARY

This chapter has explored in depth the importance of quality of life issues for public health leaders and in fact for all public health professionals. As regards healthy living as a critical component of quality of life, healthy nutrition, an adequate amount of sleep, and the importance of exercise and movement in general are important. Time management is critical in that time must be allotted for many of our healthy living requirements. Public health leaders need to practice what they preach by maintaining their health. Leaders need to be role models for the people they serve. Leaders also need to promote a culture of health orientation in their communities. The books by Rath show why wellness approaches are important and how these approaches enhance the quality of life of all leaders and their constituents.

The second half of this chapter addresses the important of emotional intelligence in our lives. Leaders spend a significant part of their work and family lives in building relationships at work and in our communities. Three approaches to emotional intelligence are presented. It is clear from this chapter that improving quality of life is important for our public health leaders. An improved quality of life increases our productivity and love of our work.

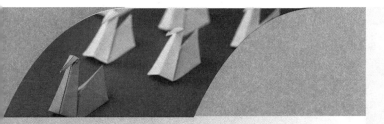

Discussion Questions

1. Discuss the major health components related to improvements in the quality of life.

2. How is the time factor related to the quality of life?

3. Discuss the 12 rules of healthy living.

4. How are the three books by Rath and his colleagues related?

5. Why is emotional intelligence important?

6. Compare and contrast the three approaches to the study of emotional intelligence.

REFERENCES

1. J. Gardner, *Self-Renewal* (New York, NY: W. W. Norton & Co., 1995).
2. R. Sharma, *The Monk Who Sold His Ferrari* (London, England: Harper Collins, 1995).
3. A. MacKenzie, *The Time Trap*, 3rd ed. (New York, NY: AMACOM, 1997).
4. S. R. Covey, *Primary Greatness: The 12 Levers of Success* (New York, NY: Simon & Schuster, 2015).
5. T. Rath and J. Harter, *Well Being: The Five Essential Elements* (New York, NY: Gallup Press, 2010).
6. T. Rath, *Eat, Move, Sleep*, (Arlington, VA: Missionday Publishing, 2013).
7. T. Rath, *Are You Fully Charged* (Arlington, VA: Silicon Guild, 2015).
8. D. Goleman, "Who Makes a Leader," *Harvard Business Review* 76, no. 6 (1998): 94–102.
9. J. M. Burns, *Leadership* (New York, NY: Harper and Row, 1978).
10. J. D. Mayer and P. S. Salovey, "The Intelligence of Emotional Intelligence," *Intelligence* 17, no. 4 (1993): 433–442.
11. D. A. Feldman, *The Handbook of Emotionally Intelligent Leadership* (Falls Church, VA: Performance Solutions Press, 1999).
12. D. Goleman, *Working with Emotional Intelligence* (New York, NY: Bantam Books, 1998).
13. Goleman, *Working with Emotional Intelligence.*
14. Mayer and Salovey, "The Intelligence of Emotional Intelligence."
15. D. Goleman, *Emotional Intelligence* (New York, NY: Bantam Books, 2006).
16. T. Bradberry and J. Greaves, *Emotional Intelligence 2.0* (San Diego, CA: TalentSmart, 2009).
17. Goleman, *Working with Emotional Intelligence.*
18. Goleman, *Working with Emotional Intelligence.*
19. L. Forman, "Directing the Heart," in K. M. Ovitsky and L. Forman (eds.), *Sacred Intentions* (Woodstock, VT: Jewish Lights, 1999).
20. Goleman, *Emotional Intelligence.*
21. Goleman, "Who Makes a Leader."
22. Goleman, *Working with Emotional Intelligence.*
23. D. Goleman, "Emotional Intelligence: Issues in Paradigm Building," in C. Cherniss and D. Goleman (eds.), *The Emotionally Intelligent Workplace* (San Francisco: Jossey-Bass, 2001).
24. Goleman, *Working with Emotional Intelligence.*
25. Bradberry and Greaves, *Emotional Intelligence 2.0.*
26. Goleman, *Working with Emotional Intelligence.*
27. Goleman, "Emotional Intelligence: Issues in Paradigm Building."
28. Bradberry and Greaves, *Emotional Intelligence 2.0.*
29. J. M. Kouzes and B. Z. Posner, *The Leadership Challenge*, 4th ed. (San Francisco, CA: Jossey-Bass, 2007).
30. Goleman, "Emotional Intelligence: Issues in Paradigm Building."
31. Goleman, *Working with Emotional Intelligence.*
32. Kouzes and Posner, *The Leadership Challenge*, 4th ed.
33. Goleman, *Working with Emotional Intelligence.*
34. Goleman, "Emotional Intelligence: Issues in Paradigm Building."
35. Goleman, *Working with Emotional Intelligence.*
36. R. K. Cooper and A. Sawaf, *Executive EQ* (New York, NY: Perigee Books, 1996).
37. Cooper and Sawaf, *Executive EQ.*
38. Cooper and Sawaf, *Executive EQ.*
39. Cooper and Sawaf, *Executive EQ.*
40. Cooper and Sawaf, *Executive EQ.*
41. Goleman, "Emotional Intelligence: Issues in Paradigm Building."
42. Cooper and Sawaf, *Executive EQ.*
43. Goleman, "Emotional Intelligence: Issues in Paradigm Building."
44. Cooper and Sawaf, *Executive EQ.*
45. M. Csikszentmihalyi, *Flow* (New York, NY: Harper Perennial, 1990).
46. Cooper and Sawaf, *Executive EQ.*
47. Cooper and Sawaf, *Executive EQ.*
48. Goleman, "Emotional Intelligence: Issues in Paradigm Building."
49. Feldman, *The Handbook of Emotionally Intelligent Leadership.*
50. Feldman, *The Handbook of Emotionally Intelligent Leadership.*
51. Bradberry and Greaves, *Emotional Intelligence 2.0.*
52. S. M. Kravitz and J. D. Schubert, *Emotional Intelligence Works* (Menlo Park, CA: Crisp Learning, 2000).

CHAPTER 6

Leadership at the Team Level

LEARNING OBJECTIVES

- Understand the characteristics of high-performing teams.
- Explain the PERFORM model.
- Learn to use the leadership wheel.
- Discover the planning documents associated with the use of the leadership wheel.
- Determine strategies for clarifying values.
- Distinguish between a mission and a vision statement.
- Understand action planning.

Leadership at the team level cannot occur without the involvement of leaders with strong personal leadership skills. In this chapter I discuss teams with the belief that team members have a leadership mindset and share leadership responsibilities within the team environment. In the 21st century, leaders find that they can no longer practice the leader's craft in a vacuum, and they need to be aware that their success depends on their ability to work with others. Because different individuals bring different expertise and skills to the problem-solving and decision-making environment, teams are created to address challenges. In teams, leadership is shared and different team members move into the leadership position at different phases of the problem-solving process.

There is a difference between groups and teams. A group is composed of two or more people with similar interests and skills. They may work interdependently but generally not in a coordinated way. Group members tend to be extremely competitive and somewhat self-serving. If the group members are asked to complete a task together, a supervisor may have to coordinate the activity. On the other hand, a team generally

has a purpose for working together. This common purpose guides the activity of the team. Working together is a positive experience. Team members help each other throughout the work. They not only share the responsibilities for the team activities, they work together as leaders to improve performance and to share in the output of the group. Team members often become work friends. The result of the team's activities is often greater than the sum total of the results that would have occurred had each member been working alone and more integrated than the activities of a group working on a similar problem.

What makes a great team? Miller[1] points to three important considerations. First, leaders need to be sure that the people they assign to a team, committee, or task force are the right people. That does not mean that they all have the same talents or strengths, but together they seem to have all the appropriate background for the task. They need to be able to take on a specific leadership role when necessary. The leader who creates the team should believe that the team members will grow as a result of their involvement. The environment that is created by and for the team should be one that allows respect, trust, and empathy to occur. Most team members will learn team skills from their experience. **Exercise 6-1** allows the class to begin to see how a team functions in working on a project.

CHARACTERISTICS OF HIGH-PERFORMING TEAMS

Many of our leadership challenges are more complex and numerous than they used to be. This requires leaders to be more creative and innovative than in the past. This is especially true for the public health leader who seems to have to

EXERCISE 6-1 The Infrastructure of Public Health

Purpose: to begin the process of seeing your team work together

Key Concepts: team, team building, teamwork, infrastructure

Procedure: Secure a box of small plastic blocks. Divide the class into small teams of five to seven people. The assignment is to build the infrastructure of public health using the blocks. You have a half hour to complete the assignment. After completion of the project, have each team answer the following questions.

1. Select one of your teams to explain the process you used to create the model.
2. Explain the team infrastructure model and why it is designed the way it is.
3. Are the members a group or a team?
4. Who were the leaders? How did you share or not share the leadership role?

address challenges constantly, from more traditional leadership problems such as annual cuts in an agency's budget to crises related to new disease entities such as the Zika virus or terrorist events and natural disasters. Leaders have to understand the entire community and organizational system for creativity to occur.[2] Creative leaders tend to be passionate about the work they do. Creative leaders know that they cannot do all the work needed by themselves. They need to trust the individuals who work for them. This trust will be the foundation for the creation of teams to help solve the challenges to health in the community. This trust helps teams improve their performance.[3] Cloud views trust as first seeing team members trusting each other as well as the agency leader. Feedback from the leader is important here. This helps motivate the team and should lead to clarity about the tasks to be performed. Third, credibility needs to be maintained and character problems need to be addressed. Cloud points out that the leader and team members have to believe that the ability, knowledge capacity, and skills of the team members are adequate for the work of the team. Finally, the past experiences of the team members also help build trust.

Leadership teams need autonomy to do their work. To be a high-performance team, the team must understand the assignment and have clarity about the specific goals of the project.[4] The goal should be elevating in that there needs to be a challenge and a learning situation built into the work. High-performing teams also require a structure that is results oriented. The end needs to be in sight. Trust will be maintained if the team sees potential results and do not think that the team will be in existence forever. Thus, there are six structural features that can readily be seen in successful teams:[5]

1. The roles of team members and methods of accountability are well defined.
2. Communication is open and information is shared.
3. Monitoring of team member performance is ongoing with both positive and negative feedback by the agency leader and other team members.
4. Results need to be based on facts.
5. Team members need not only technical skills, they need problem solving and social skills.[6]
6. Commitment to the team process is required.

There is much that we now know about how successful teams work. In the now classic work on teams, Katzenbach and Smith[7] discussed what they learned from a study of teams. There is much important common sense and uncommon sense information that will guide leaders in their work with teams. With regard to team common sense wisdom, we know that a health challenge demands a response. This challenge often requires a team to address the performance demand. A team may spontaneously come into being even without an agency director creating it. If leadership exists throughout the organization, this is more likely to happen. Team performance is affected by such factors as size, team purpose, goals developed, team approach, accountability, and commitment.

Team opportunities exist in all parts of an organization or agency. In public health, teams may exist to address clinical challenges. Middle management and supervisors may create teams to address managerial concerns. Teams at the top often need to address policy concerns. Policy challenges are very complex and can lead to major changes in an organization or agency. Agency leaders often struggle with team accountability. It is easier to deal with accountability at an individual level than a team level.

Katzenbach and Smith[8] also found a number of uncommon problems in their study of teams. Many agencies with strong quality performance seem to create more effective purpose-driven teams than organizations that use teams more generally. It also appears that hierarchical organizations use teams more readily than organizations that are less hierarchical in structure. The authors noted two other findings.

First, teams learn how to integrate their performance activities with an orientation to increasing the personal knowledge of its members. This team activity is often referred to as the learning organization. Teams can bridge the gap between their organizations and the communities that they serve. Thus team wisdom is oriented to performance and team learning.

To put this discussion of high-performing teams in perspective, Blanchard and his colleagues have developed the PERFORM model.[9] First, high-performing teams not only understand the culture of the organizations for which they work; they make sure that the **P**urpose of their teamwork is clear. Second, members of the team trust their organization leaders and feel **E**mpowered by their leaders to independently carry out the team's work. The third element involves **R**elationships. Team members trust each other, feel free to disagree on issues, and enjoy the relationship with each other. A synergy exists through the development of shared leadership and a willingness to come up with a common solution to the team's work. **F**lexibility is also important for the team. They work together and believe that team performance is a team sport. The next element is **O**ptimal productivity. The team works well together. They are extremely productive, creative, and innovative. They tend to produce more than is generally required for their work tasks. Team members get **R**ecognition and appreciation both from inside the team and organizational leadership and from community clients and partners outside the organization. Finally, **M**orale is high on the team and in the organization for which they work.

In most organizations, there are many traditional and high-performance teams that are operating concurrently. Our hero story for this chapter can be seen in **Heroes and Villains 6-1**. It is about the fourth Surgeon General of the United States, Dr. Rupert Blue, who served from 1912 to 1920.

PUBLIC HEALTH HEROES AND VILLAINS 6-1 Dr. Rupert Blue

Dr. Rupert Blue (1898–1948) was appointed as the fourth Surgeon General of the United States by President William Howard Taft in 1912 and to a second term in 1916 under President Woodrow Wilson. Dr. Blue undertook a 9-month internship in public health at the Marine Hospital Service from 1892 to 1893, followed by a commission as assistant surgeon general in March 1893. Before 1912, Blue was involved in the rat eradication and urban sanitation programs related to an epidemic of bubonic plague in San Francisco in 1902 and again in 1908, which was a result of the famous San Francisco earthquake. He was also involved in mosquito eradication related to yellow fever in New Orleans in 1905, the Jamestown Exposition in 1907, and in Honolulu in 1911 to help prepare for traffic related to the opening of the Panama Canal. Many other public health initiatives followed.

Under his leadership, many teams of researchers worked on many public health programs. He was involved in the new science of bacteriology and also continued the important work related to the practice of sanitation and public education for programs related to diseases that were linked to rural and urban poverty. During his tenure, scientists and their research teams documented tularemia's bacterial origins, discovered the extent of hookworm disease and its correlation to unsanitary soil conditions in the Southeast United States, showed the relationship of pellagra to nutritional deficiencies, and the reduced prevalence of typhoid fever. All this work led to the development of the first full-time county health department in Yakima, Washington. During World War I, there was an expansion of the Public Health Service. The Hygienic Laboratory developed vaccines against tetanus, diphtheria, typhoid fever, and smallpox. In addition, programs for venereal disease control were developed. Programs and services were funded to give medical services to workers in war plants. One act of potential villainy was the approval by Dr. Blue of supplying cigarettes to all men in service.

A major health concern during World War I was the spread of Spanish influenza. Many servicemen caught the flu. Dr. Blue showed much concern for the fact that the fatality rate was so high. After the war, he stated that the United States was unprepared for the pandemic and could not do much to aid the servicemen during the pandemic period. In 1920, Dr. Blue stepped down from his position as surgeon general. He once again took the position of assistant surgeon general and oversaw Public Health Service operations in Europe and also served as a delegate to the Office International d'Hygiène Publique (1920–1923). He retired from the Public Health Service in 1932 after a full career promoting public health. He was truly a public health hero who also saw the value of working with others in team settings.

THE LEADERSHIP WHEEL

What is the process of work? This section views teamwork within a planning model. In fact, this model is one that will be used for all the levels of leadership to follow. Good leadership depends on systems thinking and an understanding of the effect of complexity. This type of thinking focuses on ways to implement, in the short and long term, system components necessary for meeting identified needs. To ensure that systems thinking is effective, public health agency leaders must support the systems perspective and make sure staff understand what is involved in a systems approach to change. Communication must be frequent enough to allow the staff to help manage the implementation of strategic policies. The leader is responsible for guiding the implementation activities and presenting to the community the steps being taken by the agency in response to local public health issues.

Team building is a critical part of leading a public health agency. The leader creates teams inside the agency and coalitions, alliances, and partnerships outside to address the programmatic needs of the agency. Once the members are appointed, the teams need to clarify the values that will guide their activities.

Public health leaders must:

- think systemically and act strategically
- create a learning organization
- coordinate knowledge and performance management activities
- promote and support the change process
- support the values of the agency and the community
- understand the relationship between system inputs, program interventions, and outputs
- monitor and evaluate the effects of change

The remainder of this chapter covers the main stages in the systems approach to organizational change as represented by a leadership wheel (**Figure 6-1**). Strong leaders with a high level of commitment must serve as the conveners and inspirational voices for the process. These stages include values clarification, construction or revision of the agency's mission and vision, identification of goals and objectives, development of an action plan, implementation of the action plan, and assessment of the effects of the implementation. As a systems-based working model, the leadership wheel depicts the integration of planning, action, and evaluation. An important consideration in this whole process is the need to understand the assumptions that provide a foundation for

FIGURE 6-1 Systems Approach to Organizational Change (Leadership Wheel)

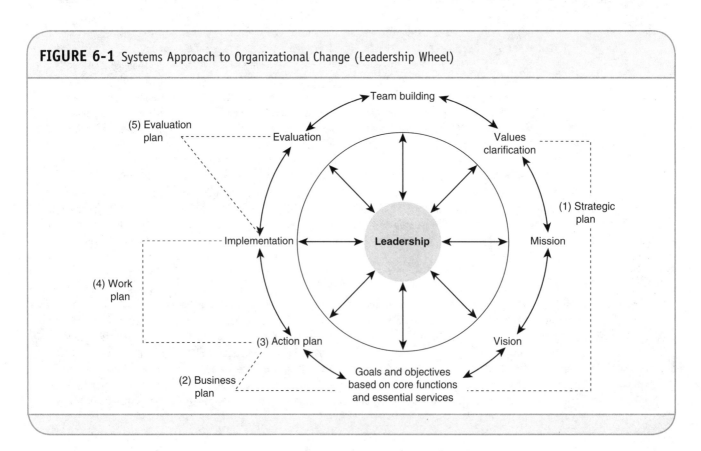

all the activities that occur as part of the systems perspective for both internal and external stakeholders.[10] In actuality, we often do not have all the knowledge necessary to the understanding of a public health or programmatic need before we start to work on it. The assumptions we make will depend on whether we take a linear perspective or a systems perspective on an issue. This assumption approach is tied to what Churchman has called an inquiry system.[11] An inquiry system involves the process of creating a system of interrelated parts or components that provide a holistic perspective on the appropriate knowledge to address a problem or challenge.

The leadership wheel leads to five specific products: a strategic plan, a business plan, an action plan, a work plan, and an evaluation plan. In the strategic planning phase, values, mission and vision, and goals and objectives are clarified. Moving from the formulation of goals and objectives, a business plan is developed in which the cost of programs that are developed to implement the goals and objectives becomes critical. The goals and business plan lead to an action plan. With implementation imminent, a work plan is devised. The evaluation plan becomes the fifth document to drive the process. Quality improvement methods and techniques are often employed as a performance measurement set of priorities. In the following subsections, we examine the stages of the leadership wheel.

Values Clarification

Blanchard and O'Connor make a distinction between the Fortune 500 and the Fortunate 50.[12] The latter are businesses in which management by values occurs. In the management-by-values process, which can take 3 years to complete, an agency goes through three stages. The first stage involves clarification of the agency's mission, values, and vision. The second stage involves communicating the agency's newly clarified mission, values, and vision to others. The final stage, which is the most complex, involves aligning the leadership and management practices of the agency with its stated values. In the case of public health leadership, the alignment of practices and values applies to the team and its members in relationship to the agency as a whole.

An agency's culture is made up, in part, of the values and beliefs that the members of the agency have in common.[13] These values and beliefs guide the members' individual and collective behavior. Also part of the agency's culture are the rituals and myths that have grown out of the agency's history. For example, a myth might be created about a former administrator, who, as an avid promoter of public health in the community, might be idealized as a public health hero. Treating the administrator as a hero has its benefits, because

it reaffirms the importance of health promotion. Yet it can also have a downside. For one thing, it may lead to organizational stasis, for the myth suggests that everything the administrator did, every policy decision made, is above question, and thus the current members of the agency may be more reluctant to make necessary changes than if they viewed the administrator as praiseworthy but fallible.

Agency rituals might include a special public health award given to a community organization each year at an annual luncheon. If this award is named after the former administrator, the ritual supports the myth. A new public health administrator with new ideas and a new vision for the agency will need to work with the agency staff to redefine its values, and thus the current myths and rituals—and even the agency's physical layout, which is a component of organizational culture—may need to be changed.

A value, according to Rokeach, is "an enduring belief that a specific mode of conduct or end-state of existence is personally or socially preferable to an opposite or converse mode of conduct or end-state of existence."[14(p.5)] Each community has a unique configuration and a unique set of values, and the local public health agency is a reflection of these values. Societies that are geographically and politically separated from each other tend to develop different community approaches to dealing with their particular problems.[15] For example, a county with a mostly rural population will have different public health priorities than a county with a mostly urban population. Rural health leaders often have to do more with less. They have less money, fewer staff than large urban health departments, sometimes geographic isolation, limited technical resources, lower salaries for staff, and often fewer external partners.[16]

Some general truths about values are worth noting. First, certain values are universal, whereas others occur only in specific locales. There is a clear recognition that there are some values that are universally held. These universal values tend to be heterogeneous in content with some tied to our human nature and some tied to living in cultural groups. Brown has connected the study of universal value systems to both human biology and evolutionary psychology.[17] Second, values tend to be organized into value systems. Third, people generally have the values they do because of the socialization they have undergone. Fourth, values are present in every social situation.

The increasing diversification in many communities has led to changes in value systems and in some cases to a confusing diversity of values. To ensure that a system of shared values evolves, a community must undertake a process of values clarification. This type of process respects diversity but is aimed at elucidating the dominant values of the community.

A vision cannot be realized unless it is built on an infrastructure of shared core values.

Credible leaders use personal values to affect their organization or community.[18] To make action activities work, leaders should align personal values with organizational and community values. When this occurs, it is possible to push a shared values agenda. Shared values lead to finding a common ground for action. Jansen Kraemer pointed out that a values orientation enhances action.[19] The prerequisites for strong leadership from a values perspective include self-reflection, the ability to see issues from many perspectives, life balance, confidence in personal abilities, and also real humility. Twenty-four leaders from around the world and from various professions were asked to address the issue of universal values.[20] They reached a consensus that the following values were universal: love, truthfulness, fairness, freedom, unity, tolerance, responsibility, and respect for life. Some widely shared values were nonetheless not universally shared, but these were listed as well: courage, wisdom, hospitality, obedience, peace, stability, racial harmony, respect for women's place in society, and protection of the environment. In the case of American culture, two other widely shared values should be added to the list: health protection and quality of life. Americans, among others, are concerned about the effect that disease can have on quality of life. Public health leaders promote a public health agenda oriented toward improving the quality of life of people in their service communities.

Public health leaders, as protectors of the values of the agency and the community, must emphasize the importance of maintaining high ethical standards inside the agency and in the community. One necessary task is to do an ethics check. Are the procedures used in the agency and the community legal? And even if they are legal, are they consistent with the values of the agency and the community? Leaders also need to examine the relationship between the science of public health, the facts that guide public health practice, and the explicit knowledge that comes from our formal learning.[21] As can be seen in **Figure 6-2**, which evolved from my discussion with Dr. Patrick Lenihan, the 2003 president of the National Association of County and City Health Officials, the science and explicit knowledge dimension of a public health system needs to be understood in relationship to the experiences, action activities, and tacit knowledge that grow out of practice and internal agency learning and operations. Tacit knowledge is difficult to communicate because it involves the internal understandings of people to the experiences they have filtered through their personal values and beliefs. The science and experience dimensions are quite interactive but derive meaning after being screened by our values positions. It is not knowledge, experience, or values alone

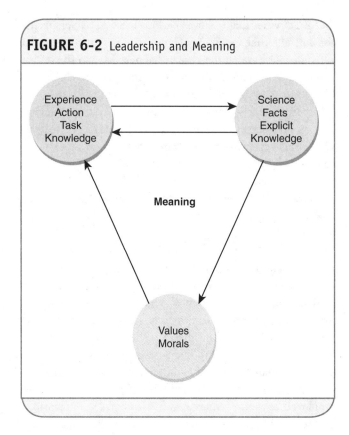

FIGURE 6-2 Leadership and Meaning

that are important—it is the meaning that is attached to these activities. Leaders and managers have the critical role of translating tacit knowledge into explicit knowledge so that there is meaning in these events for internal and external stakeholders. This translation helps the organization address similar problems in the future.

Public health leaders, besides identifying values, must consider how these values will affect the implementation of programs. They should be aware that the process of values clarification can simplify the solution of many local public health issues. Following is a list of strategies for leaders for clarifying values and promoting them in the agency and community:

- Learn which values are universal (or nearly universal) and promulgate them in the agency work teams and in the community.
- Learn which additional values prevail in the community and in the agency.
- In conjunction with agency members and community partners, integrate universal, community, and agency values.
- Evaluate prevailing values and revise those that need to be changed.
- Develop a shared values statement with the teams and in the agency.

Mission and Vision

Leaders need to be oriented toward the future and help create the vision that guides the activities of the agency. They must also inspire their colleagues to share the vision and use it to guide their activities. Therefore, the next task after values clarification for the team is to evaluate both the agency's mission and the current vision for the agency (or create a new one).

An agency's and agency-based teams' mission and vision must reflect each other. A vision is a picture of what, according to its leaders, the agency's future should be like. The agency's mission is the role it sees itself playing in the community. If the vision and mission truly reflect each other, then the agency, in fulfilling its mission, will help realize its vision (i.e., help bring about the kind of future it desires).

In addition, public health, like other areas of society, is changing rapidly, and an agency's vision and mission must change in concert. For example, disaster preparedness and response, public–private partnerships, emerging infections, drug resistance, mental health, community violence, and health reform are issues, some newer than others, that public health must address. A public health agency's mission statement must be revised periodically to take into account new problems, changing priorities, or other developments that have occurred in the public health arena. Agencies are also affected by many different constituencies as well as a number of elected officials, which makes the development of an agency vision much more complicated than it would be in the business world.[22] However, the agency mission may be defined by state or local statutes.

An organization's mission defines its purpose—its reason for existing.[23] A standard mission for a public health agency is the promotion of health and the prevention of disease. If an agency views itself as having this mission, then it should not be primarily involved in providing direct services with a strong medical orientation. During the past 2 decades, health departments have stopped doing most direct service activities. Community health centers, hospitals, drug stores, and a number of big-box stores like Walmart and Target have begun delivering immunizations and other primary care services.

A mission statement can be short or long. It can be a statement of the agency's or team's general purpose, or it can detail the agency's or team's role in several areas. According to Wall and colleagues, a mission statement needs to answer four questions:[24]

1. What is the purpose of public health?
2. How does the public health agency intend to coordinate its values and actions?
3. Who makes up the constituencies of the agency?
4. How does the agency link the present with the future?

Pearce and David claimed that a mission statement should address such things as the customer market (community), service-related issues, geographic concerns (global, national, state, or local), the level of technology, the requirements of agency survival, the personal concerns of the agency's leaders, the agency's philosophy, and the image of the agency in the community.[25] Albrecht recommended addressing the environment of competitors, economic concerns, political concerns, legal concerns, and social issues.[26] Wilson cautioned that a mission statement may leave out critical organizational activities, which sometimes shrivel financially and programmatically if not included in the mission.[27]

A mission statement should be inspiring, for the public health agency's workforce needs to embrace the mission.[28] Getting the staff members to do this could be difficult, because many of them have a minimal background in public health. Many will have been hired to perform clinical functions rather than engage in community-oriented preventive activities.

The mission is an important determinant of the agency's goals and objectives and should be closely tied to the agency's action plan. Therefore, the agency leaders must communicate the mission to community partners and constituents as well as to the agency workforce.[29] One strategy is to ask partners and constituents to read the mission statement in order to evaluate its clarity.

There is a question whether the mission or vision should be developed first. Typically, a public health agency has a clear idea of its mission but an undeveloped vision of its future. In a case like this, the mission is virtually given and the vision is what must be worked on. Sometimes an organization's mission and vision are both treated in a single statement that covers the present and the future. For example, the public health mission enunciated in *Healthy People in Healthy Communities* can also be viewed as a vision of the future.[30]

Managers are focused on protecting the integrity of their organization, whereas leaders are visionary and committed to change. Therefore, leaders can often benefit from developing their visioning skills. A vision can be likened to a blank canvas on which the leader sketches a possible future. Although a vision statement is about the future, it is often written in the present tense, which is one method of expressing the strong connection between the "now" and the "then." Lipton has developed a vision framework for leaders.[31] The core for building the vision includes organizational and/or community values, the mission of the agency, and strategy tactics. The leader should carefully select an executive team for implementing the vision. Also needed are methods that will maintain a growth-oriented perspective for the agency and techniques for managing people and getting buy-in for the vision.

Two cautionary notes: First, leaders are responsible for more than creating a vision. They need to motivate others and to play a major role in the development of action plans. Second, leaders may need to give up power in order to bring the vision into reality.[32] For example, they may be required to make changes to the organizational chart.

Following is a brief description of one method for developing a vision statement. First, the visioning team lays out the values and principles that will guide the visioning process. Second, the team develops a glossary of terms to go along with the shared mission statement. Third, it includes key constituents in the visioning process. Fourth, it describes the functions of a vision statement and how the vision statement to be created will be used. Fifth, the visioning team discusses the future and where it wants public health activities to go. (The team should consider scenarios likely to occur if the agency moves in certain directions. Scenario building is an important step in the visioning process.) Next, the team redefines terms and relates them to concepts in the glossary. Then it devises a vision statement based on the work it has done. The construction is followed by general editing, which occurs in smaller teams. The final step is to reach a consensus on the vision statement. Of course, once the vision statement is agreed upon, it is necessary to audit progress toward the implementation of the vision.

Following is a summary of the steps public health leaders need to take in order to develop a mission and vision for their agencies:

- Use a mission statement to guide the daily activities of the public health agency.
- Create a vision statement to guide the activities of the agency as it moves forward in time.
- Use visioning skills to create the vision.
- Involve colleagues and community partners in the development of a shared mission and vision.
- Develop a glossary of public health terms for colleagues and community partners.
- Review the mission and vision statements yearly.

Mission and vision are also affected by whether the leader is a traditional thinker who defines public health in a narrow sense as tied to the programmatic activities of the governmental public health agency or more systemically from the perspective of the community as a whole. Because leaders often work from the inside of their agency to the outside and also recognize the possibilities and concerns of external stakeholders as an outside-to-inside approach, the practice of action inquiry needs to occur.[33] Action inquiry is a systems activity of transformational leaders that should lead to mutual approaches to addressing public health challenges. It is through action inquiry that knowledge and action will come together.

Goals and Objectives

The next task in the systems approach to organizational change is to translate the mission and the vision into measurable goals and objectives. The mission statement is framed in general terms and does not contain the details of how the mission is to be fulfilled. Nor does the vision statement lay out how the vision is to be realized. Goals are more specific than either the mission or vision, and objectives are more specific still. They are, so to speak, the individual steps on the way to fulfilling the mission and realizing the vision.

Goals can be classified in several ways. One distinction is between organizational goals, which the activities of the organization are intended to achieve, and order goals, which are pursued as a means of preventing certain events from happening.[34] Organizational goals and team goals can be further divided into the stated goals of an organization or a team and the actual, sometimes hidden, goals of the organization. Creating a fit between organizational goals and systems goals is an important leadership activity. Goals can also be classified in terms of the areas of human activity to which they pertain, as seen in the division between economic, cultural, social, and political goals.

Objectives are the quantitatively and qualitatively measurable steps needed to achieve the goals of the organization. Along with the goals, they are used to guide the managerial processes for which public health agency leaders are responsible. The goals and objectives also need to reflect the vision of the agency and community, or the vision or goals need to be revised. Specifically, the leader then has the responsibility for:

- translating the agency's mission and vision into programmatic goals and objectives
- discovering any hidden goals that may sabotage activities (action inquiry)
- considering the budgetary requirements necessary to realize the goals and objectives
- examining goals to determine if they are translatable into action

The Action Plan

The next step is to develop an action plan for achieving the goals and objectives identified in the preceding stage. The action plan, which can include the key components of a business plan, consists of operational steps that, if performed, will lead to the attainment of the stated goals and objectives. In this step, the agency leaders or team leaders are required to be especially creative, because the action plan will almost certainly demand innovative approaches to achieving the goals and objectives. Creativity is called for by the structural tension that exists between the vision and the current reality. A creative leader looks for ways of resolving the tension in order to move the organization forward.[35]

Brainstorming is frequently used at this stage because it is an effective way of discovering worthwhile ideas. In addition, the leaders, in creating an action plan, must take into account the environment (the agency and its community) and the resources needed to carry out the plan.[36] Another set of techniques involves scenario planning, which is the development of stories to examine variations in eventual outcomes in bringing vision into reality. Scenario planning uses many tools, including forecasting, forces for change, tabletop exercises, computer simulations, environmental changes, politics, and systems tools and techniques.[37]

The creative process can be divided into three stages.[38] First comes the germination phase, in which the leader uses personal excitement to address the problems that need to be dealt with. In the second stage, the organization and its employees begin to adapt to the leader's agenda. In the third stage, the process is completed. At this time, the leader often starts the process over again.

Some management experts suggest that devising strategies for goal attainment is more effective than an action plan. Mintzberg, for example, argued that the action plan approach is too narrow.[39] For one thing, it separates strategic thinking from the goal-attainment process, and the separation prevents leaders from responding creatively to the changing environment. In Mintzberg's view, planning is an incremental process and is not something that can be done all at once. One way of proceeding is to create an action plan that addresses only a few important areas. If the plan is too complex, failure may result.[40] Note that if the strategic approach is used, the strategies chosen may in fact replace goals in the minds of the various constituencies.

One way of looking at an action plan is as a process of learning through action. Constant feedback is a necessary part of the process. If progress toward the goals is not occurring, revisions in the plan will need to be made. The leaders may have to go back to previous stages and repeat them. Feedback in systems is in actuality quite complex, as can be seen in **Figure 6-3**.[41] This diagram demonstrates that a critical aspect of action is to close the gap between a designated goal or set of goals and a series of action steps. Part of the reason for this gap is that there may be hidden goals in the system that come to the forefront when specific action steps are implemented. As action steps are implemented, unexpected occurrences may also happen that change the system. This fits the Wheatley argument that change is messy and chaotic.[42]

FIGURE 6-3 Feedback Loops in a System Dynamics Model

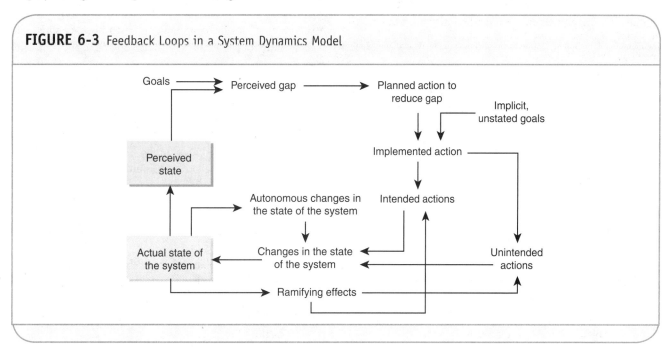

One point to mention here is that government agencies tend to be highly bureaucratic because of the legislative need for oversight and accountability. As may be expected, civil service requirements often work against organizational change, and networks are often difficult to form in bureaucratic organizations. Yet an interesting phenomenon is occurring that may help in overcoming some of the barriers caused by bureaucratization. Prior to 2012, almost all states had an in-state or regional public health leadership institute, and such institutes facilitated the development of leadership networks. Websites, forums, blogs, social media sites, chat rooms, and other forms of electronic communication are making networking easier.

The structure of any organization is multilayered, and those devising an action plan need to take account of the hidden parts of the organization's structure.[43] Furthermore, they should keep in mind that any stage in the implementation of the plan will be affected by all the previous stages. They also must pay attention to authority issues and the effect that the implementation of the plan will have on the workforce, because major changes can alter a staff member's sense of identity.

A number of strategies, including the following four, can be used to reduce the problems likely to arise from a major change. First, resulting changes in roles and relationships should be determined as the action plan is being created. Staff will worry about no longer having a job when the process is completed—and in fact, jobs may vanish as a result of the implementation. Second, the human resources office may have to be reorganized or its practices reformed in light of the proposed change. Third, an information system capable of monitoring the implementation process may have to be created. Finally, the financial management of the organization may have to be altered.

One way to measure the effectiveness of an action plan is to use the balanced scorecard model developed by Kaplan and Norton[44] This model evaluates the degree of success from the financial, internal organization process, customer, and learning and growth perspectives. What the balanced scorecard demonstrates is that developing an action plan requires awareness of the many different dimensions to action planning activities. We need to be careful to include all the dimensions in our action activities. Oversimplification can be as much of a problem as too much complexity. For an action plan to work, according to the authors, the leaders of the organization must communicate the mission and vision, the goals and objectives, and the action plan to all the relevant constituencies. Second, the leaders must understand and be able to explain to these constituencies the linkage between the action plan goals and the rewards associated with good performance—what might be called "encouraging the heart.[45] Third, the process of developing the plan must include target setting. Fourth, the action plan must include feedback and learning components.

An action plan can usher in a new era for the organization or be its death knell. It is more likely to benefit the organization if it is created by means of a well-thought-out method and is implemented using the strategies mentioned. Following is a list of guidelines that public health leaders should follow when engaged in action planning:

- Develop an action plan tied to the agency's mission, vision, and goals and objectives.
- Use strategic planning techniques for action planning.
- Formulate operational steps or strategies for each goal and objective.
- Know the resources that are needed and the resources that are available to implement the action plan.
- Explore existing barriers to successful action planning.
- Use the balanced scorecard model to measure the effectiveness of the action plan.

Implementation

The implementation of an action plan for the purpose of achieving goals and objectives and thereby realizing the agency or team's vision is the practice of public health, or at least part of it. During implementation, the leaders of the agency have the task of communicating the mission, vision, and goals and objectives of the agency to the staff and community constituents and doing this within the governing paradigm of the public health core functions of assessment, policy development, and assurance. In short, the leaders must become a bridge between the agency and the community.

Very little has been written about the implementation of action plans in the field of public health, although quality improvement techniques will work to make this occur. Yet it is clear that implementation of an action plan can involve many of the same activities public health leaders normally engage in as part of their responsibilities. These include:

- identifying community leaders and other external stakeholders
- delegating tasks to staff members and community partners
- establishing relationships with constituents
- communicating health information to the community
- working with the legislature
- working with the county board or local board of health

89

In a survey of California public health officers and executives, the respondents stated that their work encompassed budgeting, programming, disease control, staffing, environmental issues, health issues related to foreign nationals, and issues arising from undocumented care.[46] The researchers examined the lessons that the public health leaders had learned from their daily activities. These lessons included the importance of accuracy of information, flexibility, the total involvement of all stakeholders, action based on vision, patience, and providing information to the public.

Evaluation

After an action plan and work plan are implemented, the results of the implementation need to be evaluated. The object of the evaluation is to determine to what degree the goals and objectives were achieved. Although the leaders of a public health agency will not be directly involved in gathering and analyzing the evaluation data, they will use the conclusions of the evaluation to determine what steps to take next to realize the agency's or team's vision.

Leaders of an agency need data to foster a culture of evidence-based practice within the agency and among community constituents. For one thing, public health leaders are seen as sources of knowledge about community public health issues, and ensuring that evaluation data are gathered and publicized in some form confirms the legitimacy of their role as knowledge providers. In addition, the data will show the effects of the agency's activities on the residents of the community and, assuming they are mostly positive, will confirm the legitimacy of the agency's role as a protector of the community's health.

The evaluation process has been analyzed as consisting of six separate steps:[47]

1. Posing questions about the program
2. Setting effectiveness standards
3. Designing the evaluation
4. Collecting the data
5. Analyzing the data
6. Reporting the results

Not part of the evaluation process itself but an essential step nonetheless is the use of the results to determine further changes that need to be made.

Evaluation seems to frighten health professionals in the United States, who tend to think evaluation data will jeopardize their jobs. In Great Britain, in contrast, public health leaders seem convinced that evaluation helps strengthen programs.

EXERCISE 6-2   Teach the Wheel

Purpose: to practice your teaching skills as a way to increase your personal learning

Key Concepts: leadership wheel, personal learning, teaching skills

Procedure: Prepare a 30-minute presentation on the leadership wheel with 15 minutes allocated to an exercise related to the wheel. You can use five slides for your presentation.

One of the best ways to increase your understanding of the leadership wheel is to teach others about the wheel. **Exercise 6-2** gives you the chance to increase your understanding of the leadership wheel.

SUMMARY

Teams have become a critical part of the work of public health agencies today. The synergy that occurs when people work together leads to solutions that are often creative and innovative. Trust is often created when people work together. When agency leaders work closely with the teams they create, loyalty and trust become more possible. Agency leaders and team members are oriented to improving the efficiency and effectiveness of the agency. In the second part of this chapter, the main stages in the systems approach to organizational change are presented using the leadership wheel. The first step is for the organization and team to clarify its values and create a strategic plan. Once it does that, it can more easily construct a mission for itself and create a vision of its own future. The next task is to determine which goals and objectives, if achieved, will lead to the fulfilling of the organization's or team's mission and the realization of its vision (development of a business plan). The third task is development of an action plan designed to accomplish the goals and objectives. The action plan needs to be implemented during the fourth task (creation of a work plan). The fifth step is to do an evaluation to determine whether the goals and objectives were accomplished and whether their evaluation uncovers changes that need to be made if the vision is to be realized. Feedback mechanisms need to be included if the integrity of the systems perspective is to be maintained.

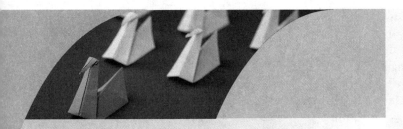

Discussion Questions

1. What is the role of leadership in team building?

2. Distinguish a group from a team and give examples.

3. What is the role of traditional teams and high-performance teams?

4. Discuss the leadership wheel and its relationship to teams and organizations.

5. How do skills at the personal level overlap or differ from skills at the team level?

REFERENCES

1. M. Miller, *The Secret of Teams* (San Francisco, CA: Berrett-Kohler, 2011).
2. M. Csikszentmihalyi, *Creativity* (New York, NY: Harper-Collins, 1996).
3. H. Cloud, *Boundaries for Leaders* (New York, NY: Harper Business, 2013).
4. C. E. Larson and F. M. J. LaFasto, *Teamwork* (Newbury Park, CA: Sage Publications, 1989).
5. Larson and LaFasto, *Teamwork*.
6. J. R. Katzenbach and D. K. Smith, *The Wisdom of Teams* (Boston, MA: Harvard Business School Press, 1993).
7. Katzenbach and Smith, *The Wisdom of Teams*.
8. Katzenbach and Smith, *The Wisdom of Teams*.
9. K. Blanchard, D. Carew, and E. Parisi-Carew, *The One Minute Manager Builds High Performing Teams* (New York, NY: William Morrow, 1990).
10. I. I. Mitroff and H. A. Linstone, *The Unbounded Mind* (New York, NY: Oxford University Press, 1993).
11. C. W. Churchman, *The Design of Inquiring Systems* (New York, NY: Basic Books, 1971).
12. K. Blanchard and M. O'Connor, *Managing by Values* (San Francisco, CA: Berrett-Koehler, 1997).
13. P. Hersey et al., *Management of Organizational Behavior*, 9th ed. (Upper Saddle River, NJ: Prentice Hall, 2007).
14. M. Rokeach, *The Nature of Human Values* (New York, NY: Free Press, 1973).
15. R. M. Williams Jr., *American Society: A Sociological Interpretation*, 3rd ed. (New York, NY: Knopf, 1970).
16. Center for Rural Public Health Practice, *Bridging the Health Divide: The Rural Public Health Research Agenda* (Pittsburgh, PA: University of Pittsburgh, 2004).
17. D. E. Brown, *Human Universals* (Boston, MA: McGraw-Hill, 1991).
18. J. M. Kouzes and B. Z. Posner, *Credibility* (San Francisco, CA: Jossey-Bass, 2011).
19. H. M. Jansen Kraemer Jr., *From Values to Action* (San Francisco, CA: Jossey-Bass, 2011).
20. R. M. Kidder, "Universal Human Values: Findings on Ethical Common Ground," *Futurist* 28, no. 2 (1994): 8–13.
21. H. Mintzberg, B. Ahlstrand, and J. Lampel, *Strategy Safari* (New York, NY: Free Press, 1998).
22. B. Nanus, *Visionary Leadership* (San Francisco, CA: Jossey-Bass, 1992).
23. S. P. Robbins and M. Coulter, *Management*, 11th ed. (Upper Saddle River, NJ: Prentice Hall, 2011).
24. B. Wall et al., *The Visionary Leader* (Rocklin, CA: Prima Publishing & Communication, 1992).
25. J. A. Pearce Jr. and P. R. David, "Corporate Mission Statements: The Bottom Line," *Academy of Management Executives* (May 1992): 109–116.
26. K. Albrecht, *The Northbound Train* (New York, NY: American Management Association, 1994).
27. J. Q. Wilson, *Bureaucracy* (New York, NY: Basic Books, 1989).
28. N. M. Tichy, *The Leadership Engine* (New York, NY: Harper Business, 1997).
29. E. Marzalek-Gaucher and R. J. Coffey, *Transforming Healthcare Organizations* (San Francisco, CA: Jossey-Bass, 1990).
30. T. Norris and L. Howell, *Healthy People in Healthy Communities: A Dialogue Guide* (Chicago, IL: Coalition for Healthy Cities and Communities, 1998).
31. M. Lipton, *Guiding Growth* (Boston, MA: Harvard Business School Press, 2003).
32. Wall et al., *The Visionary Leader*.
33. B. Torbert and Associates, *Action Inquiry* (San Francisco, CA: Berrett-Kohler, 2004).
34. A. Etzioni, *A Comparative Analysis of Complex Organizations* (New York, NY: Free Press, 1971).
35. R. Fritz, *The Path of Least Resistance for Managers* (San Francisco, CA: Berrett-Kohler, 1999).
36. E. E. Bobrow, *Ten Minute Guide to Planning* (New York, NY: Macmillan, Spectrum, and Alpha Books, 1998).
37. G. Ringland, *Scenario Planning: Managing for the Future* (New York, NY: John Wiley and Sons, 1998).
38. R. Fritz, *The Path of Least Resistance* (New York, NY: Fawcett, 1984).
39. H. Mintzberg, *Mintzberg on Management* (New York, NY: Free Press, 1989).
40. Albrecht, *The Northbound Train*.
41. A. Best, P. I. Clark, S. J. Leischow, and W. M. Trochim, *Greater Than the Sum: Systems Thinking in Tobacco Control* (Washington, DC: National Cancer Institute Tobacco Control Monograph Series, 2007).
42. M. J. Wheatley, *Leadership and the New Science*, 2nd ed. (San Francisco, CA: Berrett-Kohler, 1999).
43. P. M. Senge et al., *The Fifth Discipline Fieldbook* (New York, NY: Bantam, 1994).
44. R. S. Kaplan and D. P. Norton, *The Balanced Scorecard* (Boston, MA: Harvard Business School Press, 1996).
45. J. M. Kouzes and B. Z. Posner, *The Leadership Challenge*, 4th ed. (San Francisco, CA: Jossey-Bass, 2007).
46. J. C. Lammers and V. Pandita, "Applying Systems Thinking to Public Health Leadership," *Journal of Public Health Management and Practice* 3, no. 4 (1997): 39–49.
47. A. Fink, *Evaluation Fundamentals* (Newbury Park, CA: Sage, 1993).

CHAPTER 7

Collaboration and Change

- Determine when to collaborate.
- Describe the Himmelman matrix of strategies.
- Understand community readiness.
- Define the characteristics of a collaborative leader.
- Distinguish the three forms of collaboration.
- Explain the stages of change.
- Discuss the styles of change.
- Compare and contrast the Kotter and the Connor models of change.
- Determine what we know about adaptation to change.
- Discuss the differences between the integrated model for planned change and the integrated model for changes related to crisis events.

Collaborative leaders build high-performing teams and appoint committees and task forces inside their organizations. They build relationships outside their organizations and create linkages to organizations with similar interests. Outside the leader's organization, they build coalitions, alliances, and partnerships. Relationships are also built with elected officials at the local, county, state, and federal levels. As these relationships at all governmental levels are built, it is clear that they are built for change. Our world is one of constant change. On the surface, collaboration is employed to improve successful outcomes. Collaboration is only one method for doing this. Sometimes successful results may occur through the efforts of the leader himself or herself.

If collaboration is to be successful, a number of factors need to be included.[1] First are timing and a clear need for people to work together to accomplish some challenge. Second, collaboration may result from the influence of strong stakeholder groups with a shared agenda. For example, community groups may be concerned about a rising number of teenage pregnancies in the community and look to the local health department and local high schools to come up with a solution to the growing problem. The third factor involves multiple community groups coming together to address a community problem such as the teenage pregnancy problem. Fourth, collaboration must appear open. The leaders and organizations working together as collaborators need to seem credible. Officials at the city and county level should show support for the collaborative process. Next, agency and community leaders need to be visible in the collaborative. It should by now be clear that strong leadership is required if collaboration is to be possible at the team level or at the level of coalitions or other community structural group models.

Before starting a discussion of the benefits of collaboration, it is important to present a few comments. First, it is critical to decide whether collaboration is the best direction to follow. Second, collaboration should be used only in those situations in which working together has a synergistic effect. The issues of power, power relationships, and shared leadership often complicate any collaborative endeavor. Third, collaboration is often about the relationships between organizations, and the people relationships need to be kept in perspective. Fourth, collaboration may occur within organizations through its structure of teams and not between organizations, and vice versa. Fifth, collaboration is more about the commitment of the members of the collaboration and less about the structure of the collaboration.

With these comments in mind, collaboration can be defined as a mutually beneficial set of relationships that are well defined and that are entered into by two or more organizations in order to achieve some common goals.[2] Collaboration within an organization takes place in high-performing teams with the commitment of a collaborative organizational leader. The individuals who represent these collaborating organizations or within a specific high-performing team tend to be called members or partners. An important reason to collaborate is to achieve results that are more likely to happen when people work together than in situations where people or a specific organization would work alone.[3] Working together also creates further collaboration opportunities and builds social capital. In most circumstances, collaboration becomes a continuing set of circumstances that provides a wide range of outcomes that empower people, organizations, and systems to change. Keeping collaborations active is not an easy task. Many collaborations have to struggle with such issues as unproductive meetings, shifting members from organizations, making the same decisions over and over again, lack of accountability, difficulty of maintaining a collaboration when funding ends, and difficulty of getting agencies to implement best practices throughout the system.[4]

Ray developed a model called nimble collaboration to orient collaborative activity toward results by emphasizing the premise of the collaboration, its promise, mission, vision, outcomes, evaluation criteria, and work plan.[5] Another interesting approach has been called collaboration math, which creates a structure for the collaboration based on the participants in the collaboration.[6] Collaboration math requires a common set of definitions and categories that each partner to the collaboration identifies. A matrix is created based on the definition of the problem, key issues, available or needed data, funding issues, training needs, outside partners, and the results anticipated.

There are many reasons to collaborate.[7] Some of these reasons include a shared concern for an issue or community challenge and a strong belief that working together can address the challenge most effectively. A second reason is to pool power so the combined effect of several groups or agencies working together can have a substantial effect on the outcome. Third, when gridlock exists, working together will help the community or a specific agency get unstuck. Fourth, bringing several groups or agencies to work together increases the chances for diversity issues to be addressed. Several agencies working together can also increase the ability of the various members to handle complex community issues.

Collaboration should be viewed in relation to three other strategies for working together:[8] networking, coordination, and cooperation. Time and circumstances will affect which of these strategies will be used. **Table 7-1** shows the Himmelman matrix of strategies. Collaboration was defined as the exchange of information, or altering the way activities get done, a possible sharing of resources, and enhancing the

TABLE 7-1   Matrix of Strategies for Working Together

Definition	Networking	Coordinating	Cooperating	Collaborating
	Exchanging information for mutual benefit	Exchanging information for mutual benefit and altering activities to achieve a common purpose	Exchanging information for mutual benefit and altering activities to achieve a common purpose	Exchanging information for mutual benefit, altering activities, and sharing resources to achieve a common purpose
Relationship	Informal	Formal	Formal	Formal
Characteristics	Minimal time commitments, limited levels of trust, and no necessity to share turf; information exchange is the primary focus	Moderate time commitments, moderate levels of trust, and no necessity to share turf; making access to services or resources more user friendly is the primary focus	Substantial time commitments, high levels of trust, and significant access to each other's turf; sharing of resources to achieve a common purpose is the primary focus	Extensive time commitments, very high levels of trust, and extensive areas of common turf; enhancing each other's capacity to achieve a common purpose is the primary focus
Resources	No mutual sharing of resources necessary	No or minimal mutual sharing of resources necessary	Moderate to extensive mutual sharing of resources and some sharing of risks, responsibilities, and rewards	Full sharing of resources, and full sharing of risks, responsibilities, and rewards

Reprinted with permission of Arthur H. Himmelman, *Collaboration for a Change* (Minneapolis, MN: Himmelman Consulting).

capacity of the various partners to achieve the goals defined by working together. This latter point of mutual benefit is critical to any collaboration. Networking is the most informal of the four strategies and relates primarily to the sharing of information. Many coalitions have this networking strategy as a primary goal for getting together. The coordination strategy incorporates the major goal of networking with the additional goal of altering activities. It is hoped that this strategy will reduce barriers for those seeking to access specific services. The last strategy relates to cooperation that incorporates the strategies of networking and coordination and adds the sharing of resources for mutual benefit. The major difference in cooperation and collaboration is the willingness of organizations to enhance the capacity of the various partners for the mutual benefit of all partners and to increase the chances of meeting the goals and purposes of the relationship.

The Center for Civic Partnerships has also looked at the issue of collaboration.[9] A distinction was made between collaborative actions covering such dimensions as connectivity, continuous assessment and planning, communication, capacity building, coordination of services, and collaborative initiatives and the collaborative attitudes encompassing the six Cs:

- Commitment
- Consensus building
- Community outreach and involvement
- Conflict resolution
- Cooperation
- Change

Table 7-2 presents the details of these 12 activities. They are especially interesting when compared with the four strategies of Himmelman that are incorporated into these 12 actions and attitudes.

TABLE 7-2   Collaborative Functions: The 12 Cs of a Collaborative

Collaborative Actions:
Connection—Serving as the convener of its members to promote information sharing and networking.
Continuous Assessment and Planning—Coordinating needs and resource assessments to provide current information on service delivery gaps, existing needs, and available community resources. Another collaborative function may be to convene and facilitate ongoing strategic planning activities.
Communication—Acting as a clearinghouse for information exchange and dissemination for its members and with the media.
Capacity Building—Building the knowledge and skills of individuals and organizations through training, providing information, etc.
Coordination of Services—Coordinating services in the community to improve service delivery and availability, reduce duplication, and address service gaps.
Collaboration—Participating in joint grant proposals and collaborative projects, pooled funding, shared resources and staff, and colocated services. Organizations and community members share risks, responsibilities, and rewards by working as partners. This requires a high level of trust and commitment to the collaborative process by decision makers and collaborative members.
Important Collaborative Attitudes:
Commitment—Collaboration requires an ongoing commitment from all members.
Consensus Building—Members agree on a shared vision and participate in the development, implementation, and achievement of the collaborative's goals.
Community Outreach and Involvement—A successful collaborative stays in frequent contact with the community it serves and involves community members in planning, decision making, and other collaborative activities.
Conflict Resolution—Conflict is a natural occurrence in the collaborative process. Issues should be resolved immediately through a conflict resolution process developed and approved by collaborative members.
Cooperation—Collaborative activities promote a more cooperative approach in decision making and service delivery and enhance relationships between individual agencies and community. Information and expertise are shared, but agency resources and authority are usually separately maintained and risks are minimal.
Change—Change is both a prerequisite and a result of successful collaboration! True collaboration requires organizations and the community to think differently about how they do business and usually requires change in their current systems to achieve collaborative goals.

Center for Civic Partnerships, Collaborative Functions: The 12 C's of a Collaborative. (Sacramento, CA: Center for Civic Leadership, 2002).

It is important to evaluate whether a group of individuals or organizations in a community is ready to work together. To this community readiness issue must be added the concern or evaluation of the community's capacity to change. Thurman has used community readiness theory to explore how communities can implement successful prevention programs using a step-by-step process.[10] Communities can be defined in terms of nine stages of readiness. Once a collaborative group can define the stage in which a community can be located in the model, they can then develop the strategies to address ways to move a community to a higher level of readiness. The readiness stages start with no knowledge followed by the denial stage. Stage 3 is the vague awareness stage and stage 4 involves preplanning. The next stage is the preparation phase followed by the initiation or implementation phase. Then, stabilization should occur. The final two readiness stages include an expansion phase and then a professionalization stage. Community readiness is only part of the evaluation that is necessary. It is important to determine individual, team, and organizational readiness levels as well.[11]

There is the additional issue of a collaborative or a community's capacity to work together to build social capital and to create change.[12] First, it is necessary to clearly define the issues or the problems to be addressed. Second, the issue of leadership and who will lead the change effort is critical. It is here that power sharing and turf issues become prominent. The identification of appropriate stakeholders and partners with whom to address the issues is important. It is necessary to make sure that all key organizations and community leaders are represented in the collaborative activity. The assessment of agreement between the stakeholders must also be evaluated. All possible solutions also need to be explored. Both the issue of the community's readiness to change and the capacity of the community to change are important. In the arena of emergency preparedness and response, it is important to recognize that change will occur whether a community or collaborative feels it is ready for the change or not. If community readiness issues and community capacity for change can be addressed as part of the planning and preparedness activities of the community, some of the response events will be easier to predict.

Not all leadership is collaborative. Although all leaders need followers, all leaders do not feel that they need to share power or their decision-making authority. Collaborative leadership involves a leader who believes in engaging other leaders in working together for the common good.[13] Collaborative leaders work together, convene appropriate stakeholders in the cause for which the group is brought together,

and facilitate and find methods for sustaining their activities and interactions. Collaborative leaders also facilitate mutual enhancement of each other's activities.[14] Collaborative leaders have strong values and are clear in stating them. Collaborative leaders also see commonalities and try to find common interests that bind them to their partners.[15] These leaders are also expert in creating and refining their visions and in mobilizing others to work with them. They are also excellent mentors who work toward the development of others.

Himmelman has summarized some of the major characteristics of collaborative leaders.[16] These characteristics can be found in **Table 7-3**. These 10 characteristics can also be seen as a framework for a set of competencies for collaborative leaders. All sorts of skills are involved, such as the use of values to drive action, persuasion, mentoring and training, risk taking, information sharing through telling stories and other techniques, community-organizing skills, training other leaders, communication skills, and an ability to use humor in stressful situations. All of these competencies and characteristics are useful for all leaders. All collaboration is used for community betterment and also for the empowerment of others. Collaboration strategies are used to produce policy change and to make improvements in the local delivery of programs and services.

As part of the Turning Point Leadership Development National Excellence Collaborative in 2002, Ayre and a panel of public health department leaders discussed the topic of building understanding and information sharing. The panel believed these skills would help address the challenges to building collaborative leadership in public health. Several key themes emerged:[17]

1. Collaboration and its leadership aspects can be seen best at a local level where there seems to be greater accountability.
2. Collaboration is vital to the work of public health, which is a population-based activity.
3. Individuals define collaboration differently. Federal, state, and foundations funders also may define it differently from local leaders who practice collaboration on a daily basis.
4. Because different leadership styles are required for different situations, collaboration may not be the best approach in every circumstance.
5. If collaborations are beneficial, it becomes critical to nurture them over time by supporting the various members when they need it.
6. Collaboration can be unpredictable in that different members may have different agendas that take

TABLE 7-3   Some Collaborative Leadership Characteristics

1. A commitment to improve common circumstances based on values, beliefs, and a vision for change that is communicated both by "talking it and walking it"
2. An ability to persuade people to conduct themselves within ground rules that provide the basis for mutual trust, respect, and accountability
3. An ability to respectfully educate others about the relationship of processes to products and outcomes about the relationship of organizational structure to effective action
4. An ability to draw out ideas and information in ways that contribute to effective problem solving rather than ineffective restatements of problems
5. A willingness to actively encourage partners to share risks, responsibilities, resources, and rewards and to offer acknowledgments of those making contributions
6. An ability to balance the need for discussion, information sharing, and storytelling with timely problem solving and keeping focused on responding to action-oriented expectations of those engaged in common efforts
7. An understanding of the role of community organizing as the basis for developing and expanding collaborative power
8. A commitment to and active engagement in leadership development activities, both informal and formal, that can take the collaborative process to higher levels of inclusiveness and effectiveness
9. An ability to communicate in ways that invite comments and suggestions that address problems without attacking people and, when appropriate, draws upon conflict resolution and win–win negotiating to resolve differences
10. A very good sense of humor, especially whenever collaborative processes get ugly or boring or both

Reprinted with permission of Arthur H. Himmelman, Collaboration for a Change, Minneapolis, MN: Himmelman Consulting.

precedence to the collaborative activity, or unexpected happenings may occur.

7. It is important to deal with collaboration skeptics.
8. Collaboration skill development needs to be included as a key competency for leadership development programs.

There are many heroes in public health who practice collaboration. A number of these heroes are part of the Public Health Institute Network throughout the United States. Public health institutes are nonprofit organizations that were created to be multisectoral entities and to develop community partnerships and alliances to address population health issues and outcomes. These institutes fostered innovations in health systems. Their leadership in collaboration activities are clear. Our collaborative leadership hero is Dr. Marsha Broussard of the Louisiana Public Health Institute.

FORMS OF COLLABORATION

Citizen and community empowerment lays the groundwork for collaboration among organizations, constituencies, teams, and individuals to influence policy development. Collaboration can take many forms, and collaborative groups come in many types. Cohen and colleagues identified five.[18] Advisory committees offer suggestions and provide technical assistance to leaders, programs, or organizations. Commissions are usually composed of citizens appointed by official bodies. (The problem with commissions is that the appointments are often political.) Consortia (or alliances) are semiofficial in nature. They tend to have broad policy-oriented goals and may cover large geographic areas. A single consortium may include several coalitions. Networks, which are fairly loose in organization, are created for the purpose of resource or information sharing. Finally, task forces are short-lived groups created to address a specific issue.

To put the discussion on collaboration in a structural context, **Figure 7-1** portrays collaboration as a continuum. There are several dimensions to the continuum. First, there is the internal organization type of working together that is represented by the team. This type of working together can be collaborative, or it can be like a committee or task force in which the chair of the group guides the process. From a collaborative perspective, the second dimension shows the team model to be weak from a community collaboration approach. Teams are used in many ways, and leaders argue that they can be extremely effective in sharing leadership and responsibility.

PUBLIC HEALTH HEROES AND VILLAINS 7-1 Marsha Broussard, Hero

Marsha Broussard, MPH, DrPH, is a portfolio director for school and adolescent health for the Louisiana Public Health Institute. Dr. Broussard received her doctorate from Tulane School of Public Health and Tropical Medicine in 2012. Her career includes not only work in school and adolescent health, but she also serves as president of the New Orleans African-American Museum. At the institute, she works with an innovative program called the School Health Connection, a regional collaborative initiative to support the efforts to rebuild and expand the School-Based Health Centers in the New Orleans area that were destroyed by Hurricane Katrina. Broussard works with many collaborative partners at the local and state level on this project. The overall goal of the connection is to improve the health of school-age and adolescent students. The School Health Connection project also works with New Orleans schools on comprehensive school wellness programs.

Dr. Broussard is the director of a new effort called the Orleans Teen Pregnancy Prevention Project, which is also collaborative in nature. The goal is to prevent teen pregnancy, human immunodeficiency virus (HIV), and other sexually transmitted diseases through the use of evidence-based curricula. The project will reach 1,000 youth with curricular and safer sex interventions. Broussard is collaborating with partners from many New Orleans organizations to carry out the project.

Heroes face many challenges. Today, so much is affected by funding and changing funding priorities. Dr. Broussard is a modern leader who struggles with these issues and yet she continues to support a collaborative leadership model in all her endeavors. She is clearly a modern hero.

External to the single organization, collaboration takes three major forms. First, there is the coalition, which is created for information sharing and to bring together different community leaders and organizations to map out strategies for community change. Alliances are groups of health, healthcare, and public health organizations that combine forces to address key community or public health issues. These alliances, which are quite common, often develop informal contractual agreements to provide more comprehensive types of programs and services to their communities. Alliances may also add or delete members as programmatic needs change. The most structured organizational model is one based on written contracts, with all details of the collaboration worked out in minute detail with possible legal consequences. These collaborations are called partnerships. With a continuum perspective like the one presented in **Figure 7-1**, variations of the three major models are possible. Each major type of collaborative group is discussed next.

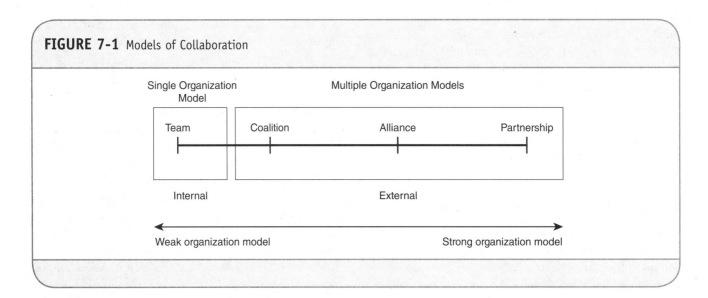

FIGURE 7-1 Models of Collaboration

Coalitions

A coalition is the coming together of people and organizations to influence outcomes related to a specific problem or set of problems. The synergism of joint action allows a coalition to accomplish a broader array of goals than could the participants acting on their own. The collaborative relationship that sometimes forms among a public health agency, other health and human service–related organizations, and various community constituencies is typically coalition like.[20] Such coalitions are created to get the organizations and constituencies involved in addressing community health needs and issues. They tend to be less structured than other types of collaborative groupings, and participants move in and out of the coalition as situations and priorities change.

To establish a coalition, a public health agency must make use of a number of strategies, including the following three.[21] First, it needs to establish a dialogue on health service delivery and policy with possible partners. Second, it needs to create a pool of groups willing to collaborate on the resolution of public health issues. This pool might include:

- at-risk groups affected by the health issues
- allies with whom the agency shares common interests
- experts knowledgeable about the issues
- associates that the agency works with on a day-to-day basis
- opposition groups that may challenge agency positions on the issues
- third-party groups indirectly affected by the issues
- state and local government officials who have influence on public policy
- media organizations

Third, the agency needs to establish a communication network for the purpose of exchanging information. Communication is essential for promoting the coalition and mobilizing the members to take action to meet the community's health needs, which is, after all, the whole purpose of creating the coalition.

Coalitions have several significant advantages:[22]

- A coalition can conserve resources, because the participants cooperate in promoting the coalition's agenda and avoid duplication of efforts.
- A coalition is an excellent communication tool, because its member organizations can send out its message to many more people than any single organization can.
- A coalition, through synergy, can achieve more objectives than could the participant organizations acting alone. For example, it possesses greater power to influence political decision makers.
- A coalition has a credibility advantage over its individual members. There is clearly strength in numbers.
- A coalition provides a mechanism for sharing information. For instance, one coalition member can provide information to others not able to attend a meeting, and the entire coalition or individual members can develop releases to provide to the media.
- A coalition typically has a lead agency that most of the coalition members provide with advice, guidance, and direction. In the case of public health coalitions, the lead agency is usually the local health department or public health agency.
- A coalition helps the representatives from member organizations by improving their self-esteem, giving them personal satisfaction, and developing their understanding of their organizations' roles in improving the health of the public.
- Finally, a coalition can foster cooperation among the members and can strengthen the community by concentrating on the community's strengths.

On the downside, a public health coalition takes some effort to sustain. Over time, the community and the community's health needs will change, and the coalition must change in concert. In addition, conflicts over turf occasionally occur, and schisms within the coalition can make it more difficult to deal with public health issues than if the coalition did not exist.

Alliances

A community health alliance is a group of healthcare and public health organizations that have combined forces to address key public health risks and problems for the population of a specific geographic area.[23] Although the participating organizations may benefit from the alliance, the purpose of the alliance is to meet the needs of the community residents. A community health alliance might include the local public health agency, healthcare providers, payers, purchasers of services, advocacy groups, community social service agencies, and neighborhood groups.

Alliances can be divided into three types.[24] An opportunistic alliance is created to increase the knowledge and expertise of organizations in a new field of operation. This new information may be used to develop a new type of program in a community. For example, a local public health agency may collaborate with a number of health maintenance organizations to learn how their managed care programs work and then use this information to develop a Medicaid managed care program of its own.

A resource dependency alliance is created to provide a needed service or resource for multiple healthcare organizations. For example, a local health department may agree to immunize all children less than 2 years of age in the community, preventing other healthcare organizations from having to develop immunization programs.

A stakeholder alliance is developed by organizations willing to work together to achieve a common objective. For example, the alliance members may jointly develop a trauma registry to better document trauma-related problems in the community.

Partnerships

The partnering process requires each partner to show respect for the other partners and put personal or organizational agendas aside. The partners, whether from the public or private sectors, treat each other as equals. That means that all partners engage as equals in the decision-making process. In an effective partnership, the partners share a vision, are committed to the integrity of the partnership, agree on specific goals, and develop a plan of action to accomplish the goals. A partnership may have a partnering agreement, which is like a contract, to guide its activities.

A collaborative leader needs to understand how to use these different collaboration models. **Exercise 7-1** gives you

the chance to experiment with coalitions, alliances, and partnerships to address a major public health problem.

CHANGE

Collaboration is about process. Change is about process and results. Although it is true that change can be planned, we do live in an age where unanticipated change events such as terrorist attacks and other crises come into our lives in an unpredictable way. Most theories of change have assumed that social change is a continuous process, but the events of the past few years clearly create discontinuities in our social structure and in our personal lives. What crisis forces us to do is view these major change events in terms of explanation rather than prediction. It is necessary to trace the event backward to garner information that will allow us to prevent or better predict similar events in the future. Chaos theories show that an understanding of how to address potential crises is tied to an awareness that unanticipated events (and the changes that occur because of them) are now part of the social fabric of our lives. All crises create messes and may lead to more crises and more complex messes.[25] Systems thinking approaches are critical in addressing emergencies and the effect of change on communities. This part of the chapter looks at the stages of change and how transition in our lives may be as important as our understanding of the process of change.

Change is a process of moving from what has become an obsolete present into a revitalized present with an eye on the future. Change also means that the old rules do not seem to be working anymore, and new rules and procedures need to be developed for the changing context in which we live today. Schein clarified the issue of change and why people are often resistant to structured and unstructured change.[26] People like equilibrium in their lives. The process of coping, growth, and survival is measured against some sense of stability in their environments. Some of this stability comes from the culture, shared values, routines, and some ability to predict how our day-to-day activities will play out. These assumptions are shared with the people with whom we interact.

Unanticipated change clearly disrupts the equilibrium of teams, people, organizations, and their communities. We now live in an age of constant and speeded-up change. The question is how to adapt to these changes or how to live in a world of unpredictable change. When change transforms a culture or community, people need to unlearn the old rules and also learn the new rules.[27] Change can be incremental or slow and intense. This latter type of change is sometimes called deep change.[28] The good news about incremental change is that the process is so gradual that people, organizations, and

---

EXERCISE 7-1   Collaboration and HIV

Purpose: to collaboratively address an increase in HIV cases in Hometown

Key Concepts: collaborative leadership, teams, coalitions, alliances, partnerships

Scenario: Hometown has seen a 20 percent increase in reported cases of HIV in the last 5 years.

Procedure: Divide the class into groups of six. Each group picks a leader. The group then decides how the growing problem of HIV cases in the community should be handled. Review the various models to determine how best to address the problem. Each group will then report how the decision was made to select the best model to deal with the problem.

communities can adapt to the changes more easily. Another advantage of incremental change is that it is possible to revert to the prechange stage more easily because the change process is so gradual. Deep change is much more profound in that it requires new ways of thinking, feeling, and behaving. It is not possible to go back. There has been a tipping point. We cannot go back to our pre–September 11, 2001, lives. Thus, deep change is a major change that breaks with the past.

Change can be seen in the context of surprises.[29] We live in a world of inevitable surprises. These surprises will continue to occur, perhaps at a much faster rate than in the past. We know now that surprise is inevitable, but we can plan for the things that are not expected. We can, even with some degree of accuracy, predict how certain types of crisis events will play out over time. One critical set of skills is creating different scenarios for different types of events. For example, it is possible to create scenarios about the effect of a terrorist event similar to September 11, 2001, from a number of perspectives.

Schwartz explored some lessons that he believed we have learned about change and these inevitable surprises.[30] First, it is important that change agents keep looking for clarifications of a surprise event. Conversations between individuals who have been involved in similar events can often provide new information, interpretations of happenings, and new understandings of the variations in outcomes of different types of surprise events. Successful leaders also become better at prediction and timing related to surprises by watching for which factors will speed up events and which factors will slow them down or stop them in their tracks. Change agents become more aware of warning indicators and are adept at developing skills related to early detection. It is possible to discard techniques and approaches that might create environments for crisis.[31]

It is also important for leaders to be careful not to deny the potential for surprise events. Leaders should understand how they judge things. Each of us has different learning and behavioral styles. Our perspectives and judgments are affected by these styles. It is worthwhile for leaders to explore these issues either through using some leadership profile instruments or through working with executive coaches who specialize in these analyses. Once again, it is important to emphasize lifelong learning for leaders. Different leadership tools and skills are required for different times and events. Leaders need to better understand how their actions are seen in their organizations and in their communities by their partners and by community residents. It is clearly critical for the public health leader to cultivate these community connections because all traditional public health activities and emergency preparedness and response activities are communitywide efforts and not just the work of one individual.

STYLES OF CHANGE

The public health leader has to be both a catalyst for change and also a reactor to change caused by unanticipated consequences. Leaders have different change styles. Musselwhite has studied the issue of styles for a long time. His organization developed an instrument to define and test change styles.[32] From more than 10 years of research, three primary change styles have emerged: conservers, pragmatists, and originators.

The Conservers

Conservers are people who are able to gauge reality in a pretty accurate way. They also like structure and tend to work well within frameworks or organizations with well-defined rules and regulations. The conservers also tend to follow continuous quality improvement techniques. When they support making changes, they want to go slow and methodically. They have many strengths in that they see the details of every situation. They are steady and reliable, they honor commitments, they encourage people to follow the rules, they investigate situations thoroughly, they see all sides of the issue when change is contemplated, and they work to protect the integrity of the organization or community. On the negative side, they tend to be so conservative that opportunities for progress may be passed by.

The Pragmatists

Pragmatists are task oriented and tend to want to get things done with clear results. They are less concerned than the conservers with maintaining the structure of the organization or with things as they currently are. They tend to focus on the action plan phase of the leadership wheel. They want strategies for change and want to see them implemented. They also support the development of scenarios of possible outcomes. Whereas the conservers take a more evolutionary and gradual approach to change, the pragmatists react to the situation and do what needs to be done in a timely fashion. As leaders, pragmatists are very practical, open to exploring different approaches to solving problems, respect other people's opinions, build teamwork, and move teams toward making decisions. They are good facilitators who also know how to tie theory to practice. These are the people who walk the walk. However, they sometimes have trouble making decisions. They straddle the middle of the road. Their indecisiveness may lead to decisions that are not made in a timely fashion.

The Originators

Originators are the people who like to challenge the process.[33] These people like to make things happen. They are innovative and creative. They also seem to search for opportunities to create change. In many ways, these leaders are revolutionaries.[34] They tend to be navigators rather than rowers or helmsmen. They are systems thinkers who are big-picture thinkers and tend to be less concerned with the details of implementation. As leaders, the originators are clearly change agents, are enthusiastic, are visionary, tend to multitask, and are analytic, in the sense that they look for unique ways to put things and situations together. However, they do sometimes threaten their organizations and communities because they are less concerned about the status quo. This disturbs many people. Musselwhite and Jones have found that the originators make up about 25 percent of the population, the conservers another 25 percent, and the pragmatists are the most prevalent and make up the remaining 50 percent of the population.[35]

UNDERSTANDING CHANGE

Over the years, there have been many theories and explanations about change and its meaning. This section reviews two contemporary approaches to change that give public health leaders two influential approaches useful for increasing understanding of the challenges facing public health in this new century. One proposes an eight-stage approach to carry out change initiatives in organizations and communities. The second approach presents change from the perspective of resilience and the ability of people to adapt to change.

In reviewing older theories of change, Musselwhite and Jones found that most of the perspectives could be boiled down to four general stages:[36]

- The first stage involves acknowledging that a threat exists or that change is needed.
- The second stage is the reaction of people to the threat or change.
- The third stage is the need to investigate and determine the kinds of change that are needed.
- The fourth stage is the implementation phase.

The challenges that our country faces seem to be increasing. There were many threats to our way of life prior to September 11, 2001. All these societal and economic factors affect our organizations as well as our communities. In 1995, Kotter pointed to technological advances, international economic policy, expansion of global markets, maturation of markets in developing countries, and the changing of the guard in many countries, especially with the fall of most communist and many socialist regimes, as factors affecting American communities.[37] To this must also be added the increase in terrorism and the potential for bioterrorist acts around the world. People change when their behavior changes, and their behavior changes because leaders speak to the feelings of individuals.[38] It is important, when change is occurring, that the solutions are seen in terms of emotions and not just changes in people's minds. Thus, the central issue in change is not just strategy, structure, culture, or systems change, but how people see the proposed change and how it affects their feelings about the changes proposed.

Kotter and Cohen[39] looked at this perspective from the vantage point of an eight-step model (which Kotter had developed earlier) for successful large-scale change.[40] Whether a change is planned or unanticipated, a sense of urgency has to be generated before any change or adaptation to an unexpected change can occur. Crises clearly increase the sense of urgency. The second step involves the development of a team or coalition to guide the change or reaction to crisis process. This means that the selection of a group must also be representative of those who will be affected by change. Third, there needs to be a vision toward which to aim. The vision will lead to the development of goals, objectives, action plans, and implementation. Next, the change, vision, or adaptation strategy has to be communicated to all affected partners and community residents. What the public health leader needs is acceptance, participation, and commitment from all the affected parties. Fifth, it is necessary to empower people to be a part of the action necessary to bring the changes into being. Sixth, it is important to emphasize short-term wins to keep people involved in the process.

Seventh, it is important to maintain the momentum of the process by showing connections between the gains and the need to produce further changes so that the projected outcomes will occur. Step eight involves making the changes stick and also fitting the changes into the cultural fabric of the community.

With regard to the eight-stage model and the behavioral changes that occur at each stage, culture and values change last and not first. In addition, the first seven stages are easy compared with step eight. Before culture can change, behavior has to change. People need to feel that the changes are necessary for the future growth of an organization or a community. It is important for behavior to change with each step of the process. **Exercise 7-2** gives you the opportunity to apply the model to a community.

It is not enough for leaders to recognize that change is necessary.[41] The critical issue is how individuals can adapt to change. Leaders are most effective and efficient when the

EXERCISE 7-2 Obesity and Change

Purpose: to use the Kotter and Cohen change model in the City of Fatville

Key Concepts: change, nutrition, obesity

Scenario: There has been a substantial increase in obesity at Fatville High School. Further research shows a 15 percent increase in the Fatville population in the last 10 years.

Procedure: Divide the class into groups of seven. Each group will define a possible way to change the eating habits of people in Fatville using the high school as a potential testing ground. Go through the eight-step model and define the behavioral changes your group wants to see at each of the eight steps.

process of change occurs at a speed at which the leader can absorb and assimilate the changes in a reasonable way. In this second perspective, the issue of changes involves the resilience of the leader and others to adapt to the changes occurring in their environment. The resilience factor is the most critical factor if successful change is to occur. Resilience is affected by seven support patterns. What the concept of support implies is that each support pattern will aid the leader or increase the capacity of the leader to assimilate or process changes that are needed in the organization or community. Changes in one part of the world affect the lives and communities of all other people and places.[42]

The first support pattern involves the nature of the change. For the leader, a concern is whether the change can be controlled. There is also the issue of whether the outcome of the change event can be predicted. The level of disruption is also a part of the nature issue and is greater for unanticipated events such as terrorist or bioterrorist events. Conner stated that all changes have associated costs. Leaders should assess their ability to assimilate the effects of change. It is possible to imagine that each person has a certain number of assimilation points and that people who are resilient have more points to use. If the change affects the individual only, it is a micro change.[43] Organizational change means each person in an organization or agency must change. Macro change is when everyone has to change whether they want to or not.

The process of change is the second support pattern. Resilient leaders see change as a process, where less resilient people see change as a yes-or-no situation, in which change is moving from one place to another over a period of time. There is a transition between these two end points. Less resilient people have difficulty with the ambiguity of the change process. Resilient people accept change as a part of life and believe that it is possible to manage that process. Leaders do not worry about the ambiguity of the process. This does not mean that the resilient leader does not feel stressed at times. Some change events are unpredictable in terms of when they occur and how they will affect all those concerned. Stress is also a part of the human condition.

The third support pattern relates to the roles of change. Resilient people are aware that the roles and relationships between people change during change events. For example, during an emergency event, the incident command system changes traditional roles and relationships into predetermined roles and relationships required during the emergency. Four special roles during change are specifically discussed by Conner.[44] First, there is the *sponsor*. This is an individual who has to legitimize and sanction the change activities whether in reaction to an emergency event or in anticipation of an intended change. *Agents* are individuals or groups who are responsible for reacting to the event or for making the change if it is a planned activity. The *targets* of change are those who have to do the changing. The final role is that of *advocate*. This is a person or group that supports the change or the implementation of a reaction procedure but does not have the power to implement the process.

Resistance to change is the fourth support pattern. Leaders expect that there will be resistance to change or the effects of unanticipated change events. Open resistance is a healthy process that brings all issues related to the change out in the open. It is covert resistance that is not healthy. Resilient people see the positives in the change process. Less resilient people see only the negative. The issue of realistic expectations comes into play in that there will be resistance if people feel their expectations are not being met. After September 11, 2001, many people became resistant to the many security measures that needed to be imposed. I remember seeing the resistance and anger of some individuals at airports who were upset with the increased security measures. It also seems as if some people become more resistant if they think increased security precautions are permanent rather than temporary.

The next support pattern involves the issue of commitment. As mentioned earlier, change has costs. If change is to be successful, all individuals must pay those costs. Conner pointed to a number of issues that affect the level of commitment.[45] First, the commitment will increase if people put personal resources such as time, money, and energy into the change process. Second, there needs to be allegiance to the goals that the change process is to achieve. This level of commitment must continue even if the changes take a long time to occur or if the proposed changes increase stress or ambiguity. Although small wins are nice, the goal should always be the prize at the end of the process. Next, there may be adversity, but it is important to be steadfast. Finally, leaders know they will need to be creative, innovative, and resourceful in removing blockages to the achievement of the end changes that need to occur.

The sixth support pattern relates to the cultural dimension, which is critical in that the outcome of any change is affected by culture, shared beliefs and values, behavior, and the ecological nature of the community and how all these factors change over time. Cultural variables are hard to change. Behavior must change first. Behavioral change will affect attitudes, which in turn will affect beliefs and values, which in turn will eventually affect the culture as a whole. Leaders must understand how their organizations and communities work. They must be willing to spend the time showing their organizations why change is necessary. Leaders should remain concerned about the values of the community and how they can be modified to accommodate the necessary changes that need to occur. Resilient leaders also know that not all people will react to change in the same way or in the same time frame that the leader is proposing.

The final support relates to synergy, which can be demonstrated in terms of four steps. First, there needs to be interaction among team and community members. All parties to the change need to communicate with each other and generate trust and credibility. Second, there needs to be "appreciative understanding," which relates to the ability to use and value diversity. The third step is integration, which relates to the blending of people with diverse backgrounds and diverse perspectives on the proposed changes. The fourth step in synergy is implementation, for which there must be successful wins. The diverse views must come together and create products of the change that add value beyond the inputs to the change. Thus, the resilient leader needs to be able to make $1 + 1 = 3$ or more.

More recently, Conner pointed out that change seems to be speeding up.[46] Organizations and communities will have to become nimble. We live in a time of potential chaos and complexity that requires constant changes to adapt to these unexpected events. An organization or community must develop strategies for success in unpredictable times and environments by implementing critical changes as effectively and efficiently as possible. The ability of the organization or community to adapt to constant change is important if these entities are to become nimble and increase their chances for successful change.

In addition to these change factors, other factors also need to be considered. As can be seen in **Figure 7-2**, resilience is an issue at many different levels. There is resilience in reaction to a disaster or emergency of some kind. Political resilience can be seen as politicians react to the constantly changing landscape of real-life issues such as a recession. Individuals have different levels of resilience depending on given events. Finally, the response to change may be organized and structured or disorganized and chaotic. The incident command system is often used in emergencies to help structure response.

CHANGE AND ADAPTATION

Much of the discussion of change relates to the effect of intended and unintended change on an organization or community. Although change affects the lives of people in these entities, there does seem to be a difference in the ability of people to adapt to change and the change process itself. There are two interesting approaches to understanding

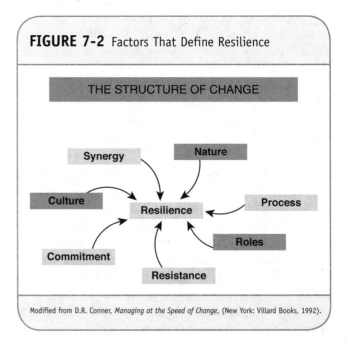

FIGURE 7-2 Factors That Define Resilience

THE STRUCTURE OF CHANGE

Synergy · Nature · Culture · Resilience · Process · Roles · Commitment · Resistance

Modified from D.R. Conner, *Managing at the Speed of Change*, (New York: Villard Books, 1992).

adaptation in people. Conner discussed what he called the adaptation reflex in terms of a four-step model.[47] Initially, there is the disturbance in the equilibrium of the environment in which the individual lives or works. This disequilibrium leads to the attempt by a person to try to adjust to the changed situation to regain personal control. An individual will explore options to regain a sense of equilibrium. The event either will appear to be strange or will appear to be somewhat familiar (conventional). Second, a decision needs to be rendered that leads to some clarification or judgment about the meaning of the event. This is followed by a response to the situation and, finally, a realignment process in which the individual develops new or modified behaviors to adjust to the change event. The response is the attempt to restore balance. The response can be adaptation with new behavior, avoidance, or assimilation of the event within the existing framework of reaction to change. In summary, the adaptation reflex involves moving from one state of equilibrium to another.

Bridges saw all adaptation as a series of transitions that occur throughout an individual's life.[48] Transitions are clearly different from the change process itself. For the individual, all change is about a loss (an ending stage), whether it be a loss of old ways of doing things or the loss of a loved one. The ending is almost like the death of someone. Endings create disengagement, sometimes a disorientation as to who the person really is, disenchantment with the way things used to be, and sometimes disorientation or perhaps denial, and a sense that life has been changed by the event. This sense of ending is clearly exacerbated when a terrorist or bioterrorist event occurs. The sense of loss is generally followed by a period of disorientation and confusion that varies in length for each person and for each type of change event. It is important for the individual to learn that this "neutral zone" is not an abnormal one but just a time in which the individual is learning to cope with the changes in his or her life and also learning to let go of the past. Recovery can thus be a long process. This recovery period eventually leads to a new perspective that Bridges called a "new beginning." As Conner previously pointed out, individuals go through adaptation in different ways. The new beginning can be very exciting in that it offers the person new opportunities and new life possibilities.

The public health leader needs to develop the skills to understand his or her adaptation responses to different types of events and to understand the three stages of transitions. The leader must also realize that each person experiences these things in different ways. Recovery and adaptation will be different for each member of the community. Simple expectations about change, adaptation, and transitions are complex and will affect the recovery effort after any change, crisis events, and other life-modifying occurrences.

PUTTING THE PIECES TOGETHER

Although there is not a perfect fit between the theories and perspectives discussed in this chapter, it is possible to attempt this integration, although imperfect, to better understand the effects of planned and unintended changes in our society. Most of the skills and perspectives discussed come into play as part of the leadership toolbox that the public health leader who wants to be prepared puts together over his or her professional career. **Figures 7-3** and **7-4** show flowcharts for the two types of change. A cursory look at the two figures shows many similar processes at play during the change process. The figures show *that changes during* (and after a crisis) are complicated by the possible effect of activating the incident command system during the crisis.

Figure 7-3 looks at the process of planned change. The need for change in an organization or community requires the leader to respond to the need. Although many may be aware that changes are needed, it will be the leader who triggers the response. It is clear from our earlier discussion that different leaders will respond in various ways. The resilience factor comes into play in that the high-resilience leader will probably respond differently than the low-resilience leader. The high-resilience leader is more flexible and willing to change. The high-resilience leader will make a decision based on need and the facts at his or her disposal to either move slowly or move more quickly and comprehensively to create the necessary changes. This leader may move incrementally but probably never looks back. If deep change is needed, this leader will take the risk and make it happen. Kotter's eight-stage model could then be followed to bring about the changes and create a new environment as a result of the changes. The leader is also aware that the changes will not be complete until most, if not all, of the affected individuals have been able to adapt to the changes by seeing that a new beginning is possible.

In contrast, the low-resilience leader will probably treat similar needs for change in a different way. This leader will explore maintaining the status quo as a viable option, because change tends to be traumatic for people, and it appears that adaptation to the change will take too long to accomplish. The low-resilience leader always seems to be looking for a way out. Even if this leader decides change is necessary, he or she finds it hard to create a sense of urgency for change.[49] If change is required, the low-resilience leader will probably opt

FIGURE 7-3 Integrated Model for Planned Change

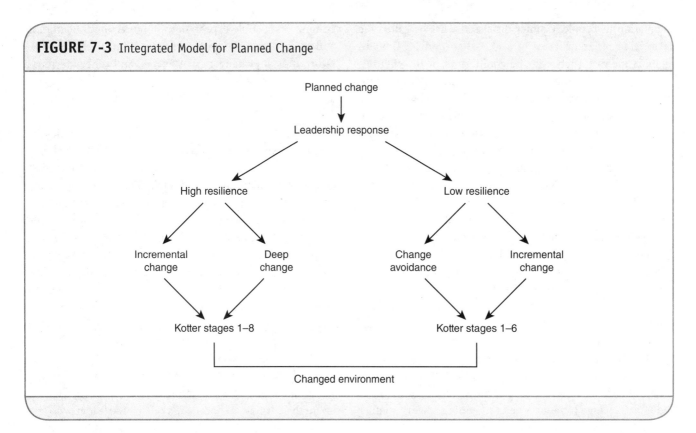

FIGURE 7-4 Integrated Model for Change during and after a Crisis

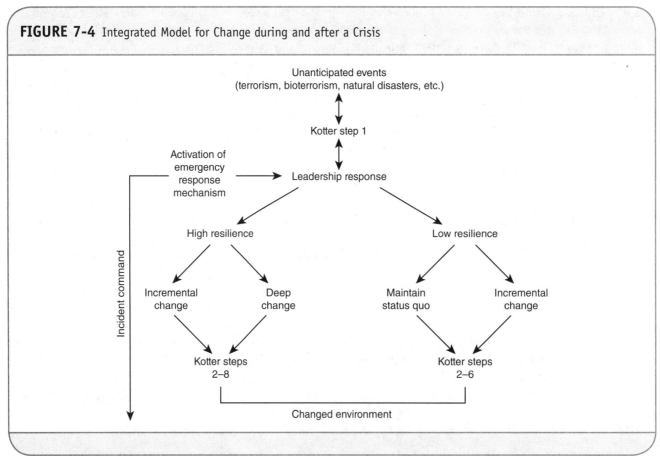

for incremental change because it allows people the chance to adapt to the change gradually. It is also possible under this model to return more easily to the starting point than it is with deep change. If change is needed, the process will begin. Using the Kotter model, steps 1–6 will probably occur. The final steps of not letting up and making the changes stick will be difficult for the low-resilience leader.

Although there are many similarities in the flowchart for change resulting from a crisis, there are still differences. As shown in Figure 7-4, the change event comes out of a chaos perspective when the status quo is destroyed by some generally unanticipated event. This emergency event triggers the need for not only adaptive responses but also further changes in the organization or community. The public health leader must respond whether or not that leader is a high-resilience leader. The change process may need to be filtered through an overlay response that is triggered by the activation of the incident command structure of the community. However, the leaders will need to respond to guide the change process in their organizations or communities while incident command is operating. The public is already feeling a loss of the way things were, and some people will already be trying to adjust to the loss and will have entered the neutral zone that Bridges discussed.

The high-resilience leader knows that further changes are inevitable. A way of life has been altered by the emergency event. This leader will have to decide whether incremental or deep change is the best strategy. The event has had major impact. Some leaders will decide that it is necessary to slow the change process because deep change will cause further trauma. However, the nature of the event may also require deep change because incremental change will not work. The sense of urgency has already occurred with the crisis event. The high-resilience leader needs to maintain the sense of urgency as the stages of change occur. The high-resilience leader knows that it is not possible to return to the precrisis event stage. Community and organization life are forever changed.

The low-resilience leader struggles with the need for further changes as a result of the emergency event. This leader may try to maintain the status quo, even though the old status has changed. This leader may opt for no further change so as not to disrupt the lives of people too much. Sometimes, the low-resilience leader recognizes that some further change is needed even though it will be painful to bring about. This leader will probably go for an incremental change approach without great enthusiasm. Kotter's steps 2–6 will probably occur without the final steps that will sustain the changes over time. The low-resilience leader will probably believe that it will eventually be possible to return to the way life was before the emergency.

The goal of this section has been to begin to create a perspective on change that builds on the multiple models of change that have been studied. As more is learned about change, it will be possible to add to the synergistic model presented in this section and begin to better understand how change occurs when it is planned and when it is unplanned. Axelrod believes that both the Kotter and the Conner models are part of what he calls traditional approaches to change management.[50] The new approach to change management needs to involve a major concern with engagement. First, it is important to increase your circle of involvement with both internal organizational and external stakeholders. Next, increase the connections with these stakeholders. Third, Axelrod argues for communities of action and stresses fairness in all change activities. In addition, leaders need to build their change activities honestly and with transparency and trust. In public health we often confront new crises—think Zika virus, contaminated water in Flint, Michigan, and earthquakes in Japan.

SUMMARY

Leaders appoint and support teams. Teams collaborate to create change. Collaboration is a mutually beneficial set of well-defined relationships between two or more people or organizations to achieve common goals. Himmelman has developed a matrix of strategies to show how the intensity of the relationship affects the work to be accomplished. Measures of readiness of communities for collaboration and change have also been developed. Collaboration outside the walls of an organization take the form of coalitions, alliances, and partnerships.

The second half of the chapter addresses the issue of change from a process and a results approach. Leaders need to understand how the process of change works. Different models were presented as a beginning orientation for leaders. Adaptive leadership is all about change and how to make change happen.

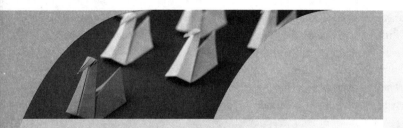

Discussion Questions

3. What are the reasons that a community readiness model will help an adaptive leader?

4. Explain the difference between the Kotter and Conner change models. What utility do these approaches have for a leader?

5. How does change affect disaster planning?

1. Compare and contrast with examples the Himmelman matrix of strategies and the Mays and colleagues models of collaboration.

2. What are the advantages and disadvantages of collaboration versus doing the job yourself?

REFERENCES

1. D. D. Chrislip and C. E. Larsen, *Collaborative Leadership* (San Francisco, CA: Jossey-Bass, 1994).

2. P. W. Mattesich, M. Murray-Close, and B. R. Monsey, *Collaboration: What Makes It Work*, 2nd ed. (St. Paul, MN: Amherst H. Wilder Foundation, 2001).

3. M. Winer and K. Ray, *Collaboration Handbook* (St. Paul, MN: Amherst H. Wilder Foundation, 2002).

4. K. Ray, *The Nimble Organization* (St, Paul, MN: Amherst H. Wilder Foundation, 2002).

5. Ray, *The Nimble Organization*.

6. L. Cohen, M. J. Aboelata, T. Gantz, and J. Van Wert, *Collaboration Math* (Oakland, CA: Prevention Institute, 2003).

7. Turning Point, *Collaborative Leadership: Collaborative Leadership Learning Modules* (Seattle, WA: Turning Point, 2004).

8. A. Himmelman, *Collaboration for a Change* (Minneapolis, MN: Himmelman Consulting, 2002).

9. Center for Civic Partnerships, *Collaborative Functions: The 12 Cs of a Collaborative* (Sacramento, CA: Center for Civic Partnerships, 2002).

10. P. Thurman, *Community Readiness: A Promising Model for Community Healing* (Washington, DC: U.S. Department of Justice, Office of Justice Programs, 2000).

11. D. Ayre, G. Clough, and T. Norris, *Facilitating Community Change* (Boulder, CO: Community Initiatives, 2000).

12. D. Chrislip and C. Larsen, *Collaborative Leadership*.

13. Turning Point, *Academics and Practitioners on Collaborative Leadership* (Seattle, WA: Turning Point, 2002).

14. Himmelman, *Collaboration for a Change*.

15. Turning Point, *Academics and Practitioners on Collaborative Leadership*.

16. Himmelman, *Collaboration for a Change*.

17. Turning Point, *Academics and Practitioners on Collaborative Leadership*

18. L. Cohen et al., *Developing Effective Coalitions: An Eight Step Guide* (Pleasant Hill, CA: Contra Costa County Health Services Department Prevention Program, 1994).

19. Cohen et al., *Developing Effective Coalitions*.

20. M. T. Hatcher and J. K. McDonald, *The Constituency Development Practice in Public Health Agencies* (Atlanta, GA: Centers for Disease Control and Prevention, 1994).

21. Hatcher and McDonald, *The Constituency Development Practice in Public Health Agencies*.

22. Cohen et al., *Developing Effective Coalitions*.

23. G. P. Mays et al., "Collaboration to Improve Community Health: Trends and Alternative Models," *Joint Commission Journal of Qualitative Improvement* 25, no. 10 (1998): 518–565.

24. Mays et al., "Collaboration to Improve Community Health."

25. C. M. Alpaslan and I. I. Mitroff, *Swans, Swine, and Swindlers* (Stanford, CA: Stanford University Press, 2011).

26. E. H. Schein, *Organizational Culture and Leadership*, 3rd ed. (San Francisco, CA: Jossey-Bass, 2010).

27. Schein, *Organizational Culture and Leadership*.

28. R. E. Quinn, *Deep Change* (San Francisco, CA: Jossey-Bass, 1996).

29. P. Schwartz, *Inevitable Surprise* (New York, NY: Gotham Books, 2003).

30. Schwartz, *Inevitable Surprise*.

31. Schwartz, *Inevitable Surprise*.

32. C. Musselwhite and R. Jones, *Dangerous Opportunity: Making Change Work* (Philadelphia, PA: Xlibris, 2004).

33. J. Kouzes and B. Posner, *The Leadership Challenge*, 4th ed. (San Francisco, CA: Jossey-Bass, 2007).

34. Musselwhite and Jones, *Dangerous Opportunity*.

35. Musselwhite and Jones, *Dangerous Opportunity*.

36. Musselwhite and Jones, *Dangerous Opportunity*.

37. J. P. Kotter, *The New Rules* (New York, NY: The Free Press, 1995).

38. J. P. Kotter and D. S. Cohen, *The Heart of Change* (Boston, MA: Harvard Business School Press, 2002).

39. Kotter and Cohen, *The Heart of Change*.

40. J. P. Kotter, *Leading Change* (Boston, MA: Harvard Business School Press, 1996).

41. Kotter and Cohen, *The Heart of Change*.

42. D. R. Conner, *Managing at the Speed of Change* (New York: Villard Books, 1992).

43. Conner, *Managing at the Speed of Change*.

44. Conner, *Managing at the Speed of Change*.

45. Conner, *Managing at the Speed of Change*.

46. Conner, *Managing at the Speed of Change*.

47. D. R. Conner, *Leading at the Edge of Chaos* (New York, NY: John Wiley and Sons, 1998).

48. W. Bridges, *Transitions* (Cambridge, MA: Perseus Books, 1980).

49. Kotter, *Leading Change*.

50. R. Axelrod, *Terms of Engagement* (San Francisco, CA: Berrett-Koehler, 2010).

Leadership at the Organizational Level

Leadership at the agency or other organizational level requires that the leader not only use the new skills and tools required to head an agency but also the tools and skills developed at the personal and team levels. For the purpose of this chapter, it is important to view the organization from an adaptive perspective. Heifetz and his colleagues discuss five qualities of an adaptive organization.[1] The first quality concerns the issue of the length of time it takes for information to spread within an organization from inside the heads of individuals to the coffee room conversation, to discussions in meeting rooms, and to the cafeteria after the meetings. The second characteristic relates to whether senior management takes shared responsibility for addressing an agency challenge or crisis. It is important for employees to ask critical questions without reprisal. Senior management also needs to work on behalf of the whole organization and not just a particular program or silo within the organization. Third, there is an expectation that senior management will have the answers or promise that they will get them. If mistakes are made, they will be seen as learning experiences. The fourth quality addresses adaptive challenges whenever they occur. Finally,

leaders need to leave time for reflection and for continuous learning experiences for all employees. **Exercise 8-1** allows you the chance to find adaptive organizations.

KNOWLEDGE MANAGEMENT

Public health leaders are major data users. Data are the basis for most of our work. However, data become useful only in the way leaders use them. Public health leaders are knowledge synthesizers. Knowledge management relates to how information gets used in the context of an organization. Through the use of a Venn diagram, Awad and Ghaziri see the use of knowledge in the overlap of the workforce of the organization, organizational processes and procedures, and information technology and infrastructure.[2] They go on to observe that most definitions of knowledge management involve how data outside the organization are used inside, how knowledge is stored and how it affects organizational processes, where the data are stored, how knowledge growth is incorporated into the work and culture of the organization, how the knowledge is attained from the data shared with others, and how the value of the knowledge is evaluated.

Regarding the issue of value, knowledge products and services have a number of attributes. There are at least six values:[3]

1. You can learn much from this knowledge, which makes you smarter.
2. The more knowledge you gain, the more improvement occurs in your work activities.
3. Knowledge gives you direction in what you need to learn next.

EXERCISE 8-1 Qualities of an Adaptive Organization

Purpose: to determine whether a public health organization is adaptive or not

Key Concepts: qualities of an adaptive organization, local health department, primary care organization

Procedures: Divide the class into groups of six. Each group will plan a visit to a local health department or primary care center to talk to staff. Investigate how many of the four qualities of an adaptive organization you can find. Report back to the class on what you have found.

4. Knowledge can help you better communicate with your colleagues.
5. Accumulating information helps in the creation of a knowledge profile.
6. You learn to customize information for different purposes

These values/attributes can be useful for the next generation of workers.

Not all organizations make knowledge management a priority. If the decision is made to do so, the leader will find that there is a systems view of a knowledge management that follows a life cycle approach. Tiwana[4] presents one such 10-step approach:

1. Look at the present organizational infrastructure for knowledge management.
2. Examine how knowledge management is aligned with agency practice.
3. Design an infrastructure for knowledge management in the agency.
4. Determine all the present sources of information in your agency.
5. Design and appoint a knowledge management team.
6. Create a blueprint or protocol for a knowledge management program.
7. Prepare and determine the staffing for a knowledge management program.
8. Implement the program with an outcome-based methodology.

9. Build in mechanisms for change, integration with agency culture, and reward structure.
10. Determine how the program is to be evaluated and refined.

Knowledge management initiatives can be a core part of a learning organization philosophy for the agency. The leader becomes a facilitator who is a promoter and steward of the collective knowledge of the agency. **Exercise 8-2** give you a chance to explore knowledge work at a personal level.

STRATEGIC PLANNING

The relationship between strategies and tactics is similar to that between goals and objectives. Both goals and objectives are ends or desired states of affairs. One difference is that goals tend to be broad in scope and objectives relatively less so. Another is that objectives are ends that are sought largely because they lead to the achievement of goals. Improving the level of health in a community is a good example of a goal. Relative to this goal, testing the community's water supply might be one objective. Note that it is relatively narrower in scope and would be one step on the way to achieving the goal.

Strategies are plans or methods that are relatively broad in scope, are often long term in nature, and often involve a significant expenditure of resources. Tactics are methods that are relatively narrow in scope and use relatively few resources. Roughly speaking, strategies are likely to be used

EXERCISE 8-2 Knowledge Work

Purpose: to determine the characteristics of a knowledge worker

Key Concepts: knowledge work, knowledge management

Procedures: Divide the class into groups of seven or eight. Each group will prepare two lists. One list will be to determine the personality and professional characteristics of a knowledge worker. The second list will answer the question of what is a knowledge worker. After the group work, the class will reconvene to come up with two integrated lists for knowledge workers from the group work part of the exercise. It would be worthwhile as a homework assignment to determine if you would make a good knowledge worker.

in attaining goals, whereas tactics are likely to be used in attaining objectives. (Be warned that there is some looseness in the use of these terms and that many people employ "goal" and "objective" as synonyms and "strategy" and "tactic" as near synonyms.)

Strategic planning is directed at the achievement of goals—significant or even ultimate ends. As such, it is an extremely important task and falls largely on the shoulders of the agency leadership. A list of strategic planning guidelines and the Bryson 10-step strategic planning model follows.[5] As in the case of any major task, those responsible for completing the task should remain upbeat in order to motivate others involved to do their share. First, the guidelines:

1. Strategic planning is a team process in which the team members need to share the leader's vision. The team members also need to be carefully selected and represent all parts of the organization. The leader should be clear about the responsibilities of the team and may want to convene a community advisory board to discuss how the plan meets the health needs of the community.

2. The team needs to set a timeline for the planning process. The process should be short enough to devise a plan and implement it before events have rendered it irrelevant.

3. The team needs to consider how to get the plan accepted after the planning process.

4. The team needs to create a schedule for the planning process.

5. The team must disseminate the results of the process—the plan—following its completion. The team must carefully determine what will be disseminated, but it is generally better to disseminate more rather than less.

6. The team must decide on the techniques that will be used to evaluate the process.

Bryson developed a 10-step procedure for strategic planning. The first step could be called the "planning to plan" stage.[6] According to Bryson, the leader needs to be clear on the reasons that strategic planning was chosen rather than some other technique. A readiness assessment occurs. The leader also needs to communicate with potential stakeholders and to lay the groundwork for a shared vision. The partners will want to know what they are "buying" and how long the planning and implementation process will take. Bryson suggested that partners might do well to start the process by going on a retreat. Strategic planning can be an expensive process, and funds will be needed to carry it out.

Step 2 involves the clarification of organizational mandates. Public health practitioners are constantly bombarded with formal mandates that take substantial time to abide by. Not only that, public health agencies are legally mandated to perform certain functions and are given funds to carry out these functions but might not be funded to implement other public health initiatives closer to the mission of public health as defined by the local health department and the community stakeholders. Stakeholders are persons or organizations that have an interest in public health programs and how they are implemented. They include concerned citizens, government representatives, other health and social service representatives, governing board members, church representatives, and members of professional associations.

It is critical to include the appropriate stakeholders in strategic planning. For example, major community employers, unions, regulatory or licensing agencies, bankers, and neighbors of the agency are often excluded from community coalitions despite the fact that they can prevent decisions from being implemented.[7] In general, stakeholders expect the agency and its leadership to be responsive to their needs and can even issue what might be called informal mandates. If the agency does not respond to these informal mandates, the stakeholders will look elsewhere for support. The local public health agency must determine whether the formal mandates prevent addressing the informal mandates. Several local public health administrators interviewed by the author said that responding to the formal mandates in their state took almost 90 percent of their agency's time. Creating innovative programs became virtually impossible because of the lack of time.

In step 3, agency leaders begin to investigate the values that will govern the agency and the agency's community relationships. The agency's mission should refer to its role in the community. By going through the values clarification process and developing a mission as shown in the leadership wheel, the agency will be in a better position to monitor the strategic planning process. This step might include the performance of a stakeholder analysis, which will clarify who the stakeholders are, what their values are, what their goals and objectives are, what issues are likely to affect them, and what their degree of commitment is to the status quo.

The fourth step involves the assessment of the internal and external environments in order to identify the opportunities and the challenges arising from the change process.[8] This has been referred to as a SWOT analysis, for it focuses on strengths, weaknesses, opportunities, and threats. The external assessment looks at forces that may affect agency programs, whether at the local, state, federal, or global level. For example, diseases or disease-causing agents that originate in one portion of the globe may eventually spread to all other parts, as did the human immunodeficiency virus (HIV).[9] The analysis should include key stakeholders who have an agenda that they wish to see implemented and major competitors, such as local managed care organizations (which may want to take over public health roles and responsibilities). Assessing external forces should be an ongoing activity and not be limited to one step in the strategic planning process[10]

The internal assessment looks at the agency's resources, the process of carrying out the agency activities, and the performance outputs. Part 1 of the Assessment Protocol for Excellence in Public Health (APEX-PH) is an assessment of an organization's internal capacity. This organizational component is not visibly present in the Mobilizing for Action through Planning and Partnerships (MAPP) assessment process, which is a system-based assessment. However, there is nothing that prevents a public health agency from doing an internal capacity assessment.

The collection of information, the clarification of values, the development of a mission, and the assessment of the agency and its environment provide the foundation for the rest of the strategic planning process. Step 5 is the identification of the issues to be addressed by the plan. In this stage, the stakeholders typically come together to define the issues, using a group process approach. The stakeholders need not only to identify the critical issues but also explain why these issues are critical and to describe what the consequences of not addressing these issues will be.

Another approach to completing this step is to define goals and objectives and then develop issues based on the goals and objectives. Still another approach is for the partners in the strategic planning process to devise ideal scenarios (descriptions of the way they would like the world to be) and present them to each other and try to come to a consensus. One problem with scenario building is that it is a complex process and requires the participants to be trained in how to create scenarios.[11] Without proper training, the participants may not be able to get results that are valid. In a fourth approach, the strategic planning team tries to facilitate the formulation of issues by slowly guiding the stakeholders through the process.

Step 6 involves the development of strategies to address the issues delineated in step 5. In short, it is during this step that the strategic plan is actually devised. Possible strategies include the setting of new policies or new rules and regulations, the development of new programs and services, and

changes in the allocation of resources. The stakeholders should determine how the chosen strategies interrelate and thus how the whole system works. Some strategies might involve both the agency and the community, some might involve just the agency or just agency subdivisions, and some might involve agency programs and services.

In step 7, the stakeholders review, modify, and adopt the strategic plan developed in step 6. Here, as in steps 5 and 6, they must consider the actions that will be necessary to carry out the plan. The plan in a sense consists of actions that are intended to achieve the goals and objectives identified by the stakeholders early in the planning process.

Step 8 is the creation or revision of the organizational vision. Strategic planning may lead to changes that affect the vision, and thus visioning is tied to each step of the strategic planning process. In fact, the vision need not be fully determined early on but can be left to evolve during several cycles of this process.[12] The vision should grow out of an integration of past accomplishments and perceptions of the future. The vision also needs to provide inspiration to other stakeholders. However, the agency's mission tends to drive the strategic planning process more than the vision does.[13]

Step 9 is the implementation of the plan. In prior steps, while developing the plan, the stakeholders need to define their roles in the implementation process. They also should try to ensure that accomplishments, even if small ones, will occur early in the process. Success tends to foster success, because the stakeholders will remain motivated and undiscouraged if they see progress. The stakeholders must allocate the necessary resources before the implementation process begins. As changes are made, the agency and the other stakeholders need to adjust accordingly and monitor the effects of the changes over time.

Step 10 involves monitoring the implementation and making necessary midcourse corrections.

Each of the 10 steps of the Bryson model is related to one of the three core public health functions (assessment, policy development, and assurance). The model is in fact compatible with the systems approach to public health leadership (leadership wheel), and all of the activities in this approach, which is based on the core functions of public health, are included in the Bryson model. The relationships between the model and the essential services of public health are more cloudy. For example, visioning is not included in typical lists of such practices and services. Montgomery has noted that the strategic process should move beyond being a distinctive set of strategies toward being a dynamic evolving proces.[14] The dynamic approach to strategic planning should create an interactive model that ties changes in the community to changes and adaptations within the agency.

As regards strategic planning, public health leaders must:

- learn the benefits of such planning
- determine the readiness of the agency to undertake the strategic planning process
- perform a stakeholder analysis
- expand the strategic planning process to include stakeholders in the community
- remain optimistic during the strategic planning process as a means of motivating other participants
- do the necessary homework to prepare for each successive step of the strategic planning process
- be realistic about what is possible
- perform an assessment of organizational capacity

Exercise 8-3 is intended to give you a chance to use or develop your strategic planning skills. The task is to use strategic thinking in the planning of a community nutrition education program designed to inform the public of the advantages of empowerment and community coalitions.

CONTINUOUS QUALITY IMPROVEMENT

Whereas strategic planning is a process that can be analyzed into a number of specific steps, continuous quality improvement (CQI) involves accepting a whole new philosophy of doing business or providing services. Public health organizations have been slow to adopt CQI methods, and where they have done so, they have not had great success.[15] Part of the explanation for the lack of success is that public health leaders have not kept up with the developments in the field of CQI. In studying public health clinics in California, Scutchfield and his colleagues found that fewer than 20 percent of the agencies performed CQI activities.[16] They also found that public health leaders were often unclear when it was appropriate to use specific tools.

Public health agencies have a reputation for providing mediocre service. One problem obstructing the improvement of service is that federal and state funding for new public health programs has been shrinking. Another is that government rules and regulations, as well as union rules, put obstacles in the way of delivering services in a timely fashion. A third problem is that public health leaders often misinterpret quality assurance as a type of CQI. Improving quality is more than an assurance issue, and it depends on viewing the public health consumer as entitled to the best that public health professionals have to offer. It requires, in other words, a whole change in philosophy.

The focus of CQI activities in a public health agency is on improving service provision and enhancing relationships with external stakeholders.[17] These activities are based on information about the public health issues to be addressed, the strengths and weaknesses of the public health agency, and stakeholder concerns.

To improve service provision, public health leaders need to use a systems perspective, promote a client orientation,[18] and engage in strategic thinking. Some public health leaders have found that they can integrate strategic planning approaches and CQI, especially if one of the strategic goals of the agency is to improve the quality of service. Quality is a personal issue as well as an agency or systems issue.[19] Each public health staff person has to be personally committed to high quality. A commitment to quality will improve performance. Having talent, knowledge, and skills to do public health's work will go nowhere without a personal commitment to do the best work possible with strong positive relationships with the public and with external stakeholders. There has been an increasing concern with the accreditation of health agencies in order to stress quality and improve the overall functioning of these agencies. Our next hero is Dr. Kaye Bender who has helped to create a system for the accreditation of public health agencies. This story is in the format of an interview.

CQI is closely related to another management methodology called "total quality management" (TQM), and in fact the terms "continuous quality improvement" and "total quality management" are often used interchangeably.[20] They are treated as synonymous here, and the term that appears in each instance in the following section is the term used by the particular author (or authors) under discussion.

EXERCISE 8-3 Community Nutrition Program

Purpose: to use the Bryson strategic planning model to develop a protocol for a community nutrition program

Key Concepts: strategic planning, leadership

Procedures: As a homework assignment, each student is given the task of developing a community nutrition program devising a 10-step strategic plan for a community nutrition program. You will present your plan in 2 weeks to your class.

PUBLIC HEALTH HEROES AND VILLAINS 8-1 Dr. Kaye Bender, Hero

Kaye Bender, PhD, RN, FAAN, is president and chief executive officer of the Public Health Accreditation Board (PHAB), the organization charged with administering the first national accreditation program for public health. Dr. Bender has more than 30 years' experience in public health practice at the local and state levels in Mississippi. She also served as dean of the School of Nursing and associate vice chancellor for nursing at the University of Mississippi Medical Center. She served on two Institute of Medicine study committees, *The Future of the Public's Health in the 21st Century* and *Who Will Keep the Public Healthy?* She is a graduate of the Public Health Leadership Institute in California. She chaired the Exploring Accreditation Steering Committee, the exploratory precursor study that led to the development of the Public Health Accreditation Board.

What is public health department accreditation, and why is it an important goal for public health department leaders to consider?

Public health department accreditation is the measurement of a health department's performance against a nationally recognized set of practice-focused, evidence-based standards. The national public health accreditation program administered by the Public Health Accreditation Board has been developed on principles of quality improvement. Accreditation is a means by which health departments can demonstrate their interest in being transparent and accountable in their operations. In today's political environment, health department leaders have to consider their image to the public. There is an increased emphasis on "good government." Accreditation is one way to demonstrate that a health department is willing to open its performance for national-level peer review.

Why has the national accreditation program for public health departments been launched now?

Two Institute of Medicine studies on public health, one in 1988 and another in 2003, both described the governmental public health system as the backbone for coordinating and ensuring a focus on population health for a given community. However, those same studies described that governmental infrastructure as being in disarray, as not being consistent in its approaches across the country, and as not being consistently funded to carry out its mission. The national public health accreditation program was developed to assist health departments with focus and with a nationally accepted framework and process for carrying out its mission. Accreditation focuses on what a health department should do, either alone or in partnership with others. The health department then decides, based on the needs of the community it serves, how it will carry out those activities.

Why do you believe that achieving national public health department accreditation is beneficial for a health department?

Public health leaders have to balance the provision of core public health functions with the essential services needed to promote a healthy jurisdiction that they serve. Health departments who are using the accreditation standards and measures have told us that it has been very helpful to have national consensus about what a health department's specific and unique role in the community is. Even though we have had the 10 essential public health services framework and the three core functions of public health for a while, health departments tell us that having accreditation standards puts it all together for them in such a way that they have a good road map to guide their work. I believe that public health is a specialty, so why would we not have a standardized framework within which to operate, and why wouldn't public health leaders want to have their health departments reviewed for accreditation? It's a good opportunity to assure the community they serve that they are doing the best job they can to protect and promote that community's health.

What are the challenges that public health leaders face in considering whether to apply for accreditation?

The first challenge is usually to convince their governing entity that it's a good idea. This is new for public health but not so for other governmental entities like schools, universities, fire departments, child care centers, police departments, and the like. So one might think that elected officials and policy makers would naturally embrace the idea of accreditation. However, these are tough economic times, and adding any new activity can be met with resistance. Public health leaders who have engaged their governing entities early in the process and who have focused on quality improvement as the rationale for embarking upon the accreditation process have been successful in obtaining governance support for their accreditation application. The second challenge is often just getting started. A commitment to performance and quality improvement involves a different way of doing business for the long term. It involves a level of intrusion and transparency that embraces a willingness to take the health department operations apart and look at every aspect. That's a threat to many leaders. What if their health department fails? What if something major is found during the review? That level of transparency involves being willing to take those risks. Public health leaders who do so, however, are moving public health into a realm of credibility that mirrors that of the healthcare system and other businesses. There is an increased level of respect for a leader who can pull that off. Finally, another challenge lies in the engagement of the health department staff. Working on accreditation in public health requires that staff at all levels understand their health department in a more detailed way than perhaps they have before. It involves knowing how their work fits into the core functions and essential services. It also involves seeing quality improvement and the "new norm" way of doing business and not as a separate public health program. That can be a real challenge for some health department leaders.

What do you see as future incentives for a health department to be accredited?

As health departments become accredited and share their experiences, I believe that the opportunity for national-level peer review will emerge as the greatest incentive. There is no other organized structure for that type of review to occur. The marketing opportunity for health departments to promote their services once they have been accredited is also an incentive. Think about how many times we have read in the headlines that a school or fire department achieved national accreditation—met national standards, as determined by an independent reviewer. That has never been the case for the health department until now. PHAB is also working with various public health program funders at the national and state levels to consider providing funding opportunities for accredited health departments. For example, if an accredited health department is applying for a competitive grant, that health department would get additional credit in that competitive process because they are accredited. The rationale for this policy is that accredited health departments have been assessed for their infrastructure soundness. Public health programs can be assured that an accredited health department can implement that public health program within a strong governmental public health system. Finally, and certainly more long term in nature, PHAB hopes that funders will eventually become comfortable enough with accreditation that they will accept the certificate of accreditation in lieu of the first section of reporting for most grants, and therefore accredited health departments would have a reduced reporting burden for most program grants.

Why does PHAB support a voluntary approach to accreditation rather than a mandate?

You really can't mandate a culture of quality improvement. When PHAB was being formed and our accreditation process was being developed, we did a lot of research into the history of other accrediting programs. Mandated programs often become routine and more regulatory in philosophy. Quality improvement, by its very nature, is about embracing a culture of routinely assessing what an agency is doing, with an eye toward doing it better. Accreditation is one important step on the journey of adopting quality improvement as a health department operating principle. Mandating that seems counterintuitive to its rationale.

Why is accreditation linked to transforming public health for the future?

In many communities, the health department is almost invisible to the public. That "out of sight, out of mind" image has, for some, created opportunities for funding cuts that create great difficulties for the health department. Accreditation as a process has been shown to help other industries define who they are and then to involve their community of interest in assessing their work. It has also been shown to help entities set priorities and focus on the most significant parts of their industry. PHAB has already heard of health departments that are preparing for accreditation that have used this window of opportunity to do the same for public health. And then, once a health department is accredited, who is going to actively participate in reducing resources that might jeopardize that accreditation?

What is your hope for public health leadership and accreditation?

Public health accreditation has been developed by more than 400 practitioners, academicians, and researchers from the specialty. The accreditation process and the standards and measures are designed to reflect the existing evidence base as well as to stretch our practice. When I was working in public health practice, it was always my hope to leave the health department better than I found it. There are many ways to do that, and some public health leaders have to spend a lot of their precious time identifying what those ways are. Accreditation is already developed and will improve considerably over time as we gain experience. Public health leaders today can partner with us to assess their health department against national standards; celebrate their accomplishment of being recognized as meeting those standards; and identify ways to move their performance to a higher level. In the world of public health leadership, it doesn't get any better than that!

Reprinted with permission of Kaye Bender and PHAB.

TQM is based on the philosophy of total quality control, first promoted by Feigenbaum.[21] According to Sashkin and Kiser, TQM uses an evolving methodologic toolkit that includes all sorts of ways of measuring quality. The two main principles are that the focus of the organization must be on the customer and that everybody in the organization, not just the leadership, must be committed to quality. In their words, "TQM means that the organization's culture is defined by and supports the constant attainment of customer satisfaction through an integrated system of tools, techniques, and training. This involves the continuous improvement of organizational processes, resulting in high quality products and services."[22(p.39)]

CQI Models

Five names are traditionally tied to the CQI movement: Shewhart, Deming, Crosby, Juran, and Feigenbaum. Shewhart demonstrated that statistical control is critical in CQI activities.[23] Deming, the best known of the CQI theorists, had to go to Japan in the 1950s to test his ideas about quality. To publicize his ideas, he devised a 14-point set of principles.[24] The focus of these principles is on training the workforce and fostering a total commitment to quality. As Deming was aware, each customer wants high-quality products and services and evaluates the quality of products and services received. Deming also developed the planning, doing, checking, acting cycle.[25]

Crosby argued that the only way to improve quality is to demand zero defects and refuse to accept anything less.[26] After all, customers define quality, and in the business world, dissatisfied consumers will stop buying defective products. The public health customer, however, has limited service choices and will grudgingly accept less than the best, so it is up to public health leaders to empower their communities and make sure that high-quality standards are maintained. Public health leaders also need to gain support for the CQI approach from both internal and external stakeholders and must be prepared to cope with resistance. Deciding to apply for accreditation may help in this process.

CQI requires total commitment and involvement.[27] Crosby outlined a 14-step process for implementing TQM in organizations.[28,29] The process starts with a commitment by the leadership to the pursuit of quality and all that this entails. Most of the steps involve the core functions of policy development and assurance. There is only one step in which assessment plays the major role.

The Crosby model applies to intraorganizational change, whereas the kind of assessment public health agencies must perform encompasses both internal operations and community needs. The focus on intraorganizational change is a characteristic of the Deming model as well. Note, however, that in the case of a public health agency, an assessment of community needs provides critical data for determining what intraorganizational changes are required and for integrating complex systems of health care in order to provide high-quality programming.

The fourth theoretician in the quality revolution is Joseph M. Juran. Juran pointed out that quality does not occur by chance.[30] It requires a planned process that encompasses planning, quality control, and quality improvement (known as the Juran trilogy). Juran also believed that leaders need to organize information for the purpose of monitoring the process. Finally, Feigenbaum held that quality is involved in every activity of an organization, from direct service activities to marketing and finance, and that an organization must determine the cost of quality improvement programs before embarking on them.[31]

Building on the work of the founders of the TQM approach, Creech identified what he called the five pillars of TQM: product (service), process, organization, leadership, and commitment.[32] According to Creech, TQM has been more effective in Japan than in the United States because Japanese businesses seem to accept the concept of quality more readily than American businesses do. Creech has further pointed out that TQM is an organizational philosophy and cannot deliver full benefits without complete organizational acceptance.

Organization is the central pillar of the five. How the organization is perceived and what its cultural orientation is will have an effect on the implementation and consequences of TQM. Also, whereas centralization has been the traditional management approach, decentralization appears to be better suited to TQM. Consequently, multidisciplinary teams play an important role. Another pillar is leadership. As indicated by the comment about decentralization, the leaders of the organization must be willing to share their power.

Organizational commitment to quality needs to occur at the border between the organization and its environment (ecological perspective). If the frontline workers do not buy the quality message, TQM will be doomed to failure. In fact, everyone in the organization needs to make a commitment to quality.

The CQI Toolkit

CQI makes use of a number of tools, including various kinds of charts and diagrams. Traditional tools include:

- control charts (for showing the results of statistical process activities)

- Pareto charts (for graphically showing defects or problems over time)
- fishbone diagrams (for tracing cause-and-effect relationships)
- run charts (for displaying trends over time)
- histograms (for showing service patterns at given time periods)
- scatter diagrams (for showing relationships between two factors)
- flowcharts (for showing input–output relationships)[33]

Seven new tools of use in CQI are shown in **Figure 8-1** and described next.[34] The first is the affinity diagram, which allows a team to organize ideas and problems into general categories. The team would first sort the items into categories then list the items in each category in a separate column. Affinity diagrams could be used for clarifying values; for constructing the organization's vision, mission, and goals and objectives; and for action and strategic planning. The affinity diagram process, like any group process, is affected by how well the team members get along.

The interrelationship digraph shows the interconnection between ideas, problems, actions, or other types of items. The arrows between the items show the direction of their relationship (e.g., cause to effect). Once a digraph is developed, it can be reworked to show new ways to relate the items. The team will want to simplify the digraph by looking for converging or diverging clusters of arrows. Constructing a digraph is especially useful for deciding on goals and objectives and during the action planning phase.

The third tool, the tree diagram, can be used in many leadership activities. For instance, a tree diagram could be used by the leadership team of a public health agency to map out how the agency's mission is to be fulfilled. The team might start by stating the mission, which, say, is to promote the health of the public and prevent disease. The next step would be to determine the goals and objectives needed to fulfill this mission, and the third step would be to decide on the tasks that must be performed to achieve the chosen goals and objectives. In CQI, the leadership team might use tree diagrams in developing quality improvement plans. In general, the process of creating a tree diagram begins with stating an overall goal (e.g., the agency's mission or an important subsidiary goal) and then breaking the process of achieving the goal into individual steps or tasks.

FIGURE 8-1 Seven Management and Planning Tools

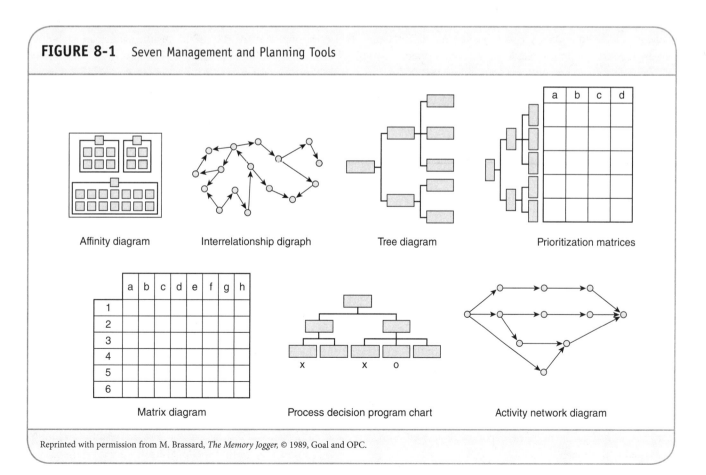

Affinity diagram   Interrelationship digraph   Tree diagram   Prioritization matrices

Matrix diagram   Process decision program chart   Activity network diagram

Prioritization matrices allow the leadership team to prioritize tasks, service activities, community activities, and so on. A prioritization matrix can be used in conjunction with a tree diagram to rank the tasks and responsibilities identified during the tree diagram process. If six activities are projected, the diagram allows the team to see what will happen if any two activities occur together. The team is able to calculate a score for each cell, and where the score falls in relation to the other scores determines the degree of importance of the conjunction of activities.

Brassard suggested that the prioritization process should encompass three steps.[35] The first step is to list and then rank the criteria that will be used in prioritizing the items (e.g., activities). Such criteria might include the speed of possible implementation, the likely degree of acceptance by staff, the effect on other parts of the agency, the cost, and the technology needed. Once the criteria are chosen, each should be assigned a percentage that reflects its perceived importance (the total percentage should, of course, equal 100). In step 2, each item is given a score in relation to each criterion. Finally, the total scores for all the items are calculated, and the results determine the priority ranking of the items.

The fifth tool is the matrix diagram, which allows the leadership team to compare two or more sets of items and explore the strength of the relationship between them.

Process decision program charts allow the leadership team to show probable events and contingencies that might occur as the action plan is implemented. For example, suppose the public health agency director wants to plan how the community will perform health assessment activities. The director might create a chart that shows how the community advisory board is to be selected, when the various activities will occur and how much time they will take, and how they will be carried out. Process decision program charts, like the other tools described here, can also be used to explore options.

The last tool, the activity network diagram, exhibits the schedule for the completion of tasks. This tool is also known as an arrow diagram. **Exercise 8-4** provides an opportunity to practice applying the seven CQI tools just described.

There has been increasing awareness of the importance of using quality improvement tools and methodology for public health agencies. These techniques have been recognized for their value in performance measurement and also as critical to accreditation of public health agencies. However, most of the tools of quality improvement, including the fishbone diagram, are limited in their application to community-wide quality improvement activities.

EXERCISE 8-4   Seven CQI Tools

Purpose: to explore the seven CQI tools

Key Concepts: continuous quality improvement, affinity diagram, interrelationship digraph, tree diagram, prioritization matrices, matrix diagram, process decision program chart, activity network diagram

Scenario: Chicago has reported an increased lead level in the water going into the buildings and residences of the city due to aging water pipes. Home owners and building owners have a year to address the problem. In concert with the city, the health department develops a plan of action for monitoring the problem and its results.

Procedures: Divide the class into groups of six or seven. Which of the tools will help the groups monitor the project and see progress as it occurs?

CQI requires a total commitment by public health leaders and all their constituencies if it is to be successful. The professional staff of the public health agency must buy in to the total quality approach. To get staff to do this, public health leaders must:

- develop a commitment to quality and best practices
- incorporate CQI into a systems framework
- become educated about CQI
- master the seven CQI tools
- educate the public about CQI
- inspire staff and others to see the value of the CQI approach
- train the public health workforce
- integrate strategic planning techniques and CQI techniques

PUBLIC–PRIVATE PARTNERSHIPS

A public health agency, although it must lead the way, cannot carry out all the public health activities needed to protect and improve the health of a community. Consequently, it must foster new types of alliances and partnerships, including joint ventures, research sharing, community-based projects and programs, and semistructured alliances.[36] For example, a local public health agency might contract with a local federally qualified health center to provide childhood immunizations at a price that the local health department cannot match—an interesting example of what the business community calls outsourcing.

Because trust is a critical component of any partnership, the public health agency must know both its agenda and the agendas of its partners, whether from the public or private sector. Possible partners include businesses, hospitals and managed care organizations, community health centers, private healthcare providers, local community organizations, local community clubs, churches and synagogues, schools, and police and firefighter groups, among others.

A local health leader told the author that a good way to involve the private sector in public health is for public health leaders to become involved in local organizations, such as the Kiwanis or the local chamber of commerce, which will create opportunities for them to network with other leaders on community issues. Public health leaders need to become known in the community if they are to gain credibility. Their goal should be to create an integrated system of care that will provide every resident of the community with the care they need and at the same time promote a healthy lifestyle among the residents in order to prevent disease.

Public health leaders must:

- develop public and private relationships to improve the local community
- health system

- share power and responsibility with other community members who have an interest in improving the community's health
- become involved in the activities of the community
- join local community groups and organizations
- act to gain the trust of the community

SUMMARY

Leadership at the organization involves the use of knowledge and skills developed at the personal and team levels of leadership. This chapter looks first at how leaders adapt to challenges. In order to adapt to these challenges, leaders need to develop knowledge based on factual data. Knowledge management helps leaders to use appropriate tools for these activities. In addition, strategic planning tools and CQI tools are useful, individually or jointly, for turning a vision or adaptive challenge into programs and services,

Public and private alliances and partnerships are needed at the planning stage as well as the program implementation stage. Developing and maintaining collaborative relationships require leadership skills, and public health leaders must master these skills and the planning skills necessary to formulate strategies for improving the community's health.

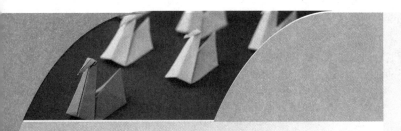

Discussion Questions

1. Why is adaptive leadership important in public health agencies?

2. How are data converted into knowledge?

3. Compare and contrast the leadership wheel with Bryson's strategic planning model.

4. What is the relationship between strategies and tactics?

5. How can we use the CQI tools in strategic planning?

6. What are some of the ways to open doors to public–private coalitions, alliances, and partnerships?

REFERENCES

1. R. Heifetz, A. Grashow, and M. Linsky, *The Practice of Adaptive Leadership* (Boston, MA: Harvard Business Press, 2009).

2. E. M. Awad and H. M. Ghaziri, *Knowledge Management* (Upper Saddle River, NJ: Pearson, 2004).

3. J. Botkin, *Smart Business: How Knowledge Communities Can Revolutionize Your Company* (New York, NY: Free Press, 1999).

4. A. Tiwana, *The Knowledge Management Toolkit* (Upper Saddle River, NJ: Prentice-Hall, 2000).

5. J. M. Bryson, *Strategic Planning for Public and Nonprofit Organizations*, 3rd ed. (San Francisco, CA: Jossey-Bass, 2004).

6. L. Goodstein et al., *Applied Strategic Planning: A Comprehensive Guide* (New York, NY: McGraw-Hill, 1993).

7. P. R. Scholtes, *The Leader's Handbook* (New York, NY: McGraw-Hill, 1998).

8. Bryson, *Strategic Planning for Public and Nonprofit Organizations*.

9. Bryson, *Strategic Planning for Public and Nonprofit Organizations*.

10. Goodstein et al., *Applied Strategic Planning*.

11. H. Mintzberg, *The Rise and Fall of Strategic Planning* (Englewood Cliffs, NJ: Pearson, 2000).

12. Bryson, *Strategic Planning for Public and Nonprofit Organizations*.

13. Goodstein et al., *Applied Strategic Planning*.

14. C. A. Montgomery, "Putting Leadership Back into Strategy," *Harvard Business Review* 86, no. 1 (2008): 54–60.

15. E. A. Scutchfield et al., "The Presence of Total Quality Management and Continuous Quality Improvement Processes in California Public Health Clinics," *Journal of Public Health Management and Practice* 3, no. 3 (1997): 57–60.

16. Scutchfield et al., "The Presence of Total Quality Management and Continuous Quality Improvement Processes in California Public Health Clinics."

17. G. P. Mays et al., "CQI in Public Health Organizations," in C. P. McLaughlin and A. D. Kaluzny (eds.), *Continuous Quality Improvement in Health Care*, 2nd ed. (Gaithersburg, MD: Aspen Publishers, 1999).

18. C. P. McLaughlin and A. D. Kaluzny, "Defining Quality Improvement: Past, Present, and Future," in C. P. McLaughlin and A. D. Kaluzny (eds.), *Continuous Quality Improvement in Health Care*, 2nd ed. (Gaithersburg, MD: Aspen Publishers, 1999).

19. H. V. Roberts and B. F. Sergesketter, *Quality Is Personal* (New York, NY: Free Press, 1993).

20. McLaughlin and Kaluzny, "Defining Quality Improvement."

21. A. V. Feigenbaum, *Total Quality Control* (New York, NY: McGraw-Hill, 1961).

22. M. Sashkin and K. J. Kiser, *Putting Total Quality Management to Work* (San Francisco, CA: Berrett-Koehler, 1993).

23. W. A. Shewhart, *Statistical Method from the Viewpoint of Quality Control* (Mineola, NY: Dover, 1986).

24. W. E. Deming, *Out of the Crisis* (Cambridge, MA: Massachusetts Institute of Technology, 1986).

25. M. Walton, *Deming Management at Work* (New York, NY: Pedigree Books, 1991).

26. P. B. Crosby, *Quality without Tears* (New York, NY: Penguin Plume, 1984).

27. P. B. Crosby, *Completeness* (New York, NY: Penguin Dutton, 1992).

28. P. B. Crosby, *Quality Is Free* (New York, NY: McGraw-Hill, 1989).

29. P. B. Crosby, *Let's Talk Quality* (New York, NY: Penguin Plume, 1990).

30. J. M. Juran, *Juran on Leadership for Quality: An Executive Handbook* (New York, NY: Free Press, 2003).

31. Feigenbaum, *Total Quality Control*.

32. B. Creech, *The Five Pillars of TQM* (New York, NY: Truman Talley Books and Dutton, 1994).

33. Sashkin and Kiser, *Putting Total Quality Management to Work*.

34. M. Brassard, D. Ritter, F. Oddo, and J. MacCausland, *The Memory Jogger II* (Methuen, MA: Goal and QPC, 2010).

35. M. Brassard, *The Memory Jogger Plus* (Methuen, MA: Goal and QPC, 1996).

36. P. Drucker, *Managing in a Time of Great Change* (Boston, MA: Harvard Business School Press, 2006).

CHAPTER **9**

Boards of Health and County Commissioners

Public health has a strong political aspect. In fact, all local, state, and national programs and services involve public oversight. Public oversight involves appointed or elected representatives of the public. That is where our challenges begin. These representatives often have personal agendas that are not necessarily compatible with the views and positions of all the people. Boards of health members and county commissioners are often seen as adversaries by the professionals who operate our local health departments. The state health department has the governor and elected representatives who provide oversight and controversial positions. The directors and some of the deputy directors are often political appointees. What obviously needs to change is the adversarial position to one that is more collaborative The outside directors and commissioners can become the agents for supporting the health agendas of the health departments. An interesting example is one of the first public health heroes. In 1799, Paul Revere of the famous midnight ride was named the chairman of one of the first boards of health, in Boston.[1] The board's task was to address the "filth and offal" that was believed to be the cause of illness in the city.

THE POLITICS OF PUBLIC HEALTH POLICY

Policy development is a complex process in which the participants consider alternatives for action and decide which alternatives to implement. It is a team process, and many individuals and organizations can be involved, including state and local boards of health, elected officials, community groups, public health professionals, healthcare providers, and private citizens. Factors that the participants typically should take into account in their decision making include budgetary considerations; federal, state, and local regulations; and program and organizational operating procedures.

The infrastructure of public health is currently at risk because of the general attack on social and public health programs in Congress and in state legislatures throughout the United States. The discontent with social programs in the United States can be traced back to the 1960s, when many of them were created. Since then, the American public seems to have grown increasingly disenchanted with such programs, largely because of the supposed negative effects of the welfare state as well as doubts about the effectiveness of current programs.[2] There is evidence that the public will no longer tolerate increases in taxation to support health and social programs, including public health programs, and indeed from the mid-1990s and into the 21st century, public health programs appear to have come under special assault.

Part of the discontent with federally operated social programs is based on skepticism regarding the competency of the federal government. "Decentralization" was a watchword of the 1990s, and state and local governments took over many programs that had been run by the federal government.

However, part of the discontent is probably based on the idea that social programs act as replacements for traditional groups devoted to problem solving and helping people live better lives.[3] Furthermore, so goes the thinking, social programs, by weakening the authority of traditional groups and encouraging people to become dependent on the government for help, create a demand for more social programs, which foster a higher level of dependency, and on and on in a vicious circle.

It is easy to see the appeal of the view that communities should redefine themselves, reestablish traditional values, and become less dependent on government. Yet it is also easy to see that public health programs are significantly different from other programs. Whereas individuals arguably should assume more responsibility for protecting their own health, surely some type of public health system is necessary to assess the effects of terrorism and disasters on health, control health hazards, educate the public about these hazards, and provide population-based services designed to help individuals shed harmful behaviors. Public health leaders must become advocates for their own agencies and for a population-based approach to health promotion and disease prevention. They also need to distinguish public health programs from other types of social programs and make a strong case that public health programs should be supported no matter what other programs the public chooses to dispense with.

According to one definition, politics is the process of putting the moral consensus of the community into practice.[4] In democratic politics at its best, interested parties discuss the issues face to face, reach a consensus, and develop and implement policies. Yet in this country conflict always enters the picture, because the ideology of self-interest (the American ethic of individualism and search for personal success) is at odds with the strong concern Americans have for promoting and protecting the community. The ideology of self-interest leads to the development of special-interest coalitions, and one of the challenges faced by public health leaders is to find ways to promote the community and satisfy special-interest groups at the same time.

Among the strategies that can be used to meet this challenge are the following:[5]

- Community leaders and organizations and special-interest groups should be involved in policy development.
- The policies developed and implemented should include some that tie together medical care and public health activities. Health promotion is a shared responsibility that calls for interagency collaboration in the pursuit of population-based goals.

- The policies should also include some that will help build a community-oriented continuum of care. Primary prevention programs clearly need to be community based. Examples include programs to reduce the prevalence of lead paint, provide acquired immune deficiency syndrome (AIDS) education, and get people to stop smoking.

Some guidelines related to the politics of public health policy development include:

- Consider national health and social policy trends when developing local policies.
- Make a case for the importance of having a governmental public health presence in the community. Moore has called this the process of creating public value.[6]
- Use special public health interest groups in public health policy development.
- Develop integrated and interdependent health and social policies for the community.
- Partner with elected officials to promote public health programs.

GOVERNANCE

Governance is a process that is married to the core functions of public health. Governance and leadership are also closely related. In public health we expect our agency leaders to work closely with oversight boards that make the rules and regulations that guide action at the agency level. We hope this relationship is collaborative in nature. This is not always the case. Thus, politics are about the creation of the rules whereas governance is an administrative and process-oriented approach to making the system of laws, rules, and regulations work. The next story (with the county name changed) is a story of villainy related to public health.

A number of principles affect governance at the policy level.[7] Members of boards should not be seen as volunteers but rather as trustees who represent community constituencies. A difficulty in public health is that board members are often appointed by county commissioners who appoint friends or individuals for political reasons. Second, decisions should be made in a positive way by the board and not in an adversarial way by a specific board member who disagrees with the decision that was made. Third, board decisions are policy decisions and not public health practice decisions made by the health department director and his or her staff. Fourth, policy decisions are value driven and should be stated in the broadest way possible. Broader decisions should be

PUBLIC HEALTH HEROES AND VILLAINS 9-1 A Story of Villainy in Nicholas County

This story begins in 1997 where a high school teacher (Villain no. 1) sends a girl of 15, with whom he was having sex, into a local public health clinic for contraceptives. The girl was injected with a birth control medication. The teacher remained in the car. The clinic staff (Villains no. 2) never reported the girl's request as required by county law. A U.S. House committee was informed of this occurrence and asked a Nicholas County commissioner to come to Washington to testify about this incident because a federal grant was to be given to the county. The commissioner later stated that he was happy that the county would have the courage to decline the grant. At about this time, the Nicholas County Health Department director was informed that they were eligible to receive a grant from the federal government that requires the county government to provide family planning and birth control to minors regardless of whether they tell their parents. The county commissioners informed the county health board that the county board refused to accept the grant (Villain no. 3). The Nicholas County health department director (Hero) contested the decision because it put a critical public health program in jeopardy. The director resigned soon after. Other local family agencies were concerned because part of the grant would go to them. Eventually family planning money from the state went to the local agencies and not to the county health department. This story demonstrates antagonism between the county commissioners, the county health board and the director of the county health department concerning an important program of benefit to the public.

made before narrow ones. Next, boards of health should help define service priorities and then delegate the practice of programs to address these priorities to the health department or other related departments. Sixth, the board should be more interested in the results of programs and priorities and leave the practice and process of carrying these out to the health professionals. Next, the board's control function is more on limiting what can be done programmatically and not on the way the staff thinks is the best way to run the program with the board limits in place. Eighth, a board may undertake projects of its own that may lead to future programming and funding decisions. The board and the health department director need to develop a positive working relationship. The final principle involves the evaluation of the director using criteria related to service priorities and programs. Thus, the county commissioners or the local board of health is responsible for protecting the public's health by monitoring the performance of the appropriate agencies and also collaborating in achieving public health goals and services. In the end, the board should be able to help in creating a culture of health for their municipality or county.

Carver now adds a new governance perspective of 15 additional principles to guide board work.[8] I have added some changes to this new model.

1. The board of health develops the vision for health in the community in concert with the health department director. The board protects and markets the vision widely. The director works with agency staff to create a shared vision within the agency.

2. The board and the director use the health values that they have created for the community in support of the implementation of a culture of health orientation for all programs and priorities.

3. Whereas the health department executive staff often has to focus on the internal management of the agency, the director and the board must maintain an external community focus.

4. The board of health is interested in results and must work to have the agency employ appropriate means to reach the results.

5. Boards must work on big issues and leave the smaller ones to the agency director and staff. Board members have limited hours to carry out their work.

6. Boards should be oriented toward the future and not spend too much of their time on present issues. Boards should not, for example, micromanage the agency budget.

7. Board governance should be more proactive and less reactive.

8. The board membership needs to be representative of the community demographics.

9. Boards should be careful to address the concerns of different constituencies in the community.

10. Boards ought to develop protocols for delinquent board members as well as guidelines for evaluating the health department director.

11. The roles and expertise of board members needs to be determined relative to topics discussed by the board.

12. The board should determine the type of data that are required and develop some kind of knowledge management system.

13. Governance requires a balance related to oversight of the health agency relative to control.

14. The board should use its meeting times efficiently.

15. The board needs to work out a realistic approach to power sharing with the health department director and the county commissioners.

Exercise 9-1 helps you see how a board of health meeting occurs.

In concert with the Centers for Disease Control and Prevention, other agencies and partners, and public health experts, NALBOH (National Association of Local Boards of Health) have developed their own list of six functions for public health governance.[9] First, policy development itself is seen as one of the functions of public health governance. It is the task of boards of health and elected officials to develop internal and external policies that support the activities of the local health agency. Boards should also develop and ensure the enforcement of rules and regulations that support a culture of health orientation in communities. As a policy-oriented body the board also will update mission, vision, goals, and objectives statements. I believe

EXERCISE 9-1 Board of Health Meeting

Purpose: to observe how the local board of health or county commissioners follow the 15 principles

Key Concepts: board of health, county commissioners (county board), governance

Procedures: First, prepare a checklist of the traditional leadership and the new governance principles. Attend a board of health or county board meeting and see how the meeting progresses. Document which governance principles are used and whether the board is doing something contrary to a given principle.

that this latter set of tasks should occur in concert with the health department director.

The second public health governance function involves resource stewardship. Resources include legal, financial, human, technological, and material sources necessary to carry out the core functions and essential services of public health. Boards will have to work closely with elected official responsible for funding to make this happen. Health boards thus will eventually approve the budget of the health department. Boards also will engage in long-term planning as they tend to be future oriented. Boards of health will advocate for additional funding when necessary. Finally, these health boards develop agreements with cross-jurisdictional units involving the sharing of resources.

Third, boards will also carry out legal authority as required by law. These boards must always act in an ethical manner in relationship to the laws that guide their actions. Boards and other entities must ensure that high-quality services are given to those in need. They must engage legal counsel when it is called for or when it is appropriate.

The fourth public health governance function relates to partner engagement. Collaboration is critical in public health because the health of the public is a communitywide or countywide activity. The board's partners should include people and organizations throughout the community or county. The board needs to engage in communication that is community or countywide. The board serves as a link between the health agency, community or county, and other stakeholder organizations. The overall governance function here involves building the linkages that will help improve the health of the public. A strong culture of health is an end goal.

Fifth, boards must support continuous quality improvement protocols. Boards are looking at measures of improved community health status as well as measures that show the board and health department are carrying out their responsibilities. The board and the agency need to engage in a community health assessment process at regular intervals. Targets should be set for quality and performance improvement. Performance standards and overall quality improvement warrant support from the board as well as the health agency. It is important in governance to examine structures, compensation, the core functions, and the roles of the governing body and health agency at regular intervals. Finally, it is necessary to offer orientation for new board members and professional development during the tenure of board members, who are seen by others as community or county leaders. The board also must ensure that agency staff receive training as well.

The final public health governance function relates to oversight. The board and its members are leaders who have the ultimate responsibility for high-performance and high-quality programs. This oversight supports the achievement of measurable outcomes by the local health department. It is also necessary to demonstrate the active participation of individual board members to help carry out core board functions as well as to ensure that the core functions and essential public health services are being carried out. The board has the responsibility of evaluating the health department director using criteria defined by the contract with the director. This is why it is not legitimate to use director evaluation forms developed for other agencies or jurisdictions. Each board needs to develop its own evaluation forms. Good relations between the health director and board members are exceedingly important. As part of its oversight function, the board act as a go-between for the health agency and other elected officials.

As can be seen in this section governance is very important for organizations and their boards. Governance and leadership go together. Many directors of health departments will take on different board roles during their professional careers. In many states, former public health professionals take on political roles through elections to city, county, and state offices.

TYPES OF BOARDS

From the previous discussion, it is clear that the governance process is quite complex. It is also true that not all boards have complex governance functions. The board model with the most governance activities is the governing board.[10] This type of board has ultimate accountability to the public and to the board of elected county commissioners. Most of the governance functions in public health would apply to the governing board. The local health department director reports directly to this board on a regular basis. In some cases, the director has an ex officio position on the board. A governmental board of health has jurisdictional governance responsibility or district-based jurisdiction. This board gets its revenue from taxation, user fees, or state grants and contracts. These boards thus help define the mission, vision, and goals and objectives for their organizations,

The second type of board is the advisory board, which does not really serve as a governance body. This board or body gives counsel to the director of the health department or to some governing entity. The advisory board is not involved in the hiring of the department director. However, this board can make recommendations to a governing entity for potential policy considerations. The third type, the line

board, is rather rare. This board has limited jurisdiction. It is a board put together to oversee a particular grant or contract required program. It may have either a management function or have some governance activity if required by a grant program. The final type of board is the workgroup board is a board that is involved in carrying out the work of a program, grant, and contract. Thus, this board manages, leads, governs, and ultimately does the work. **Exercise 9-2** gives you the chance to experiment with the first two boards.

The next question relates to the ways that a given board is most effective. First, a board and its members require an excellent understanding of how their local area, county, and state function at social, economic, and political levels. They need to understand the culture and values of their jurisdiction. For public health boards, members should come from outside the agency and not be agency employees. The board should not be too large or it will be almost impossible to get effective work done. Absenteeism should be kept at a minimum. The membership of the board should be representative of the community or county and have diverse professional backgrounds. Although a board chair has added responsibilities, he or she should not control all agenda concerns. All members must participate. The relationship between the board and the health department executive should be collaborative in nature. Relationships between the board and

---

EXERCISE 9-2 Boards in Action

Purpose: to contrast governing and advisory boards and the ways they solve problems

Key Concepts: governing board, advisory board

Scenario: The County of Columbia is a small county in the state of Oceon. There is only one high school in the county. The county has both a county board of elected officials and a board of health composed of appointed members by the county board. An increasing number of students have been getting tattoos. Two students got extremely ill from getting tattoos. There are 10 tattoo parlors in the county.

Procedures: Divide the class into groups of six. Sort the groups into either a governing board of health or an advisory board of health. How will each group address a solution to the problem of underage students getting tattoos?

the county commissioners need to be positive as well. The board must acquire all data that are required to expedite policy decisions.

It is believed that all members of the board of health are leaders. The chairperson or the president of the board has special responsibilities.[11] Some of these responsibilities include:

1. In concert with the health department director, prepare the agenda for meetings. The chair has final decision on the agenda items.
2. The chair runs the meetings and keeps the agenda moving forward.
3. Parliamentary procedures are to be followed.
4. The chair works to keep the relationships on the board congenial and positive if possible.
5. The chair needs to keep all meetings focused because time is often limited.
6. The chair will honor the open meetings act if required by law. Guests will be entitled to speak during the time allotted by the agenda.
7. The chair will provide the board of timely issues of a positive or negative basis.
8. The chair will bring in experts or tap into the knowledge of board members on issues of interest.
9. The chair will coordinate relationships with the county commissioners.
10. The chair will give board members access to the senior health management team as necessary.

BOARD-BUILDING CYCLE

Boards go through a growth cycle on an ongoing basis. This is true of newly formed or well-established governmental or not-for-profit boards.[12] The first step in the cycle involves the identification of what the board requires in terms of types of members, types of information to guide action, and reasons for existence. In other words, what is the board's purpose? The second stage is a cultivation step in which attempts will be made to convince potential members to join the board. Getting people to join the board is sometimes a difficult task because the time commitment may be great and the financial commitment for not-for-profit boards may be high. The third step, recruitment, is closely related to the second. Why particular people are wanted needs to be well stated. Interviewing potential members with discussion of board roles and responsibilities will occur in this step. It is important to answer any questions that a potential member may have.

Once an individual commits to being on the board (step 4), he or she should be introduced to both to the board and to the health department and perhaps to the county commissioners. The orientation will include committee structure, responsibilities of each board member, issues of attendance at board meetings, and any key staff of the agency or the board. A workshop on governance may also be necessary. Step 5 is the actual engagement step in which to discover the interests of the new members. Assignment to committees occur at this step in the cycle. The availability of time for this committee work should also be discussed here. Step 6 involves the continuing education of board members. Because there are always new threats in public health, board members need to understand the consequences of these threats. The threats can severely affect the agency budget. Regular retreats may also be useful here. Some boards are specific about creating a learning organization model for their boards.

Step 7 is the rotation of board members. Term limits should be established. Most members do not want to make a lifetime commitment to a particular board. The board needs change and possibly different types of members. Step 7 may require the board to go back to step 1 again. Step 8 involves the issue of evaluation of both the board and the public health agency. Evaluation of individual board members may also be required. Evaluation forms can be developed to expedite this evaluation process. The last step in the cycle involves the celebration of the accomplishments of individual board members, staff of the agency, and the board itself.

Exercise 9-3 asks your help in an evaluation project.

EXERCISE 9-3 Evaluation of Board Meetings

Purpose: to determine the effectiveness of board of health meetings

Key Concepts: board-building cycle, evaluation

Procedures: Divide the class into groups of six or seven. You have been hired by the board of health to develop an evaluation instrument to determine the effectiveness of board meetings. Present your form with copies for all your classmates. Pick the best evaluation form and give a prize if possible. Celebrate the occasion.

THE BOARD MANUAL

As a former chair of a local health department advisory board, I found it useful to have a board of health manual that included information related to the state and local areas of the state. This manual was developed by a leadership team of the Mid-America Regional Public Health Leadership Institute (MARPHLI). The team developed the first edition, which was updated every 2 years by the MARPHLI director and staff. This section gives you an outline for creating a manual for a local health board in your state. It is also useful to put your manual on the Internet for use by other local boards in your state. It is also easier to update in the Internet approach. Some boards prefer hard copies of the manual that can easily be downloaded.

Here is a basic outline for a board of health manual:

1. Introduction and support letters
2. Organization charts for the state health department and other related state agencies. Organization charts for the local health department and other related local organizations
3. Mission and vision statement of the board of health and the health department. The two statements should be complementary
4. Short section on "What is public health?"
5. Listing of core functions and essential services of public health
6. Legal authority/powers and duties
7. Functions of boards and board member duties
8. Local board information
9. Parliamentary procedure in a simplified form
10. State statutes and regulations in a copied format. They should not be rewritten for the manual because mistakes can be made.
11. Board bylaws
12. Copies of open meetings act (if relevant) and any other acts
13. Board member profiles
14. Board minutes
15. Information on recruitment of health administrators
16. Evaluation forms for board or health department
17. Special topic information

SUMMARY

Boards of health provide a linkage between the local health department and the community, the public, and elected political leaders. Board members need to be seen as trustees and not as volunteers. Trustees represent all of their community. Thus, it is important that board of health members recognize that they represent the public and not only themselves or special interests. Governing boards have legal authority to make laws, make funding decisions, set community health priorities, and work on a health agenda with both the health department and community partners. As has been demonstrated in this chapter, governance is complex and has many components. Governance in public health focuses on developing a long-term vision for public health. The health department vision is more short term and tied to budgetary decisions. As part of its governance activities, the board helps define public health values and promotion of a culture of health for the community. Governance is also about establishing rules and structures that are consistent with these values and ensuring programs that result in the desired health outcomes.

This chapter also looked at the board-building cycle and what boards must do to stay up to date. The importance of a board of health manual as an important tool was also discussed. The responsibilities of the board chair or president were also listed.

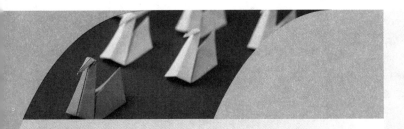

Discussion Questions

1. Why are boards of health important?

2. Distinguish between governance and management.

3. What are the responsibilities of a board of health member?

4. What evaluation questions would you require for the board to improve their performance?

5. What are the potential barriers to good governance?

REFERENCES

1. Massachusetts Association of Health Boards. www.mahb.org. Accessed April 15, 2016.
2. N. Glaser, *The Limits of Social Policy* (Cambridge, MA: Harvard University Press, 1988).
3. L. A. Aday, *At Risk in America* (San Francisco, CA: Jossey-Bass, 1993).
4. R. N. Bellah, "The Quest for the Self," in P. Rubinow and W. M. Sullivan (eds.), *Interpretive Social Science* (Berkeley, CA: University of California Press, 1987).
5. M. H. Moore, *Creating Public Value* (Cambridge, MA: Harvard University Press, 1995).
6. M. H. Moore, *Creating Public Value*.
7. J. Carver and M. M. Carver, *Basic Principles of Policy Governance*, The Carver Guide Series on Effective Board Governance, no. 1 (San Francisco, CA: Jossey-Bass, 1996).
8. J. Carver, *Boards That Make a Difference*, 3rd ed. (San Francisco, CA: Jossey-Bass, 2006).
9. National Association of Local Boards of Health, www.nalboh.org/?page=GovernanceResources.
10. Carver, *Boards That Make a Difference*, 3rd ed.
11. R. Charam, *Boards That Deliver* (San Francisco, CA: Jossey-Bass, 2005).
12. S. R. Hughes, B. M. Lakey, and M. J. Bobowick, *The Board Building Cycle* (Washington, DC: National Center for Nonprofit Boards, 2000).

Leadership at the Community Level

- Understand the factors that affect community growth.
- Define the Human Sigma model and its components.
- Understand the idea of "fit."
- Determine where to find community leaders.
- Describe the steps in stakeholder analysis.
- Apply the Leadership Wheel to communities.
- Become aware of multicultural considerations in community building.
- Determine the advantages of an assets-planning model in community building.
- Describe the principles of community engagement.

The public health leader spends more of his or her time in the community that he or she serves than inside the agency he or she leads. Public health today is about community and community relationships. It is also about building social capital and about new partnerships. The positive orientation of the leader will serve as a guide through the good times and also through the times of crisis. In a book of reflections on his leadership experiences told as short vignettes, Magee, who is a physician, stated that positive leaders stand on principle, and these principles then have a visible effect on all those with whom they interact.[1] Positive leadership is clearly needed in times of crisis. Leaders must see beyond the crisis to recognize the lessons to be learned and the important tasks related to healing. The goal of leadership is to learn the skills necessary to make our communities safe and to always respect every individual who lives in these communities. This chapter looks at additional skills that leaders require as they face the challenges of public health in the 21st century in a positive way.[2]

OVERVIEW OF COMMUNITY BUILDING

There has been much discussion in recent years about the importance of building communities. It is believed that a strong community is one that can address any attack on its infrastructure. There has also been discussion about the concern that our communities are disintegrating because people who live within a jurisdiction do not relate to that community in anything other than a superficial manner. It is clear that communities grow when there is collaboration with and commitment to that community. The public health leader needs to work with all community groups to create an environment for positive social change through collaboration. Mattessich and Monsey have enumerated 15 factors that can help the process of community growth and development:[3]

1. It is important to get widespread community involvement and participation.
2. Good, if not great, communication skills are critical to successful community building.
3. Collaboration to support community development is better than competition.
4. It is important to develop a community identity and agreement on community priorities.
5. Community residents must see and feel that they are benefiting from any changes that occur.
6. Community development is tied to building relationships with others and offers events and accomplishments that support relationship-building activities.
7. Communities that succeed have relationships with organizations and communities other than themselves.

8. Community growth begins small and simple and becomes bigger and more complex over time.

9. It is important to monitor changing needs of community residents and any other gauge of community reaction or concern.

10. Community residents and leaders should be offered training and informational meetings so they can learn and better understand what is occurring.

11. Community organizations with long tenure in the community need to be involved in any community-building activity.

12. Technical assistance and consultation should be used to expedite change and to help residents to better understand why changes and growth are necessary.

13. It is important for communities on the move to grow new leaders.

14. Residents and their trustee community leaders must be able to control any decisions that are required.

15. Internal and external resources to promote community growth should be balanced.

COMMUNITY RELATIONSHIPS

If organizational staff are not engaged in their agency work and do not feel motivated by managers and leaders, work with community clients and residents will be adversely affected. The external environment is also critical in defining the service community for human services agencies. If public health is all about the system, the public health agency is embedded in its community and needs to be seen relative to its customers (residents of the community), its agency competitors (other community stakeholders), public pressure groups (also community stakeholders as well as elected officials), and suppliers (public health technology and public health experts external to the community) (see **Figure 10-1**).[4] The specific community is also strongly influenced by its neighbors, the state, the federal government, and the global public health community. Broad economic, political, social, legal, and technological concerns affect the local community.

For public health agencies, the relationship with community customers is a primary relationship. The concept of Human Sigma has been formulated to show the importance of this relationship.[5] There are five key components or rules that define the Human Sigma model. The first rule requires good management of public health agency staff by local administrators and good relationships with community clients and all community residents. Staff and customers need to be seen in terms of the relationships that are generated between them. In fact, these relationships should be regarded as primary to the work of public health. If the agency staff are not engaged in their work, then the community clients will also be affected. This rule and the other three rules work synergistically in that staff and customer interactions

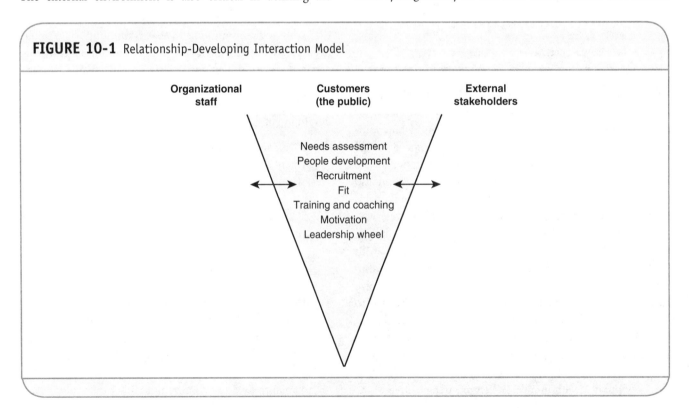

FIGURE 10-1 Relationship-Developing Interaction Model

Organizational staff — Customers (the public) — External stakeholders

Needs assessment
People development
Recruitment
Fit
Training and coaching
Motivation
Leadership wheel

are affected by the positive and negative consequences that come from the interaction as well as customer feedback. It is often impossible to predict these synergistic outcomes, but it is possible to learn from them to help in future encounters.

If I take my child to the public health agency to be immunized and my child and I are kept waiting for several hours for the nurse, then I will be upset. If the nurse is patronizing, my negative experience gets compounded. I will complain and I may also tell others in the community about my negative experience. The second rule of Human Sigma is the necessity of paying attention to the emotions aroused in an encounter between an agency staff member and a community resident. Emotions become facts in relationships.[6] The third rule addresses the issue of thinking globally and acting locally. Public health is a local phenomenon but is clearly affected by health issues in other parts of the world. If staff and customer interactions are mostly positive, then the chances increase that these positive occurrences can affect future budgeting considerations. The fourth rule points out that successful staff and customer relationships will affect the financial bottom line of the organization. These solid relationships will lead to the better use of the finances of the agency. The final rule states that intentions are not enough. Action will be the criterion for success. Despite these rules, all people have good and bad days.

There are many factors that can help to build customer loyalty. In addition to building good relationships between agency staff and community residents, leaders look for such things as consistency in service provision, caring and helpfulness, authenticity, positive attitude, professionalism, orientation to detail, responsiveness to complaints, good communication and follow-up, knowledge of other service providers to address special needs of clients, humor when appropriate, and community health days to celebrate improvements in the health of the community.[7] Good customer relationships are affected by always knowing why and for whom you are doing your work, treating your clients the way you want to be treated, supporting staff as discussed previously, and providing leadership in support of the public health enterprise.[8]

Part of the responsibility of the local public health agency is to monitor the health needs of the public and provide the technology and programs necessary to address those needs. Sometimes, things do not work out as expected. In addition to the needs assessment process, public health agencies have to determine how to help community residents understand public health and how their behavior affects their health. Education of the public is one way to increase knowledge of the public about public health. Recruitment of community residents to serve as volunteers in public health is also a useful process. Another interesting approach used by business is to use satisfied customers as spokespeople for successful public health programs. The development of the Medical Reserve Corps to address a community crisis is another example.

The issue of "fit" requires that there be a solid relationship between the engaged staff member and an engaged community resident. Not all residents choose to go to a public health agency for service. It is necessary to point out that the public health agency is only one partner in the public health enterprise. Fit needs to be expanded to all the community agency and hospital resources. The goal is to strive to find appropriate access to service for every resident somewhere in the community and even to extend the service option to other agencies outside the community when necessary. In many ways, public health is about education. People need to learn how to help make themselves more healthy. Public health leaders should use their skills to create teachable moments. Community residents require motivation and support for their health. Finally, strategic and action planning requires that the public be involved in public health activities. Their needs and concerns must be addressed as part of all planning activities.

COMMUNITY LEADERS

As public health leaders extend their work into the community, the involvement of residents becomes more and more important. Most leaders with positional authority are not willing or lack understanding of the ways to interact with community people in a collaborative way. Part of the challenge relates to that abstract phenomenon referred to as *sharing power*. Because many community people lack leadership training, it is important for the public health leader to work with the community in developing leaders who will become trustees in the sense that they will represent other community residents. Empowering the community to train its representatives as leaders involves working with people rather than doing the work for them.[9] These grassroots leaders will often be part of a community-based coalition or organization. They also need to see themselves as community trustees.

A trustee becomes involved in what has been called community ownership. Community ownership involves taking responsibility for the challenges that a community will face. Community leaders will thus define the issues of concern for community health. Not only will they help to define the issues, but these grassroots leaders, in collaboration with public health leaders, will help to define and implement the solutions and strategies for carrying them out. These leaders require the training and tools necessary to make these solutions work. Trust can easily erode when community leaders are not involved in the implementation of the strategies or when the professionals take over and disenfranchise the community leaders.

Leaders in the community come from several places.[10] Formal community leaders include elected or appointed officials, heads of community agencies, direct service providers, and civic leaders. These leaders often represent specific constituents in the community and have the power to speak for a group or groups of residents. A second key group of leaders are volunteers. These leaders are community residents with grassroots constituencies. They clearly have the trust of their constituencies, where formal leaders may not have the same level of community trust. The third group of community leaders are informal leaders. This often includes people with high community respect but without an active constituency. They include those people who know the history of the community, people who will always give advice when you have a problem, and the person who will just listen to you and not give advice.

All communities have organized sectors with people who are seen as leaders in those sectors. It is possible to create a list of these organized sectors in a specific community. These sectors include leaders from police and fire departments, elected offices, youth and senior centers and agencies, healthcare organizations, and so on. Because many communities are in a state of flux, there may also be developing community sectors from a variety of places, including new industry, new gangs, a new church, and so on. **Exercise 10-1** gives you the opportunity to explore community sectors and some ways to increase community outreach.[11] Some community outreach strategies for the public health leader include the following:[12]

1. Identify and reach out to community leaders in all three sector groups.
2. Contact organized and developing community sector groups through public and house meetings and door-to-door contact.
3. Perform street outreach by going to the sector sites.
4. Set up information tables at community meeting sites, such as supermarkets.
5. Attend community meetings and speak at the open portion of a meeting, if possible.
6. Do community assessment or community participatory research.

Another dimension of working with community leaders relates to why a community leader may want to participate in the endeavors being supported by public health leaders. Kaye and Wolff stated that there are six reasons (the Six Rs)

EXERCISE 10-1 Attacking Gangs in a Big City

Purpose: to identify community sectors and organizations to address increasing gang violence in a large urban area

Key concepts: community sectors, gang warfare, community building, collaborative leadership

Scenario: The mayor of BigTown is concerned about the growing number of murders in by gangs in the city. The mayor appoints Dr. I. M. Helping, the director of the Big Town Health Department, to address this problem and find possible solutions.

Procedures: Select a student to be the leader of this initiative. Identify potential community health sector leaders to serve as task force leaders. Using role playing, develop potential solutions to the gang problem. Discuss the results and then demonstrate what community-building strategies were used.

---

that people participate in all types of groups or community-based endeavors:[13]

1. People participate for *Recognition* of their leadership. Recognition can be shown through such activities as award dinners.
2. People want *Respect* from their peers or neighbors. Involvement also needs to occur in nonwork hours when community people who work during the day can attend.
3. Community leaders like to have a specific, defined *Role* in a community initiative. These roles also should have some power and authority associated with them.
4. Community leaders will become involved in community activities because they have a *Relationship* with others who are involved.
5. There need to be *Rewards* for being a member of a coalition or involved in a community-based activity that outweigh the costs of involvement.
6. Community leaders want to see *Results*. As business people will state, a demonstrable product should be produced through the interaction.

There are many tools available for evaluating community involvement. In addition to the two sources described in this section, Ayre, Clough, and Norris have developed a manual that examines change in communities from the vantage point of community readiness for change, the importance of energy in team activities, the importance of building successes into the program, motivation of the community, direction setting for the change that is proposed, and implementation of the change.[14]

An interesting set of issues relates to the self-determination part of community leadership. The Community Toolbox website is used by many community leaders. Axner has studied the issue of learning how to be a community leader.[15] People who become community leaders have strong concerns about where their communities are going. They also want to improve their communities. Community leaders must think they can make a difference. Leadership development is a growth activity, and there is not really a limit on how many leaders there can be in a community. There are several issues for potential community leaders to consider, including the following:[16]

1. It is important to create a personal vision for a community in a *big picture* way.
2. Listening skills are important because the community leader needs to know what the concerns of other community members are.
3. It is critical that the potential leader agrees to serve a community in a leadership role.
4. Leaders need to turn their vision into a set of goals.
5. Leaders must protect the interests of other people in their community group.
6. Leaders also have to look at their collaborative in terms of what is best for the community as a whole and be able to justify their position to others.
7. Leaders guide the process of developing and proposing programs and policies.
8. Follow-through is important—the work must get done.
9. Leaders should nurture the leadership potential of other community residents.

COMMUNITY STAKEHOLDERS

Public health leaders know that they have to work with other community partners if the public health enterprise is to work. These decision makers outside the public health agency must be involved in the overall public health planning and agenda if there is to be successful implementation of public health programs and services.[17] These stakeholders will have to make a commitment and also provide financial resources to the enterprise.

Public health leaders also need to view the community with a systems thinking orientation. The public health system includes the local public health agency and the population of the community; it also includes many stakeholders such as other health and social agencies from the private, public, not-for-profit, and volunteer sectors who will work with the local public health agency in carrying out the essential services. **Figure 10-2** views the public health system as a network of interacting partners that includes public health agencies, healthcare providers, public safety agencies, human service and charity organizations, education and youth development organizations, recreation and arts-related organizations, economic and philanthropic organizations, and environmental agencies and organizations.[18] Community residents have many relationships with these organizations and influence policy through these relationships with community stakeholders.

In strategic planning, stakeholder analysis is one of the techniques involved. Public health leaders need to study stakeholders to see what the local public health system is like and to determine if gaps exist in the service system. There are three steps in stakeholder analysis.[19] The first step involves a determination of the services available. This step involves an enumeration not only of resources but also of what each stakeholder resource can contribute to the overall public health enterprise. Second, a determination should be made about the level of organizational performance by potential public health partners. Finally, public health leaders need to determine how public health stakeholders will perform relative to the goals and objectives for public health in a given community.

One important dimension that is often ignored is the necessity of stakeholder development. Stakeholders do not always understand what public health does. They need training in public health and need to develop a virtual public health stakeholder learning community if a face-to-face community is difficult to sustain. Public health leaders also should be on the lookout for new or emerging resources as they develop. Partners from outside the service community are also important. At the transactional leadership level, recruitment of new stakeholders will address reciprocity concerns.

Fit is clearly important as well. A few years ago, a small local health department in a Midwest state applied for a state grant to develop a special maternal and child health program. A local community agency also applied for the same grant. The directors of the two agencies were extremely competitive and did not work well together. The state gave the grant to the community agency, requiring the two agencies to work together on the program. The staff of the two agencies tried to collaborate, but the fit was not a good one. Many conflicts ensued.

FIGURE 10-2 The Public Health System

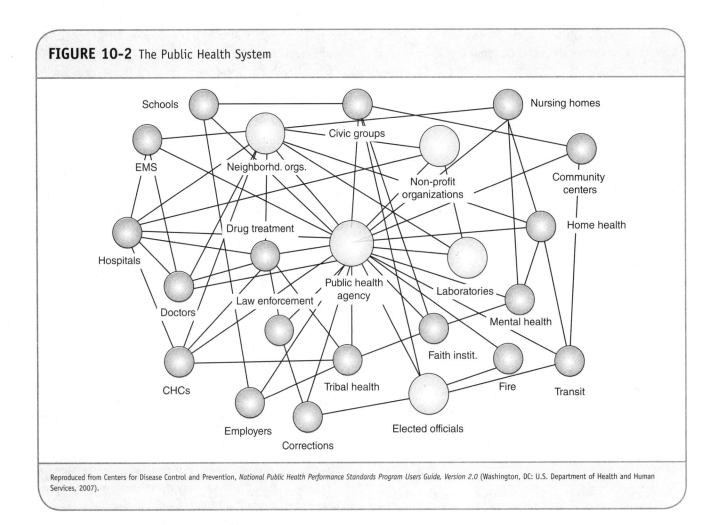

Schools

EMS

Civic groups

Neighborhd. orgs.

Nursing homes

Non-profit organizations

Community centers

Home health

Drug treatment

Hospitals

Public health agency

Laboratories

Doctors

Law enforcement

Mental health

Faith instit.

CHCs

Tribal health

Fire

Transit

Employers

Corrections

Elected officials

Because leaders are often dealing with leaders in stakeholder situations, motivation strategies still remain important. Relationships need to be on a person-to-person level. Relationships that are always or mostly position to position tend to be conflictual. There have to be both transactional and transformational gains if collaboration is to succeed. Decisions must be made about carrying out the 10 essential public health services. Whenever strategic planning activities occur or the public health assessment process is undertaken, community partners need to be involved in the process. Public health planning both strategically and in terms of action requires a partnership among the local public health agency, its customers, and its partners.

The complexity of stakeholder relationships often extends outside the community and gets tangled up in politics at a county and state level. The following public health leadership story addresses how a public health issue can become politicized and lead to many villainous acts. When these political actions are seen as external to the state, the situation can become more complex. The Flint, Michigan, water contamination with high lead levels presents such an example.

LEADERSHIP WHEEL APPLIED TO COMMUNITIES

Elsewhere, I introduced a systems approach to the tasks of leadership in organizations in a model called the *Leadership Wheel*, and it can now be expanded to include the tasks of leaders in communities. The wheel not only uses the activities of groups in communities but applies these activities to the core public health functions of assessment, policy development, and assurance. A community challenge, crisis situation, or community-building process brings the public health leader together with community leaders and all the emergency preparedness and response officials. In a collaborative group, these leaders will form themselves into a coalition, alliance, or partnership. It is usually some community need (assessment) as defined qualitatively or quantitatively with some policy considerations that brings the collaboration into being. Skills in collaboration with a strong commitment to

PUBLIC HEALTH HEROES AND VILLAINS 10-1 Villains in Michigan[20]

The governor of Michigan has been seen as a villain in a water contamination case in Michigan beginning in 2014. Many have argued that Governor Richard Snyder should have taken action before 2016 to address this public health crisis. He has tried to apologize for his actions, but many have thought his apologies have come too late. Calls for his resignation have been made. It took Snyder almost 2 years to declare that there was a crisis in Flint.

Mr. Wynant, the director of the Michigan state environmental agency, resigns. In April 2016 three people from the Michigan Department of Environmental Quality were indicted with criminal acts. in the Flint water contamination crisis by Michigan Attorney General William Schuette. The three were charged with misconduct in office, tampering with evidence, a treatment violation of the Michigan Safe Drinking Water Act, and a monitoring violation of that same act. The former Flint water plant operator Michael Glasgow was also charged with willful neglect of his office and the felony on evidence tampering. Glasgow accepted a plea deal. The villains were increasing.

Between 1901 and 1920 water service lines with cast iron water mains were installed in Flint. These lead pipes eventually leached lead into the water. By 2011, Flint was primarily a poor city with a large minority population. The city went into receivership under emergency managers appointed by Governor Snyder. In late April 2014, Flint switched the source of its supply from the treated water from Lake Huron purchased from Detroit to water from the Flint River in order to save about $5 million. After the switch, Flint residents noticed the color of the water was changing. The taste was different and there was an odor. High levels of lead were being leached into the water supply. By August 2014, boiling water advisories were occurring. Detroit offered to reconnect water to Flint in January 2015. Emergency Manager Ambrose refuses the offer and another villain enters the case.

In March 2015, an Environmental Protection Agency (EPA) expert finds that lead levels in Flint have been underreported. A private consulting firm hired by the Flint mayor says this is not the case. There is an on-again off-again dialogue between EPA and Flint about the lead levels. Other 2016 events happened. In September 2015, the Michigan Department of Environmental Quality disputes a water expert from Virginia Tech who said that corrosiveness of the water was causing lead to leach into the water supply. These differences in opinions continued throughout 2015 with the governor still refusing to take action. Flint declares a public health emergency in December.

In January 2016, the Michigan legislature authorizes funds to assist Flint. Additional funds were allocated the following June. Flint became a national issue. The Michigan Democratic presidential primary in Michigan features talks about the Flint water problem. Celebrities like the Reverend Jesse Jackson came to Flint. The actors Matt Damon and Mark Ruffalo called for the governor's resignation. A rapper wrote a song about the crisis. Lawsuits were initiated by Flint residents affected by the crisis. The Genessee County Health Department reported on an increase in cases of Legionnaires' disease. The news media has covered the story extensively. Donations of bottled water were made by individuals such as Cher as well as businesses and organizations. Congressional hearings occurred. As of this writing, the crisis has not yet been completely resolved even though the governor made a media event related to drinking a glass of Flint water. The villains in this story are numerous. The heroes are harder to find.

Information for this story was adapted from http://en,Wikipedia.org/wiki/Flint_water_crisis and http://www.nytimes.com/2016/01/21/us/flint-lead-water-timeline.html. Accessed June 1, 2016

address the community need serve as catalysts for the leadership process required.

The wheel represents a strategic and action planning approach, with the addition of a values-clarification stage and potential for feedback at every stage of the wheel. Values clarification is often ignored as a stage in community collaboration. It is important to understand the cultural and organizational diversity that every collaboration entails. If your community stakeholder group or other community collaborative takes the values-clarification task seriously, then the job of developing a mission and vision statement will be greatly simplified. Mission and vision are also part of the public health core function of policy development. Once the mission and vision are discussed and agreed upon, then specific goals and objectives to make the vision a reality are developed. Goals and objectives are the link between the mission of today and the vision of tomorrow. If the goals and objectives do not reflect this linkage, then the mission and the vision are disconnected. Goals and objectives also connect the core function of policy development with the assessment function, as goals and objectives are often tied to information gleaned from the needs assessment that brought the collaborative group into being.

The steps thus far are often where strategic planning ends and action begins. It is possible to develop a series of action steps for each goal and objective. Action planning is closely related to the important considerations related to goals management, performance measurement, and performance standards. Goals management and performance measurement tell us how effective we are in tying our action steps to addressing goals and objectives. Performance standards are benchmarks to measure our progress and successes and failures. This step is often not given the time and effort required to create a viable implementation.[21]

Action planning requires a series of steps for the creation of an action plan. The first step is determining the underlying reasons for the plan by relating it back to both vision and overall goals and objectives. Next it is important to develop a framework based on the core functions and essential public health services. A series of design meetings can then be held to create the plan. The plan should be written down so there will be no confusion about its components. Validation will be needed not only from members of the collaborative but also from any other affected stakeholders. Finally, the plan should be disseminated to the community as well as to all the agency partners.

When the plan is implemented, the core function of assurance comes into play. Here is where the real action occurs. All activities should be evaluated as well. The next stage is for the group to begin discussions about next steps and whether the group should continue, disband, or restructure itself and start the planning and implementation process again. It is difficult to determine how long the entire cycle will take. It will vary from community to community.

MULTICULTURAL CONSIDERATIONS

It is important to consider the multicultural diversity of a community in any community-building process. Multicultural representatives should be part of any community-based activity. It is important to have different social and cultural groups involved in shaping a community collaboration, making decisions that will affect the community in which these groups live and making sure the collective interest is supported and nurtured.[22] If public health leaders want to build

effective community coalitions, alliances, and partnerships, several steps should be followed:[23]

1. Create a vision for any collaborative activity, taking into account that trust needs to be built through values clarification.
2. Be as inclusive as possible in membership recruitment—making a conscious effort to do this is critical.
3. Respect cultural differences and create rules for the collaboration that do not undermine these differences. A safe and nurturing environment is required.
4. Ensure that whatever structure is created for the collaboration reinforces social and cultural equity.
5. Develop communication rules that reflect language differences as well as cultural etiquette so people do not feel threatened.
6. Create leadership opportunities for every member of the collaboration regardless of gender, race, or ethnic identity.
7. Make sure all action plans and program implementation strategies are culturally sensitive.

ASSETS-PLANNING MODEL

Especially in this age of the fear of terrorism or bioterrorism, the prepared public health leader needs to better understand the strengths of our communities and how to use these strengths in confronting all types of crises. Public health leaders have traditionally taken a problem focus in their data collection activities. A negative approach slows the process of effecting change. In working with communities, it is important to build on the strengths and resources of the community. If these resources are mobilized effectively, then all sorts of community challenges can be addressed.

There are differences between a problem-oriented focus and an assets-based focus.[24] If we were to map the problems in a community, we would have to consider such things as unemployment, school truancy, rates of literacy, lead paint in old buildings or in the water supply, school dropouts, gang activity, adult crime, domestic and child abuse, broken families, the number of people on welfare, and on and on. Each of these problems creates a community need for a solution. If we were to determine the assets of the community in terms of individuals, community collaborative efforts, associations, and public and private organizations, it would be possible to determine an interesting balance of resources against needs. On the assets side, we would create a map of resources such as schools, churches, libraries, parks, businesses, community colleges, healthcare providers, local health departments, citizen organizations, cultural groups, artists, and so on. To these assets can be added the personal gifts of community people, in terms of talent or money, and special gifts of people in different age groups.[25] It is important not only to recognize the assets of the community but also to mobilize the resources in such a way that community growth becomes more possible.

There are five steps involved in assets planning.[26] First, it is necessary to create an assets map of the community that delineates the capacities and gifts of individuals in the community, citizens' organizations and other entities, and local institutions. Once this mapping process is tentatively completed, the next step involves the building of new community relationships between local assets in order to better develop strategies and programs to address community needs. In reality, assets maps are constantly changing as the community changes. It is important to mobilize these assets for community-building activities. The third step in the process is to expand mobilization activities for economic and social development. It is also important to increase information-sharing activities with all community assets. Fourth, community leaders need to convene a group of people from all assets categories to build a community vision and plan for community growth and development. Finally, it is important to leverage internal community resources with likely external resources, possibly through grants, contracts, and gifts to support the assets-based planning and development activities.

Communities should develop a toolbox of techniques for community-building activities.[27] There are several tools to help in carrying out assets-planning and development activities. First is the assets map just discussed, with the addition of a capacity inventory of information about the given assets and ways that different individuals and groups can better work together. The important question is whether a given community has enough assets and capacity to address all the needs that exist in that community. A second set of tools is based on self-help techniques similar to the 12-step program of Alcoholics Anonymous, where peer groups form to address needs using some self-help model. A third tool employs a circle of support, a technique used in Canada to help people in need find support in difficult times. A fourth tool is also an expansion of the map to discover any small associations or groups in the community that were not caught in the mapping process but are

groups that can address community needs. Finally, a business inventory is useful for helping community residents address employment issues in the community. Ayre and his colleagues would add some sort of civic index process that would specifically pull together the preferred vision for the community, governance factors, strategies for collaboration, and information needed to help the community to better address community needs.[28]

COMMUNITY ENGAGEMENT

In the second decade of the 21st century, there is once again belief that the community working together is best qualified for promoting the health of the public. Community engagement approaches and strategies are being pursued for these renewed activities. Community engagement has been defined as a process in which individuals and community organizations promote programs that will benefit the community.[29] With a community benefit philosophy, community engagement through collaboration is the goal, with a common vision of health promotion and disease prevention. Specifically, community benefits refer to programs and services that are designed to improve health in a community and also to increase access to a comprehensive array of community services.[30] The definition of community will vary depending on the type of jurisdiction covered.

SUMMARY

This chapter presented a number of techniques related to building the community and improving community engagement activities. Public health leaders are often not aware of many of these skills. The issue of developing and working with community leaders and community stakeholders was discussed, as was the importance of assets planning. In the Flint, Michigan, water contamination with lead story, it was demonstrated that negative leadership can affect the resolution of a community crisis. Villains come from many places including the political sector. Multicultural considerations were also discussed. The Leadership Wheel was used to show the various activities leaders use in working in collaborative relationships. The advantages of an assets-planning model were presented. The principles of community engagement were also discussed.

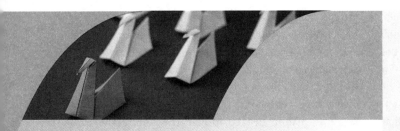

Discussion Questions

1. What is social capital? How is it related to community building?

2. What is Human Sigma?

3. Check the Community Toolbox website. How is the website useful to the public health leader?

4. What is stakeholder analysis?

5. What are the leadership lessons to be learned from the Flint water contamination story?

6. Compare and contrast the use of the Leadership Wheel in public health agency work and also in community-building activities.

7. How does community engagement work?

REFERENCES

1. M. Magee, *Positive Leadership* (New York, NY: Spencer Books, 2000).
2. Magee, *Positive Leadership*.
3. P. Mattessich and B. Monsey, *Community Building: What Makes It Work?* (St. Paul, MN: Amherst H. Wilder Foundation, 1997).
4. S. P. Robbins and M. Coulter, *Management*, 11th ed. (Upper Saddle River, NJ: Prentice-Hall, 2011).
5. J. H. Fleming and J. Asplund, *Human Sigma* (New York, NY: Gallup Press, 2007).
6. Fleming and Asplund, *Human Sigma*.
7. J. Brandi, *Building Customer Loyalty* (Dallas, TX: Walk the Talk, 2001).
8. K. Blanchard, J. Ballard, and F. Finch, *Customer Mania* (New York, NY: Free Press, 2004).
9. W. K. Kellogg Foundation, *Sustaining Community-Based Initiatives: Developing Community Capacities* (Battle Creek, MI: Author, 1995).
10. Kellogg, *Sustaining Community-Based Initiatives*.
11. Kellogg, *Sustaining Community-Based Initiatives*.
12. Kellogg, *Sustaining Community-Based Initiatives*.
13. G. Kaye and T. Wolff, *From the Ground Up* (Amherst, MA: AHEC Community Partners, 1997).
14. D. Ayre, G. Clough, and T. Norris, *Facilitating Community Change* (San Francisco, CA: Grove Consultants International, 2000).
15. M. Axner, *Developing a Plan for Building Leadership, Community Toolbox*. http://ctb.ku.edu/en/tablecontents/sub_section_main_1119 .aspx. Accessed September 2005.
16. Axner, *Developing a Plan for Building Leadership*.
17. J. M. Bryson, *Strategic Planning for Public and Nonprofit Organizations*, 3rd ed. (San Francisco, CA: Jossey-Bass, 2004).
18. Centers for Disease Control and Prevention, *National Public Health Performance Standards Program Users Guide, Version 2.0* (Washington, DC: U.S. Department of Health and Human Services, 2007).
19. Bryson, *Strategic Planning for Public and Nonprofit Organizations*.
20. Information for this story was adapted from http://en.Wikipedia.org/wiki/Flint_water_crisis and http://www.nytimes.com/interactive/2016/01/21/us/flint-lead-water-timeline.html. Accessed June 1, 2016.
21. K. Johnson, W. Grossman, and A. Cassidy (eds.), *Collaborating to Improve Community Health* (San Francisco, CA: Jossey-Bass, 1996).
22. Kaye and Wolff, *From the Ground Up*.
23. Kaye and Wolff, *From the Ground Up*.
24. J. P. Kretzmann and J. L. McKnight, *Building Communities from the Inside Out* (Evanston, IL: Northwestern University ABCD Institute, 1993).
25. Kretzmann and McKnight, *Building Communities from the Inside Out*.
26. Kretzmann and McKnight, *Building Communities from the Inside Out*.
27. J. P. Kretzmann and M. B. Green, *Building the Bridge from Client to Citizen: A Community Toolbox for Welfare Reform* (Evanston, IL: Northwestern University ABCD Institute, 1998).
28. Ayre, Clough, and Norris, *Facilitating Community Change*.
29. www.cdc.gov/nphpsp. Accessed December 10, 2011.
30. www.chausa.org/communitybenefits. Accessed December 10, 2011.

CHAPTER **11**

The Community in Crisis

Since September 11, 2001, it seems as though most of our conversation in public health relates to bioterrorism, emergency preparedness, and our response to it. There is also conversation about the critical role of public health during any crisis. Public health preparedness is all about the need to be ready for any health crisis that a community may face. The major responsibility of public health in a crisis or other emergency that includes terrorism events similar to those of September 11, 2001, or the anthrax letters bioterrorism events in the months following, must be seen in the context of the overall mission of public health to promote and protect the health of the public. If this is the case, then emergency preparedness is to be seen as an extension of the public health mission and integral to public health.

A crisis is a disruption in the normal activities that guide the daily work of public health. Crisis is an abnormal event or series of disruptive events that threatens the total operation of an organization or threatens the functioning of a community or country. Thus, crisis and its aftermath are examples of system failure. It is the crisis event that triggers community emergency response activities. I use the words *crisis,*

disaster, emergency, and *hazard* interchangeably, although the meanings of these terms do show subtle differences, as discussed later. In terms of other relevant definitions, the World Health Organization (WHO) and Pan African Emergency Training Centre made a distinction between a disaster and an emergency.[1] A disaster refers to the occurrence of an event that disrupts the normal conditions of existence and causes a level of suffering that exceeds the capacity of adjustment that is usual for a given community. It is important to remember that people are the most affected by a disaster, although structural damage may also occur. WHO defined an emergency as a time in which normal procedures for dealing with events are suspended and extraordinary measures must be taken to avert further disastrous events. WHO further distinguished between a hazard that is a natural or human event that threatens to adversely affect human life, property, or activities to such an extent that a disaster occurs and vulnerabilities in a population or community that may make a crisis event more severe. Vulnerabilities then refer to predispositions to suffer damage in a population or community from external events. A disaster occurs when hazards and vulnerabilities meet.

The United Nations has used the following definition to refer to disaster preparedness:[2]

> Disaster preparedness minimizes the adverse effects of a hazard through effective precautionary actions, rehabilitation and recovery to ensure the timely, appropriate and effective organization and delivery of relief and assistance following a disaster.

TYPES OF CRISIS

In two excellent books on crisis and crisis management, the discussion of crisis and its aftermath is seen as related to the type of crisis that is involved.[3,4] Bioterrorism events relate to only one type of crisis situation. Crisis falls into several different groups. Each major type of crisis requires different response patterns. Mitroff developed a typology of crisis that delineates at least seven different classes of crisis.[5] The first group of crises is economic in nature and includes such things as labor strikes. In public health, an economic crisis relates to cutbacks in budget or loss of staff without an ability to hire replacements. Although there have been increases in funding for emergency preparedness and response activities, other programs in public health have suffered from budget cuts and budget shortfalls.

The second group of crises is informational in nature. These crises deal with things such as tampering with public records, computer viruses that affect an entire agency's computer system, false information in files, privacy issues, and so forth. The potential information crises in public health are numerous and complex. Sharing information across agencies is a problem. Different methods for collecting data as well as different data classification schemes all add to the potential for information crises in the governmental public health sector. Federal and state guidelines related to the sharing or disclosure of health information to outside parties also create data problems. Misinterpretation of data is also important because it can create an inadvertent series of reactions to the report that can have crisis consequences.

Next, there are physical crises that involve the loss of property or key equipment through breakdowns or theft. This can lead to disruption in the normal flow of operations in an organization. Many universities report the loss of computers and laptops from staff offices, for example. A power outage can affect activities. A lack of flu vaccine, as occurred during the fall of 2004, during a potential influenza outbreak in a community is another crisis possibility. Public health agencies often struggle with a shortage of physical resources to carry out their work. The fourth group of crises relates to the human resources needs of organizations. These are the crises that occur when there is a sudden budget cut in programs and programs and staff must be eliminated or cut on short notice. These types of crises occur when a health administrator resigns or takes ill and the organization flounders because of a lack of competent leadership. A crisis occurs if there is a flu epidemic in the community that leads to a rise in absenteeism in the agency because the primary program staff are out sick.

Many people ignore reputational crises, but they can severely cripple an organization or community. Here we are dealing with the effects of gossip, slander, misinformation during a crisis, rumors, and so forth. This is in many ways an extremely important group of potential crisis events. They cannot be ignored. For example, a rumor that a health administrator may be leaving or a health administrator is accused of sexual harassment by one of his employees can create agency problems. Thus, it is possible that a reputational crisis can occur even when the public health agency is operating to protect the rights of the public. Crises and their occurrence are unexpected happenings.

Most of our discussions in public health in recent years have been related to psychopathic crises, which include bioterrorism events, hostage taking in domestic and foreign places, workplace rage and violence, product tampering that affects the health of the public, foreign substances in the mail, and so-called weapons of mass destruction (biological warfare). The importance of the present typology is that psychopathic crises are only one group of crises, although much of the attention of public health is turned toward this class of abnormal events. The funding that public health agencies is receiving today is tied to this class. Public health preparedness models build on the military preparedness model related to these types of events. Preparedness models are not limited to psychopathic crises but rather can be expanded and applied to all the crisis categories discussed in this section.

Public health has been most comfortable with the natural disaster form of crisis. We have dealt with these events on many occasions and have developed effective emergency preparedness and response plans for dealing with these natural disasters. For example, during the Florida hurricanes of 2004, the way agencies worked together to address the aftermath of one hurricane after another reaching landfall in Florida and other affected areas of the South is an excellent example of agencies working together. Following the earthquake and tsunami in southeast Asia during Christmas week of 2004, the emergency response was slow at first but eventually involved worldwide response to the events.

Although public health agencies have worked well with fire departments and other emergency response groups during natural disasters, these relationships have tended to be jurisdictional in nature. Difficulties still exist when federal, state, and local entities must work together. The situation becomes even more complex when the relationships cross state or national boundaries or involve federal agencies and international organizations, entities, and personnel as partners.

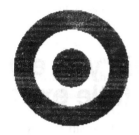

PUBLIC HEALTH PREPAREDNESS TODAY

There is growing evidence that public health and its leadership are still not prepared to manage a large-scale emergency. In 2002, Congress enacted legislation as a response to the events of September 11, 2001, and the anthrax attacks that occurred later that year. The Public Health Security and Bioterrorism Response Act of 2002 was passed. This act was intended to provide guidance to public health officials at the federal, state, and local levels through cooperative agreement funding mechanisms to increase the ability of public health agencies to be prepared for potential bioterrorism activities through strengthening the public health system in the areas of emergency preparedness and response. State and local governments, including municipal health departments, were given funding to develop bioterrorism and other emergency response plans; purchase and upgrade equipment, supplies, and staff to manage national drug stockpiles necessary to enhance preparedness and response activities; conduct exercises and drills to test emergency response capabilities; improve surveillance methods; and train personnel in the use of early warning and surveillance networks to provide early detection.

Trust for America's Health reviewed our state of readiness at the end of fiscal year 2003[7] and for a second time in 2004.[8] The Trust noted progress in the area of completed bioterrorism planning documents, improvements in laboratory capabilities and upgrades, and improvements in communication systems. However, the Trust felt that there were many concerns with our progress in improving our public health preparedness activities. Their concerns related to such factors as increasing state deficits and budget declines for public health, unspent federal aid, lack of preparation for pharmaceutical stockpiles, local health departments often left out of decision-making activities, and an increasing public health workforce crisis. In fiscal year 2010, the Trust presented a state preparedness evaluation process using the following 10 indicators:[9]

1. Increased or maintained level of funding for public health over previous fiscal year.
2. Sends and receives currently electronic data information.
3. Has an electronic syndromic surveillance system that can send and receive information.
4. Has the ability to activate an emergency response team within 1 hour.
5. Was able to activate its emergency operations center at least twice in the previous fiscal year.
6. Developed at least two after-action reports from exercises or events in the previous fiscal year.

7. Requires childcare facilities to have a multihazard written emergency plan.

8. Able to identify foodborne illnesses and submit results within 4 days.

9. Has necessary laboratory workforce to work five 12-hour days.

10. Increased Laboratory Response Network for chemical events.

In 2010 it was found that some states miss a number of criteria. Clearly a major success has been in the improvement in laboratory capability. Half the states did not meet the childcare facility requirement of a multihazard written evacuation and relocation plan. Some states met only half the criteria (Iowa and Montana, for example) and some states (Arkansas, North Dakota, and Washington) met all 10.

Clearly, the Trust report indicated the importance of strengthening the public health system in the United States. Strong public health leadership is required to make this happen. By the 2011 report, much deterioration in readiness was noted.[10] Key programs related to our disaster and emergency preparedness were in jeopardy of major cuts in federal and state funding. Specifically, 51 of the 72 cities that had received Cities Readiness funds were slated for elimination. These funds had been allocated to distribute and administer vaccines and medications during emergencies. All 10 states with laboratories with high-level chemical testing status may lose their status, leaving only the laboratory at the Centers for Disease Control and Prevention (CDC) with this Level 1 funding. CDC may have difficulty responding comprehensively to nuclear, radiological, and chemical threats because of these funding cuts. Twenty-four states were also in jeopardy of losing their career epidemiology field officers. It is possible to maintain a core and basic level of preparedness and response, but our public health leadership must develop strategies to make sure this core response coverage is developed and maintained even in the shrinking economic environment.

MANAGING A CRISIS

As discussed earlier in this chapter, a crisis is an unstable time. Normal activities are disrupted. The outcomes are unpredictable. Usual agency or organizational processes are affected. Much of the writing about crisis and its effects relates to the effects of crisis on an organization and its levels of functioning. The rationale is somewhat easy to explain. Whether we are discussing the effects of a natural disaster such as a hurricane or a terrorist event, it is the various governmental, nonprofit organizations, and other community

organizations that are called upon to handle these events. Thus, the management of the crisis becomes critical to its amelioration or solution. Being a prepared public health leader may also mean being an effective manager as well.

Most discussions on management of a crisis see crisis management techniques as being different during each stage of a crisis. Crisis planning has a precrisis stage; a stage in which the crisis or disaster, either natural or human made, occurs; a recovery phase; and some return to a new level of normality phase, which can start the entire planning and reaction cycle again. In discussing some of these issues, the time between crises seems to be shortening.[11] There seem to be many more crises today than in the past. In addition, crises sometimes overlap, or sometimes one crisis leads to another crisis. Thus, multiple crises may be occurring simultaneously. Fink saw crisis management in the context of a four-stage cyclical model.[12] Stage 1 is the prodromal crisis phase, which is basically a warning or precrisis phase. The important question to be answered is whether clues to a potential crisis exist. The events of September 11, 2001, have put Americans on constant alert for the possibility of an impending human-made disaster. The increases in crises since 1979 probably mean that we should be constantly on the lookout for warning signals.[13] Signal detection may be one of the most important components of crisis management. If public health leaders and their partners are vigilant in their signal detection efforts, many crises may be preventable.

The second stage is the acute crisis stage.[14] At this stage, the crisis has occurred. The major concern at this stage is how to control the crisis. It is at this stage that fear levels increase. Deaths may occur. Organizational structures collapse. It is here that the incident command system or its variations come into play to handle the crisis. This system is simply the model for the command, control, and coordination of a response to a community emergency that provides a well-defined structure for the coordination of the activities of community agencies and partners for dealing with the crisis.[15] These partners often include Federal Bureau of Investigation agents, local and state police, fire departments, local governmental agencies, public health leaders and their staffs, emergency medical system personnel, and many other community groups. The critical point here is that this system is basically a quasimilitary model that is management based. Each participant knows his or her place in the system and his or her responsibilities in it.

The third phase in the model is the chronic crisis phase.[16] Crises do not end abruptly. They have both short-term and long-term effects. This is also the phase in which the crisis management team tries to lessen the long-term effects of the crisis. With September 11, 2001, and the anthrax letters in our background, this phase is also one in which major preparedness planning occurs to try to prevent future crises. In fact, it almost seems that there is a feedback loop at play here with the management strategies of the prodromal phase of activity. Fink talked about the importance of recovery and the need for people to get back to normal activities. An additional concern in this stage is the possible legal action that may occur as a result, which lengthens the time required for any final resolution of the crisis. An important example of the activities at this phase of a crisis included a law passed by the U.S. Congress in 2002 to establish the National Commission on Terrorist Attacks Upon the United States. President George W. Bush appointed the commission, which held hearings in 2003–2004 and presented the final 9/11 Commission Report in 2004 with recommendations for changing the way the United States handles potential terrorist activities.[17] (The recommendations were controversial and led to a number of changes in the U.S. national security system.)

The fourth and final stage in the model is the crisis resolution phase. It is hoped that the crisis is eventually resolved and life returns to some semblance of normality. However, the reality is that things are never quite the same. All crises leave some scars. New levels of adaptation must occur. Crisis resolution may actually trigger a new prodromal phase of awareness in which there is a need to prepare for other potential crisis or emergency events.

Fink also presented a model for crisis forecasting that is useful for evaluating crisis events.[18] The tool that he used is called the crisis impact scale. For any category of crisis, it should be possible to determine the potential for the crisis to escalate in intensity, the media or governmental scrutiny of the event, the effect of the event or potential event on the operation of agencies or organizations or the community, the effect of the crisis (if it is an organizational one) on the image of the organization, and the financial effect of the crisis. To develop a crisis impact scale, a score is determined for each of these variables or any others that are determined to be relevant from 0 (the lowest impact) to 10 (the highest). The scores are then added together and divided by the number of variables included in the index. The final score from 1 to 10 gives a rough index of the impact of the crisis or the potential crisis on the agency or community.

Fink took this scale and tied it to a probability scale to create something he called a crisis barometer.[19] For each crisis or potential crisis, it should be possible to tie the crisis impact score to a probability of occurrence score. The combination of these two scales can give an indication of the severity of the crisis or potential crisis. For example, a crisis such as a terrorist event would probably fall in the red zone, which would be a high score on crisis impact and probability. It could also fall in the amber zone if the probability is lowered due to good preparedness activities. Although the barometer can be a useful tool, there are some cautions to keep in mind. It is important to plan for at least one potential crisis in each of the seven major crisis categories presented earlier, regardless of the low probability of that crisis category leading to a disaster in the near future.[20] The public health leader can learn much about disaster preparedness from simply being ready for any possible set of circumstances coming into being.

Although a prediction about the potential for a specific disaster may be useful to have, most disasters are unpredictable in terms of the time they will occur. For this reason, the crisis severity index may be more useful in that it adds a severity score to Mitroff's major crisis types. It is useful to develop a series of scenarios for each type of crisis at different severity levels. Then communities will be prepared for more crisis types at different severity levels. **Exercise 11-2** gives you the opportunity to experiment with the crisis severity index.

EXERCISE 11-2 Crisis Severity Matrix

Purpose: to learn how to use the Crisis Severity Matrix tool to make an initial evaluation of the severity of a potential crisis

Key Concepts: crisis, crisis severity matrix, crisis impact, terrorism

Procedure: To learn to use the Crisis Severity matrix, divide the class into groups of 8 to 10. With your group, plot the following crisis events by type and severity and have the group discuss its reasons for plotting them in the way the group did. What types of considerations ought to occur for a crisis of this severity? What would be different if the crisis were more or less severe?

1. Sudden death of the health director
2. Spread of the Zika virus into the United States
3. Terrorist attack at a New York City airport
4. Forest fires in California
5. Damage to a local health department's reputation.

A MODEL OF DISASTER PREPAREDNESS

To understand the management concerns related to a crisis, the preparedness or planning phase is explored next, followed by a discussion of some of the management activities related to recovery. There are many different approaches to disaster preparedness. Many of these approaches take an organizational management perspective to demonstrate the factors and procedures that need to be taken into account in preparing an agency or company for a possible crisis of whatever type. Other approaches take a more systemic view of disaster. Whatever perspective is taken, there are clearly overlaps in the approaches. This section views an approach taken by an organizational consultant.

In preparing for a possible disaster, Blythe discussed how organizations plan for potential disruptive events in their organizations.[21] One important distinction that was made involved the need to create two different crisis teams to address different aspects of a disaster. The first is a crisis management team for which seven steps were enumerated in putting this team together. The team should be multidisciplinary so that it represents all aspects of the organization. As a team, they need to develop decision-making strategies. As an organization sets up this special team, it is important to first decide the parameters by which the team will do its work. This becomes the scope of work. Second, the team requires two types of leaders—a senior-level supporter of the team's work and also a logistical person who can lead the team through the planning process in an orderly manner. The selection of members is an important third step because the team needs to represent all interests of the organization. Fourth, a planning agenda and a planning budget for the team are created. An important limitation related to local planning activities in health departments is that there are often no specific budgets for the agency's planning activities. For example, some local health departments have told me about the difficulty of getting local funding bodies to financially support the critical activities related to carrying out community health assessment activities. The sixth step in planning the work of the crisis planning team is establishing a schedule of regular meetings and also a process for running these meetings.

The crisis planning team may need to be restructured when the crisis management team has been designated. A crisis command center must be set up. Procedures for handling the crisis are included in crisis plans and crisis procedure manuals. If the crisis is primarily one that the organization handles, procedures differ from a crisis that has strong community effects. More is said about these issues when we discuss crisis response. There is a critical need for an organization to consider the development of a humanitarian response team.[22] The crisis management team often does not have the time during a crisis to deal with all the issues related to working directly with the families of victims or injured people during a crisis. Thus, the creation of this humanitarian team is an important consideration in crisis planning and response activities.

Blythe presented a six-step preparedness process that he named the "A,E,I,O,U, and Sometimes Y" approach.[23] The A step involves the analysis of vulnerabilities. One of the tools for this activity could be the Fink crisis barometer discussed previously. This step is concerned with the determination of foreseeable risks. If a crisis type has occurred previously, procedures and strategies may already be in place for dealing with it. Reality tells us that some crises or disasters are not predictable, and a process should be developed to address these events. There are ways to handle different crisis types.[24-26] Even though the crisis itself is unique, certain strategies can be developed to handle a crisis event that has not happened before. In determining vulnerabilities, all crises involve people, finances, and reputation.[27] Reputation involves the issue of blame and how the organization will be viewed relative to the way it handles these unexpected happenings.

The E step involves the evaluation of existing procedures for crisis management. A four-dimensional evaluation strategy for a crisis was suggested.[28] First, there would be a determination of the foreseeable risks of a particular event. Second, a determination would be made of the types of controls that are already in place for handling this special type of risk. Third, it would then be necessary for the crisis planning team to determine if these controls could be enhanced in any way. Finally, a determination could be made of any new or additional types of controls that might be needed. Relative to the issue of controls and new methods that might be required, an organization should consider the issues of time required to become prepared, money needed to implement the controls and other strategies, and the effort that these activities may require. One important strategy that is often used today to check these controls and strategies involves the use of exercises, drills, and other simulations.

The I step refers to the identification of new primary and secondary prevention preparedness procedures. This step involves a determination of types of possible incidents. For example, it is possible to use the crisis typology model as a guide. Next, ways and strategies to prevent these events are determined (primary prevention). A good example of this relates to airport security measures. Because it is possible to screen all airline passengers before they board a plane, the chances of an explosion in the air due to a passenger carrying explosives on his or her person is greatly diminished. Secondary prevention activities involve the creation of strategies for what happens if a crisis occurs so that further damage is prevented. If we take the anthrax letter example, primary prevention activities would entail the screening of all mail in the mailroom before it is delivered to the staff of the organization. Secondary prevention techniques might be to give all staff biobags if a suspected letter is delivered to a staff member.

Next, it is important for the crisis planning committee to organize the plan (the O step). The issue of the relationship between the culture and values of an organization and the ways that the various controls fit that culture is an important consideration.[29] With this step the issue of educating and training the staff of the agency becomes critical. The implementation of controls as well as the person who will be responsible for monitoring that implementation need to be determined. Values clarification in an organization is a necessary early step in the process. The values clarification activity can be used by organization leaders to work with staff to modify the organizational structure to accommodate these new crises protocols. It may well be necessary to modify the mission and vision of the organization to accommodate these changes. For example, a simple change in vision might be made. If the vision of the local health department is "Healthy people in healthy communities," it can be changed to "Healthy people in healthy and safe communities."

The U in the preparedness process refers to utilization of the plan. Utilization involves the creation or change of the crisis planning team into a crisis management team. It is here that the use of all those drills and tabletop exercises becomes important as a way to determine readiness. The debriefing and the lessons learned activities are important here. As it is not possible to determine when and if a disaster will occur, these drills and exercises should become a routine part of the activities of the agency or organization. Crisis leaders may be different people from those who lead in noncrisis times. Some leaders handle stress better than others. It is important to determine who the right leaders may be. Leadership is a complex phenomenon in that some leaders shine in crisis yet seem to be less effective in other times. An interesting example is Rudolph Giuliani, who was mayor of New York City during the crisis of September 2001.[30] Although there had been criticism of Giuliani's effectiveness as mayor prior

to September 11, 2001, most people agree that he became effective as a crisis leader during and after the terrorist events of September 2001.

The final planning step in the Blythe model refers to the need to scrutinize "yourselves," the Y step. This involves checking at regular intervals how well prepared the organization is for a potential crisis. It seems that the further away an organization is in time, the less the organization seems to be concerned about a potential crisis. What September 11, 2001 and the ISIS attacks of the last several years have taught us is that a crisis can occur at any time. It is always necessary to monitor our organizations to determine preparedness and readiness. This approach needs to become a critical part of the culture of the organization. If these preparedness activities are to occur, top management of our organizations must support them. Without this support, the plans will remain on the shelf, and preparedness will not become a reality.

PUBLIC HEALTH RESPONSE

When an emergency occurs, planning activities should have been completed. Public health response is about management strategies and addressing the emergency in a constructive way. Blythe discussed the immediate aftermath phase of a crisis.[31] The effects have to be determined quickly. It is best to imagine that the worst has happened and then figure out what needs to be done. The crisis management team and the crisis structure have to be called into action. Plans have to be implemented to handle the events over the first 72 hours. This has to occur even prior to receiving the information on what happened specifically, how bad the event or events were, what has been done and what needs to be done, and the ultimate question of whether the crisis can escalate.

Ten immediate actions should be taken in any crisis:[32]

1. Evaluation of potential for continuing danger
2. Verification of the availability and quantity of emergency vehicles
3. Availability of information to determine the severity of the emergency
4. The cordoning off of the incident area and its perimeter, if appropriate
5. Implementation of a notification process for the families of the wounded or deceased
6. Implementation of strategies to prevent escalation of the crisis
7. Following of protocol for notification of individuals to assist in the emergency

8. Implementation of communication procedures for the media
9. Determination of the legal and regulatory compliance process
10. Contact of any specialists that may be required

When a crisis occurs, it is important to contain the crisis as soon as possible. In an organization, this involves the activation of the crisis management team and a crisis command center. At a community level, the activation of the incident command system is comparable to what occurs at the organization level. The community response activity are discussed further later. What the crisis management group should do is determine and accurately document the emerging facts of the event. The development of a log of evolving facts itemizes what the emerging fact is, the time each fact was verified, and the person who discovered it. The crisis team should also prioritize its activities with the determination of who takes the lead on addressing any priority. There should also be a determination of an end time for a priority to be carried out. The goal of all response activities is to restore order as soon as possible.

Whereas preparedness is a planning and proactive stance, response is about reaction. Public health's involvement in response has often been tied to the issues of emerging infections and bioterrorism. Landesman discussed nine specific roles for public health in response situations:[33]

1. Developing and using multidisciplinary protocols for collaborative activities between public health agencies and their community and health agency partners
2. Determining the specific symptoms of various emerging infections and activating public health surveillance systems
3. Increasing laboratory capacity, upgrading public health laboratories, and developing communication criteria for a laboratory response capability that distributes information on suspected bioterrorism agents to the appropriate sources
4. Developing methods to deliver diagnostic and bioterrorism treatment protocols to the medical service community
5. Making sure response protocols are in place to reduce morbidity and mortality from a crisis event by stockpiling antibiotics and other drugs, using quarantine procedures if necessary, delivering medical services as necessary with surge capacity procedures available, using humanitarian notification procedures, and implementing a well-considered crisis communication network

6. Developing, testing, expanding, and implementing the Health Alert Network (national network to link state and local public health agencies and community and governmental partners through the Internet to get information on crisis events quickly)
7. Implementing procedures for handling victims
8. Developing training programs for the public health workforce
9. Implementing procedures for the resolution of public health legal issues relating to disasters

In the United States, the major process for response is tied to the activation of an incident command system or a number of variations of it. The models are built on a military approach to the handling of a crisis. A number of online courses on the incident command system are available to managers and leaders from the Department of Homeland Security and the Federal Emergency Management Agency (FEMA).[34] The following comments on the system come from the basic incident command system (ICS) course offered online. The incident command system is an organizational structure using command, control, and coordination approaches to response. The ICS model provides a means to coordinate the efforts of individual agencies (for our purpose, public health agencies as well) as the system works toward the primary goal of stabilizing the incident and protecting life, property, and the environment. The ICS has proved over time to be effective in the response to hazardous materials (HazMat) incidents; planned events; natural hazards response; law enforcement incidents such as potential riots outside a political convention facility; lack of a comprehensive resource management strategy; fires; multiple casualty incidents; multijurisdictional and multiagency incidents; air, water, and ground transportation incidents; search and rescue missions; pest eradication programs; and private sector emergency management programs.

As can be seen in **Figure 11-1**, the basic structure of the ICS system has five components. The command function is directed by the incident commander, whose job it is to manage the response to the crisis event. For many incidents, the commander is the senior first responder to the event. Because ICS is a management system with the roles and responsibilities of all participants well determined, it is worthwhile to list 12 of the management process activities involved in the system:

1. Establishment of command structures
2. Assurance of responder safety
3. Assessment of incident priorities
4. Determination of operational objectives

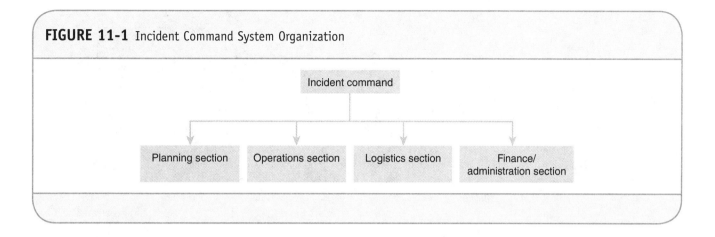

FIGURE 11-1 Incident Command System Organization

Incident command

Planning section   Operations section   Logistics section   Finance/administration section

5. Development and implementation of an incident action plan
6. Development of an organizational structure appropriate to the incident
7. Maintenance of a manageable span of control for all levels of the system
8. Management of incident resources
9. Coordination of overall emergency activities
10. Coordination of partnership activities
11. Authorization and management of the communication of information
12. Maintenance of cost and financial records for the incident

The second component of the basic ICS is the planning section, which collects, evaluates, disseminates, and uses the information about the development of the incident and the status of resources. This section may also develop the incident action plan that lays out the response activities and the use of resources for a specified time period. The third component is the operations section, which has the responsibility for carrying out the response activities described in the incident action plan. This section also directs and coordinates all ICS operations, assists the incident commander in the development of response goals for the incident, requests needed resources from the commander, and keeps the commander informed about the state of the response operation and the use of resources.

The next component in the basic structure is the logistics section, which has the responsibility for providing facilities, services, personnel, and materials to operate the requested equipment for the incident. The logistics section often has a medical unit to provide care for any incident responder who is injured. The final component of the system is the finance/administration section, which is responsible for tracking incident costs and reimbursement accounting. The five components of the ICS can be and often are expanded with the appropriate delegation of authority.

There is much discussion these days about an expanded model of ICS called *unified command*. This system brings together the incident commanders from all major organizations in the community or the state for the purpose of coordinating the response to a crisis event. This coordination does not preclude separate ICS activities related to specific jurisdictions. The unified command links the various ICS activities and allows the commanders to make consensual decisions. The unified command becomes responsible for the overall response and the overall management of the event.

To conclude this chapter, I want to tell you about a classic crisis case. The case involves Mary Mallon, George Soper, and Josephine Baker.

SUMMARY

A major purpose of this chapter is to give an overview to the whole field of emergency preparedness and response. As a field of practice, public health has many new responsibilities. Although much discussion of emergency preparedness and response has been about terrorist acts, the issues in a crisis are more complex. Types of crises have been reviewed and commentary given about the need to plan for different classes of crises. The planning-and-response approaches differ depending on the type of crisis. The one sure fact is that crisis and disaster events seem to be increasing. Readiness is clearly an important area of concern for the prepared public health leader. Crises go through a series of stages in which different activities occur. Discussions of the preparedness phase were viewed from the vantage point of an organization

PUBLIC HEALTH HEROES AND VILLAINS 11-1   The Reluctant Villain[35]

Mary Mallon was born in Ireland in 1869. She came to the United States at age 15 and settled in the New York City area. She took a job as a domestic worker. In the summer of 1906, Mary was engaged as a cook in the house of a banker named Charles Warren and his family on Long Island. In the late summer, 6 of the 11 people in the house were diagnosed with typhoid fever. Warren hired one of our leadership heroes George Soper. Mallon was hired by three other families and typhoid outbreaks occurred in those households as well. In 1907, Soper published his findings arguing that he believed that Mallon might be the source of the outbreak. He approached Mallon who rejected his conclusions and his requests for tests to determine if she was the carrier.

Mallon had now become known as Typhoid Mary. In 1907, the New York City Health Department sent our second leadership hero, Dr. Sara Josephine Baker, to talk to Mallon. Baker brought the police with her and they took our villain into custody. Mallon continued to deny any complicity in the typhoid outbreak. Tests were done and it was found that she had a nidus of typhoid bacteria in her gallbladder. Under a New York City charter, Mary was put into isolation until 1910. In 1910, she was released with the stipulation that she should change occupations.

By 1915, Mary had changed her name to Mary Brown and became a cook again. Wherever she worked, more typhoid cases occurred. She was arrested again and put into quarantine for the remainder of her life.

J. W. Walzer, *Typhoid Mary: Captive to the Public's Health* (Boston: Beacon Press, 1996).

---

as well as from the perspective of a community or country. The discussion of response was viewed from both an organizational perspective and a community one. The incident command system basic model and its extension into a unified command model was discussed as a model that is used in the United States. It does seem clear that many approaches to emergency preparedness and response fit into traditional management perspectives. The chapter ends with the story of a public health series of outbreaks caused by Typhoid Mary.

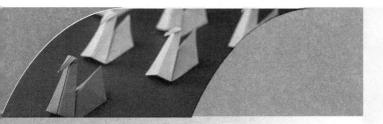

Discussion Questions

1. Discuss Mitroff's crisis types and different approaches to addressing each type of crisis.

2. What happened to U.S. readiness between 2003 and 2012?

3. Describe the stages of a crisis.

4. Why is it important to have a separate humanitarian response team during a crisis?

5. What makes Mary Mallon a public health villain?

REFERENCES

1. World Health Organization and Pan African Emergency Training Centre, Addis Ababa, *Disasters and Emergencies: Definitions* (Geneva, Switzerland: World Health Organization, 2002).
2. United Nations Disaster Management Training Programme, *Disaster Preparedness*, 2nd ed. (New York, NY: UN Disaster Management Training Programme, 1994).
3. I. Mitroff, *Managing Crises before They Happen* (New York, NY: Amacom, 2001).
4. I. Mitroff, *Crisis Leadership: Planning for the Inevitable* (New York, NY: John Wiley and Sons, 2004).
5. Mitroff, *Managing Crises before They Happen.*
6. Mitroff, *Crisis Leadership.*
7. Trust for America's Health, *Ready or Not? Protecting the Public's Health in the Age of Terrorism* (Washington, DC: Trust for America's Health, 2003).
8. Trust for America's Health, *Ready or Not? Protecting the Public's Health in the Age of Terrorism* (Washington, DC: Trust for America's Health, 2004).
9. Trust for America's Health, *Ready or Not?*, 2004.
10. Trust for America's Health, *Ready or Not? Protecting the Public from Diseases, Disasters, and Bioterrorism* (Washington, DC: Trust for America's Health, 2011).
11. Mitroff, *Crisis Leadership.*
12. S. Fink, *Crisis Management: Planning for the Inevitable* (Lincoln, NE: Authors Guild, Backinprint.com, 2002)
13. Mitroff, *Managing Crises before They Happen.*
14. Fink, *Crisis Management.*
15. B. Turnock, *Public Health: What It Is and How It Works* (Burlington, MA: Jones & Bartlett Learning, 2012).
16. Fink, *Crisis Management.*
17. National Commission on Terrorist Attacks Upon the United States, *The 9/11 Commission Report* (New York, NY: W. W. Norton & Co., 2004).
18. Fink, *Crisis Management.*
19. Fink, *Crisis Management.*
20. Mitroff, *Managing Crises before They Begin.*
21. B. T. Blythe, *Blindsided* (New York: Portfolio Penguin Putnam, 2002).
22. Blythe, *Blindsided.*
23. Blythe, *Blindsided.*
24. Mitroff, *Managing Crises before They Happen.*
25. Mitroff, *Crisis Management.*
26. C. M. Alpaslan and I. I. Mitroff, *Swans, Swine, and Swindlers* (Stanford, CA: Stanford Business Books, 2011).
27. Blythe, *Blindsided.*
28. Blythe, *Blindsided.*
29. Blythe, *Blindsided.*
30. R. W. Giuliani, *Leadership* (New York: Hyperion Books, 2002).
31. Blythe, *Blindsided.*
32. Blythe, *Blindsided.*
33. Landesman, *Public Health Management of Disasters.*
34. Department of Homeland Security, FEMA, *Basic Incident Command System (IS 195)* (Emmitsburg, MD: Department of Homeland Security, 2004)
35. J. W. Walzer, *Typhoid Mary: Captive to the Public's Health* (Boston, MA: Beacon Press, 1996).

CHAPTER **12**

Leadership at the Global Level

LEARNING OBJECTIVES

- Discuss the importance of global leadership development.
- Understand the principles at the intersection of global and domestic leadership.
- Recognize the importance of partnership in the solution of global health challenges.
- Describe SCOPE.
- Define the requirements and traits for successful global leadership skill development.
- Understand social entrepreneurship.

The fifth level of leadership becomes extremely important because public health has a global mission to improve the health of all humankind. The skills required at this level can be adapted from the skills, tools, and strategies learned at the first four levels of leadership. With a global perspective, there are a number of factors that can have an effect on health.[1] First, travel has become easy. People are able to travel from place to place in a short time. People migrate to new places to live. Health workers can be ready to aid in the prevention and treatment of diseases. Then, the health workers can return home as carriers of some of these diseases. Second, the diffusion of health-related information has accelerated. Medical and scientific information can cover the world in a short period of time. Third, technology, social media, telemedicine links, and new technologies that affect health move quickly. Other factors also affect health such as commerce and the move of goods and services, environmental factors, wars and terrorist acts, and crime. A final set of factors include those related to religion and culture. All these factors will affect the adaptive skills of a public health leader.

The requirements associated with successful leadership seem to present leaders with a moving target. Our world is ever changing at the same time that it appears to be flattening. As the world changes and flattens, public health leaders need to be flexible enough to adjust to these changes. Not only is public health important for building the infrastructure of public health in the United States, but leadership is important for building the infrastructure of public health around the world.[2] With the health issues of the world becoming more complex, the number of agencies addressing these issues appears to be increasing as well. Leadership is critical for this growing response to health and disease around the world. Public health leaders are needed for policy development, development and formulation of innovative public health and primary care programs, monitoring of global health issues, and evaluation. Leadership development programs similar to those in the United States are required throughout the world. If these programs can collaborate with the leadership development programs in the United States, coordinated global public health initiatives become more possible. As we look forward, we discover the necessity of understanding people throughout the world.

With an understanding of the importance of broadening our view of leadership and the recognition that being a leader on a global level may be different, it is worth briefly looking at the GLOBE Project (Globe Leadership and Organizational Behavior Effectiveness Research Project), begun in 1991 by Robert J. House of the Wharton School of Business. The GLOBE Project became a 62-society, 11-year study involving 170 researchers throughout the world. The respondents included more than 17,000 middle managers from about 950 organizations in the food processing, financial services, and telecommunications industries. The 62 societies were classified into 10 cultural clusters: Anglo Cultures, Latin Europe, Nordic Europe, Germanic Europe, Eastern Europe, Latin America, Sub-Saharan Africa, Arab Cultures, Southern Asia, and Confucian Asia. The GLOBE work was guided by the implicit leadership theory, which states that from childhood, people gradually develop beliefs about the characteristics and behaviors of leaders.[3] House and his colleagues reported that across all societies included in the GLOBE study, people expect their leaders to be trustworthy, just, honest, decisive, encouraging, positive, motivational, able to build confidence in others, and dynamic, and having foresight.[4] And yet leader effectiveness is clearly contextual and may vary in its presentation in different cultures and societies. With the flattening of the world, however, our overall expectation of our leaders may coalesce across cultures.

At the intersection of domestic and global leadership, it is possible to find eight principles at work.[5] First, the principle of reciprocity is important. Most leadership involves negotiation of something for something else. Leaders want to be treated with respect by other leaders and will return the respect to the leaders with whom they interact. Second, the principle of fidelity is critical. With fidelity comes trust and the opportunities provided by the small things that occur between leaders. Third, change is a guiding principle in most relationships. Leaders grow and require new approaches and strategies over time. Status quo is not a viable option. Fourth, the principle of investment is important. Leaders commit to lifelong learning for themselves and others. The next principle is service. If you serve, you put yourself on the road to greatness. Next is the principle of responsibility. By being responsible, we get positive returns and sometimes more than we expect. The seventh core principle involves perseverance, which leads to positive results over time. The final principle is unity, which helps an organization to grow and survive over time.

With a shift from a domestic look at leadership to a global look, public health issues such as global warming, pandemic influenza, child survival initiatives, human immunodeficiency virus/acquired immune deficiency syndrome, and other emerging and reemerging global infections become more and more important.[6] Public health leaders need to remove the barriers between countries to work in partnership with our public health colleagues all over the world. Hesselbein has stated that the time for partnership is now.[7] A world vision related to healthy families and children, excellent schools, decent and available housing and work opportunities, and health equity is necessary for international and global public health to become a reality.

It will not be possible to attain global health equity without partnerships. Collaboration becomes critical if we are to make these partnerships productive. In order to make collaboration work, it is important to move from a business-as-usual approach to a new stage of transformation that makes collaboration lead to positive change. In real collaboration, the partners become an integrated team that discusses and debates health challenges on a global level in order to come up with potential solutions to these challenges.[8] Rosenberg and his colleagues discuss the partnership pathway as going from its beginning or genesis through the first mile, the journey, and the last mile. In the genesis comes the realization that positive changes can occur. After the right partners come together during the first mile, a shared goal or goals are set, an appropriate structure is created, system-based strategies are created, and organizational roles are defined. During the journey, management issues predominate, necessitating a disciplined and flexible approach that guides the partnership. The individuals who compose the partnership also must take leadership roles at an individual level to bring about change. In the last mile, there will need to be adaptation to sustain the momentum created, transfer of control in a supportive way, understanding and communicating of the lessons learned, and finally a method for dissolving the partnership when the goal or goals are reached. One of the public health heroes demonstrates many of these important partnership issues.

A cautionary note is necessary here. Public health is not the same everywhere. It has different meanings from country to country. For example, leadership is practiced differently in countries where health service is provided at the national level. In these countries, there is a clinical focus, and almost all the leaders are physicians. Public health does not extend to social and behavioral scientists and other professions in the same way. In Asia, Africa, and some European countries, public health leaders put public health and clinical health together with a primary care focus. In the United States, we tend to separate the clinical focus from the public health focus. There are strengths and weaknesses in all of these systems. In partnerships, the cultural differences must be dealt with first before the partners can ever deal with collaboration and discover ways to work together.

There is the important question of what motivates people to become involved in these important partnerships or to become involved at an individual level in improving the health of the peoples of the world. Former President Bill Clinton explored some of these issues.[10] He pointed out the increasing involvement of private citizens in doing public good. With the end of the Cold War, Clinton believes that citizen advocacy has increased, specifically in democratic

PUBLIC HEALTH HEROES AND VILLAINS 12-1 D. A. Henderson, Hero[9]

Donald Ainslie Henderson, who was born in 1928, was an American physician, public health epidemiologist, educator, and dean of the Johns Hopkins School of Hygiene and Public Health from 1977–1990. He directed a 10-year initiative that led to the eradication smallpox throughout the world. As the chief of the Centers for Disease Control and Prevention during 1960–1965, Henderson worked with the epidemiologist Dr. Alexander Langmuir on a U.S. Aid for International Development program aimed at the elimination of smallpox during a 5-year period in 18 countries in western and central Africa. This study and other programs led Dr. Henderson to Geneva in 1966 to become director of the campaign to eradicate smallpox. Henderson worked with the World Health Organization staff and advisors from 73 countries. The last case occurred in Somalia in October 1977. In 1980 the World Health Assembly recommended that smallpox vaccinations could cease.

Henderson is clearly one of the major public health heroes of the 20th century for his work on smallpox and his ability to work globally with so many partners. In the 1980s, he served as dean at Johns Hopkins and in the 1990s he worked with the Office of Technology Policy, Executive Office of the President, and later as the deputy assistant secretary and still later as senior science advisor to the Department of Health and Human Services. In 1998, he became founding director of the Johns Hopkins Center for Civilian Biodefense Strategies. After the terrorist attacks on September 11, 2001, Henderson became director of the Office of Public Health Preparedness in Washington, DC. He left the post in 2004. Dr. Henderson died in 2016.

http://en.wikipedia.org/wiki/Donald_Henderson and http://www.smithsonianmag.com/science-nature/30-who-made-a-difference-d-a-henderson. Accessed June 15, 2016.

societies with elected governments. Second, he argues that the explosion of information technology and the globalization of commerce have made many individuals wealthy. Finally, charitable giving has also been democratized and has increased the number of people willing to help the rest of the world. Giving takes many forms, including the giving of money, time, things, skills, and so on. Another term for when individuals become involved in these international and global activities is *social entrepreneurship*. In spite of all the barriers that can be established to block change, social entrepreneurs make positive change and create model programs.[11]

GLOBAL HEALTH LEADERSHIP

Public health leaders gain from lifelong learning. Global public health cannot do its job effectively without a well-trained public health workforce. The best next step is a strong commitment to public health professionals who dedicate their lives to serving others in the international arena. It is not that leaders in the domestic arena have different leadership traits and abilities. The public health tasks of leaders domestically and globally are quite similar (see **Exercise 12-1**). According to Gundling and his associates, the differences are in the strategies used, business processes, and personal style changes related to different cultural environments.[12] The authors use a five-stage model called SCOPE. S is for seeing differences in the practice of leadership in different cultures. C is for closing the gap and building intercultural relationships. O is for opening the system in order to expand the ownership

EXERCISE 12-1 Applications of Domestic Leadership Tools to a Global Problem

Purpose: to apply strategic planning and continuous quality improvement techniques to a global malaria problem

Key Concepts: strategic planning, continuous quality improvement, leadership teams, malaria

Procedures: Divide the class into small groups of six to eight. Half the leadership teams will use the tools of strategic planning to address the development of a malaria eradication problem at a global level. The second half of the teams will use continuous quality improvement tools to address the eradication issue. The teams will report back to the class as a whole. Discussion will include any modifications of the tools for international work.

and involvement in the public health enterprise. By expanding ownership and promoting approaches to health that may have been developed elsewhere, future leaders from the local communities can be trained in many of these new strategies. P is for preserving balance and knowing when to change and when not to. Flexibility becomes critical. The idea of resilience becomes important, as does transparency. E is for establishing solutions and results that matter. The authors present the idea of a three-pronged process beginning with a recognition of past results, building intercultural trust, and promoting lifelong learning, leading to cocreation of solutions and then their implementation.

Global work is more than complex—it is multiplex.[13] Some requirements for the successful development of global leadership skills include the importance of becoming comfortable with the new environment and its culture. Second, knowing the language of the new culture will increase your ability to work in the new environment more quickly. Third, taking vacations in different countries will clarify differences between your personal experiences and the experiences of people in these other countries. Finally, volunteer abroad during your college years to increase your ability to adapt to other countries and cultures.

Gundling and his colleagues argue that there are 10 traits necessary to be a successful global leader.[14] Some of these traits are not required for domestic leadership activities. Coaching for global activities is very beneficial. The obvious first behavior is cultural self-awareness, which includes cultural issues related to health behavior. The second behavior looks for the unexpected or approaches in the environment that are unexpected for you as a new global leader. With a personal commitment to lifelong learning, there is also a strong readiness to learn new things. The third behavior relates to the skills tied to building relationships and the awareness of the importance of these relationships in building a solid public health agenda. Transactional leadership skills are the essence of this third behavior. The fourth behavior involves frame shifting. This behavior is more than paradigm busting. It involves flexibility in addressing health issues that may require leaders to change visions and directions from the way they have developed programs in the past. Expanding ownership is the next behavior. The community owns the programs and services. Agencies respond to community need with an awareness that ownership is a shared activity. The sixth behavior relates to the importance of the future development of leaders. Questions arise as to how to do this. Is it through formal training programs, mentoring and coaching, some other technique, or a combination of approaches? The seventh behavior involves the skills of adaptation and the adding of value tied to local public health practice. To do this well, leaders need to be totally self-aware and to have good judgment and perhaps restraint. These traits should be combined with cultural and contextual awareness. The eighth set of skills involves the learning of the values of the new culture in which you work and live and the flexibility to adjust to living in the new culture and developing relationships around the values of the community. Next, global leaders have to help generate solutions to public health problems in the new country and to generate solutions across functional boundaries. By putting organizational needs and consumers up front, the final behavior involves third-way solutions, which are integration of the same behaviors discussed previously.

SUMMARY

There is increasing concern about public health challenges and practice on the global stage. This chapter has begun a discussion of leadership challenges of growing concern in the 21st century. This chapter addressed some of these issues, including the GLOBE study, social entrepreneurship, giving at a global level, the SCOPE model, and the 10 global leadership behaviors.

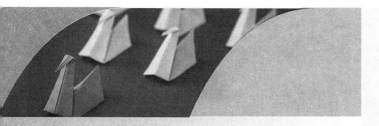

Discussion Questions

1. How would you develop a global public health leadership training initiative?

2. Compare and contrast public health leadership in the United States with leadership in other places.

3. Give domestic examples of the 10 behaviors discussed by Gundling and his colleagues.

4. Why is collaboration important in the eradication of diseases at a global level?

5. Discuss social entrepreneurship.

REFERENCES

1. J. I. Boufford, "Leadership Development for Global Health," in W. H. Foege, N. Baulaire, R. E. Black, and C. E. Pearson (eds.), *Global Health Leadership and Management* (San Francisco, CA: Jossey-Bass, 2005).

2. J. W. L. Roper and J. Porter, "Creating Public Health Leaders: Public Health Leadership Institutes," in W. H. Foege, N. Baulaire, R. E. Black, and C. E. Pearson (eds.), *Global Health Leadership and Management* (San Francisco, CA: Jossey-Bass, 2005).

3. http://www.grovewell.com/pub-GLOBE-leadership.html. Accessed March 1, 2012.

4. R. J. House, P. J. Hanges, M. Javidan, P. W. Dorfman, and V. Gupta, *Culture, Leadership, and Organizations* (Thousand Oaks, CA: Sage Publications, 2004).

5. J. L. James, *SHAPE: The Business of a Meaningful Life (Dust Jacket, 2013)*.

6. W. H. Foege, "Preface," in Foege, Daulaire, Black, and Pearson (eds.), *Global Health Leadership and Management*.

7. F. Hesselbein, "Leadership and Management for Improving Global Health," in Foege, Daulaire, Black, and Pearson (eds.), *Global Health Leadership and Management*.

8. M. L. Rosenberg, E. S. Hayes, M. H. McIntyre, and N. Neill, *Real Collaboration* (Berkeley, CA: University of California Press, 2010).

9. http://en.wikipedia.org/wiki/Donald_Henderson and http://www.smithsonianmag.com/science-nature/35-who-made-a-difference-d-a-henderson. Accessed June 15, 2016.

10. B. Clinton, *Giving* (New York, NY: Alfred A. Knopf, 2007).

11. D. Bornstein, *How to Change the World* (New York, NY: Oxford University Press, 2007).

12. E. Gundling, T. Hogan, and K. Cvitkovich, *What Is Global Leadership* (Boston, MA: Nicholas Brealey Publishing, 2011).

13. http://www.huffingtonpost.com/tayo_rockson/how-to-develop-global-leadership-skills. Accessed June 15, 2016.

14. Gundling, Hogan, and Cvitkovich, *What Is Global Leadership*.

CHAPTER **13**

Cross-Cultural Communication

Leaders require many tools and skills in carrying out their responsibilities. This chapter is concerned with communication skills. These skills are important at all levels of leadership. This chapter covers the use of these skills at the global level. Leading, after all, is an interactive process involving leaders and followers, and good communication among all participants in the process is absolutely essential.

Communication is the transfer of information and meaning,[1] and it has become even more important over the past decades—the start of the so-called information age—than it was previously. Information makes situations orderly, promotes change and growth, and defines reality. Meaning and how the messages are perceived and processed by the recipient of the message are extremely important. Communication plays an important part in the leadership process, as does the transfer of information in all the various forms that such communication takes, from face-to-face conversation to electronic transfer of data. In learning organizations, it is communication that drives the process. Leaders are teachers as well as learners. Their personal experiences lead the way

into their vision of the future. Tichy and Cohen stated that ideas, values, and energy drive the learning and teaching process.[2] These three skills give leaders an edge in solving problems and making decisions. This energy and passion gets communicated through many mechanisms that are discussed in this chapter.

THE COMMUNICATION PROCESS

It may be difficult to communicate effectively, but it is impossible not to communicate at all.[3] Each person's life is based on developing and using language to interact with other people. A communicative act involves the transmission of two messages. The first message is about the topic of the communication. The second message concerns the hidden or real agenda of the parties to the communicative act. Communication is an ongoing process throughout our personal and professional lives. It does not solve all our problems itself but must be accompanied by action.[4]

Barriers to Communication

There are many barriers to effective communication.[5] Communication can be blocked by forces within the participants as well as external forces. Nonverbal behavior—in the form of facial and hand gestures—can influence how a message is received, as can conscious and unconscious thoughts and distractions such as noise and motion. In addition, men and women have different conversational styles that can either enhance communication or create barriers to communication. The intended recipient's state of mind can be a major barrier to receiving a message. How many of us have found ourselves daydreaming in a public health agency staff meeting when the agency director or our supervisor asks our opinion on an issue? Other reasons for not listening to a conversation include anxiety about talking, lack of interest in the topic, thinking about what to say, confusion from trying to make sense of overly complicated discourse, lack of understanding of the professional lexicon, dislike of the speaker and his or her principles, and a desire to be somewhere else.[6] Lencioni has warned of the problems of boring and uninteresting meetings.[7] We need to be wary of death by meeting.

Sometimes a person says things in order to upset the listener, and the message does not completely reflect the ideas of the sender.[8] This type of behavior can create tensions in a marriage—or an agency. Suppose the director of a program says to a staff member, "John, I need further infant mortality data from the state. Please call the state epidemiologist and get me the infant mortality data for the last 5 years for our county. Would you also ask her to evaluate the data for us?" The true message might be this: "I don't trust John's interpretation of the data. John probably did it wrong." John may understand the underlying message, and his response—"I'll do it immediately"—might have as its underlying message, "Why doesn't he do it himself? I did the analysis correctly."

Other barriers include injecting into the communicative process a judgment that discredits the other party to the process and avoiding the concerns of the other party. Barriers can also be put into a number of categories including physical barriers as a group, cultural, perceptual, motivational, experiential, emotional, linguistic, nonverbal, and competition based.[9]

Communication Skills

Table 13-1 lists the communication skills needed by leaders at the six levels of leadership. A public health leader requires at least 20 communication skills. To be effective communicators, public health leaders must:

- fully develop their communication skills as part of their lifelong learning agendas
- respect the different agendas that coalition members or partners bring to the table

TABLE 13-1 Communication Skills and Levels of Leadership

Skill Categories	Personal Leadership	Team Leadership	Agency Leadership	Community Leadership	Professional Leadership
Interpersonal communication	X	X	X	X	X
Active listening	X	X	X	X	X
Public speaking	X	—	X	X	X
Interviewing	X	X	X	X	X
Written communication	X	X	X	X	X
Computer skills	X	X	X	X	X
Media advocacy	X	X	X	X	X
Cultural sensitivity	X	X	X	X	X
Feedback	X	X	X	X	X
Delegation	X	X	X	X	X
Framing	X	X	X	X	X
Dialogue, discussion, and debate	X	X	X	X	X
Meeting skills	X	X	X	X	X
Health communications	X	X	X	X	X
Social marketing	X	X	X	X	X
Coaching, mentoring, and facilitation	X	X	X	X	X
Conflict resolution	X	X	X	X	X
Negotiation	X	X	X	X	X
Storytelling	X	X	X	X	X
Journaling	X	—	—	—	—

- use the core functions and essential services of public health to guide communication with others
- use their communication skills to guide the transfer and management of knowledge
- be on the lookout for barriers to communication

CROSS-CULTURAL COMMUNICATION

As American society becomes more and more culturally diverse, it becomes important to develop skills that allow us to work with people born in other cultures. New technologies such as the Internet and social media have increased the connections between people from diverse backgrounds both in the United States and globally.[10] Even people from different English-speaking cultures still face problems in communication. For example, handshaking is acceptable in the United States but acceptable in some other cultures. In teamwork with people from different cultures, there needs to be awareness of cultural differences. Displays of humor may also be an issue.

If individuals have the opportunity to take an overseas leadership assignment, Shepard identifies three major stages to the expatriate experience.[11] First, it is important to address the actual process of changing countries. Second, there is the adjustment phase of moving to a new country and eventually determining what reentry to your birth country may be like. The third stage involves the complexity of reentry to the home country. The first stage of expatriation includes several phases:

1. Predeparture orientation
2. Selection protocols with preparation and possible counseling
3. Language and cultural training
4. Stateside mentor to help assignee in adjustment to new country
5. Relocation issues (involves what to do with U.S. house or apartment)
6. Concern for impact on family of the assignment (those who stay and those who go)
7. Relocation problems
8. New country mentor or cultural advisor

Exercise 13-1 is an interesting way to look at cultural differences with a communication twist.

INTERCULTURAL COMMUNICATION

As a graduate teaching assistant in 1960, I was introduced to the now classic book, *The Silent Language* by the cultural anthropologist Edward T. Hall.[14] This is the book that introduced the concept of "intercultural communication." Not all

---

EXERCISE 13-1 The Meal[12]

Purpose: to explore cross-cultural issues by eating at an ethnic restaurant

Key Concepts: world meal, cross-cultural communication

Procedure: Divide the class into small groups of four or six. Choose a restaurant that is not one that you usually attend. Arrange a lunch or dinner. Talk to the restaurant ahead of time to see if a staff member is available to talk to your team, and role play with different cultural rules to talk about cultural differences. Have the class discuss what is learned about the country and any communication concerns that arose.

Other possible exercises can involve the meaning of your name as discussed with others, discussion of unique family experiences with food, and role play with different cultural rules.[13]

http://www.wilderdom.com/games/MulticulturalExperiential-Activities.html. Accessed July 11, 2016.

---

communication is tied to words. Much communication is nonverbal. The nonverbal form of communication is often out of our immediate consciousness. Intercultural communications accept that cultures vary by context. Hall also introduced the idea of proxemics, which relates to how space is used to affect communications. His other concept was chronemics, which relates time to communication. All of this early work was developed as part of the training of individuals in the Foreign Service Institute.

More clarification of these communication concepts is needed.[15] Intracultural communication relates to communication between people of the same culture. Intercultural communication involves communication between people of different cultures. International communication involves communication between nations and governments. Public health communication can occur in all three of these. Perhaps these communication issues become clearer if we see them as part of a communication continuum. **Figure 13-1** is an example of an communication continuum. At the interpersonal level, cultural issues are diminished. The intimacy associated with a close personal relationship between the participants guides action. As pointed out cultural elements begin to affect relationships and interaction as we become involved in interactions at the intracultural level. Students in this class interact in the context of public health nursing, and other

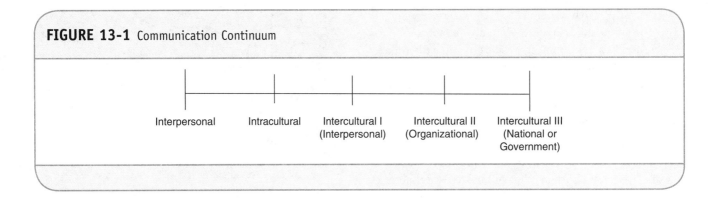

FIGURE 13-1 Communication Continuum

Interpersonal   Intracultural   Intercultural I (Interpersonal)   Intercultural II (Organizational)   Intercultural III (National or Government)

human services with the communication governed by rules of the field of study and/or the cultural rules of the classroom.

The center of the continuum involves intercultural communication in which individuals may be guided in their interactions by differences in the cultural orientations of the participants. Conflict and competition are often factors in this type of communication. When we take these intercultural differences into an organization with its own cultural orientation, there are often new challenges that affect the communication strategies of the different participants. When our communication moves to the national or international level, the challenges increase exponentially. As we advance through the continuum, leadership and the leadership mindset become more and more important.

The element of identity affects communication at all parts of the communication continuum. Identity is partially ascribed to you by demographic and role designations.[16] Ascribed designations include age, gender, race, religious affiliation, your name, and class standing, for example. The other aspect of identity is avowed or achieved identity resulting from life experiences. In order to understand the dynamics of intercultural communication, it is important to understand how ascribed and avowed identity of the participants affects communication and social action. These identity designations are demonstrated in the context of communication and social interaction.[17] Identity is seen in language used, nonverbal signs, clothing, and personality traits. Hecht and colleagues have identified three dimensions at work relative to cultural identity performance: the scope of performance, intensity of communication, and the salience of the performance.

At the national level, Hofstede argues that it is critical to understand the underlying cultural principles that guide the day-to-day communication and activities that affect that nation.[18] This is not to imply that there may not be cultural variation within that nation. It is possible to increase a leader's understanding of another nation by observing life along six cultural dimensions:

1. Is the nation individualistic or collective in orientation?
2. Does the nation tend to avoid uncertainty?
3. How much or how easy is it to relate to power in the nation (power distance)?
4. Is the nation competition oriented (masculine) or cooperation based (feminine)?
5. Is the nation oriented to short-term or long-term outcomes?
6. Do people feel in control of their lives or not (a happiness factor)?

The following hero story involves the public health professions and its leadership as strong believers in support of climate change arguments that have a negative impact on the health of people.

INTERCULTURAL COMMUNICATION TOOLS AND SKILLS

All the tools discussed in this text can be adapted for use at the global level. Effective intercultural communication ability is critical in global public health initiatives and activities. To be effective intercultural communication should be constructive and not suffer from ineffective action, misunderstandings, and breakdowns. Much of the interaction requires negotiation and an awareness that no one type of negotiation works in all situations. Up-to-date knowledge and skill for managing it are necessary. Emotional intelligence skills, especially empathy skills, are also required. Language skills are definitely important with some additional understanding of cultural gestures and nonverbal cultural cues. Different cultures not only have different customs, social mores, and thought patterns but different laws and social standards.

In addition to the study of language both verbal and nonverbal, the application of this knowledge needs to take

PUBLIC HEALTH HEROES AND VILLAINS 13-1 Public Health Leaders as Heroes

One of the most contentious social and health issues relates to climate change and whether it is occurring. The World Health Organization (WHO) has reported that social and environmental determinants of health affect health.[19] It is predicted that deaths caused by changes in climate will accelerate between now and 2050 to about 250,000 more per year. Associated costs will also increase substantially. Improvements in the control of greenhouse gases will affect health status. Thus, climate change will increase extreme heat problems, increase the number and severity of natural disasters and rainfall patterns, affect waterborne diseases and other diseases. Everyone will be at risk. WHO argues that much can be done from building global partnerships, raising awareness, more scientific work, and major support at a global level for the work of public health.

In 2008, WHO began a work plan on climate change and health that was completed and approved in 2009.[20] The plan listed several priority areas:

1. Support health systems in all countries.
2. Develop strategies and action plans to protect human health.
3. Share knowledge and good practice methods.

This all sounds good. Public health professionals and agencies internationally have taken a lead in arguing about the importance of recognizing the reality of climate change and the need to address the importance of immediate action. Public health leaders are our heroes in this fight. However, there are a number of entities working against public health:

1. Politicians in many countries believe climate change is a myth and argue that any changes in environmental states are temporary. Climate change is natural and has occurred for millennia.
2. Arguments are made against scientists who support climate change. Research funds for the study of environmental factors or surveillance of environmental change are significantly reduced or abolished.
3. Public health concerns are often ignored including successful programs to prevent these changes.
4. Public funding for prevention programs tends to disappear routinely especially during economic crises.
5. There are strong arguments made by the business community that environmental controls hurt businesses and lead to the loss of jobs.

Our public health leaders are heroes who struggle each day to improve the health of the public and are stopped by many enemies (villains) who have agendas that prevent public health from carrying out its work. What can we do to change this? This question is critical as a new generation of public health leaders enters the profession. Rimal and Lipinski argue that communication is an important part of the solution.[21] However, there are three important intervention concerns in communication. First, communication is received and processed by others through different social and cultural perspectives. Second, public health messages may be received with discrepancies between the sender and the receiver. We do not all process information in the same way. Third, communication is dynamic where sender and receiver change roles. Public health leaders must be aware of how their messages are received.

place in as positive an environment as possible. In intercultural work, the use of the language of other people at the beginning of a conversation is beneficial. Beforehand, discuss with your agency partners whether there are any cultural traps and problems that must be avoided. You can also gain cultural understanding by watching television in the new country you are visiting. As a leader, the burden is upon the outsider to adapt his/her behavior to the new cultural situation if at all possible. The leader should check understanding at several times during the interaction. It is fine to apologize if a misunderstanding occurs. For leaders, it is always beneficial to reflect on your experiences and if possible discuss your reflections with others.

SUMMARY

In this chapter, the importance of communication at the global level was discussed. With the breakdown of borders as diseases spread, the cultural and intercultural level was discussed. Tools, skills, and strategies for doing global work at the communication level were also discussed. Diseases seem to move freely from place to place. Public health has become a global enterprise. Communication at the cross-cultural and intercultural level were also discussed.

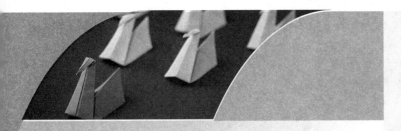

Discussion Questions

1. Why are communication skills important in international work?

2. What are examples of nonverbal communication in the United States?

3. Using Table 13-1, give examples of how these tools would be used at the international level.

4. What are the problems that one may encounter on reentry to the United States after an international health assignment?

5. Give examples of avowed identities of students in this class?

REFERENCES

1. S. P. Robbins and M. Coulter, *Management*, 11th ed. (Upper Saddle River, NJ: Prentice Hall, 2011).

2. N. M. Tichy and E. Cohen, *The Leadership Engine* (New York, NY: Harper Business, 1997).

3. R. B. Adler and J. M. Elmhorst, *Communicating at Work*, 5th ed. (New York, NY: McGraw-Hill, 1996).

4. Adler and Elmhorst, *Communicating at Work*.

5. J. G. Liebler and C. R. McConnell, *Management Principles for Health Professionals*, 4th ed. (Sudbury, MA: Jones & Bartlett, 2004).

6. D. Walton, *Are You Communicating?* (New York, NY: McGraw-Hill, 1989).

7. P. Lencioni, *Death by Meeting* (San Francisco, CA: Jossey-Bass, 2004).

8. D. Tannen, *That's Not What I Meant* (New York, NY: Ballantine Books, 1986.

9. R. Bolton, *People Skills* (New York, NY: Touchstone, 1986).

10. http://www.mindtools.com/CommSkll//Cross-Cultral-communication.htm. Accessed July 10, 2016.

11. S. Shepard, *Managing Cross-Cultural Transition* (Bayside, NY: Aletheia Publications, 1998).

12. http://www.wilderdom.com/games/MulticulturalExperientialActivities.html. Accessed July 11, 2016.

13. http://www.wilderdom.com. Accessed July 11, 2016.

14. E. T. Hall, *The Silent Language* (New York: Doubleday, 1959).

15. L. H. Chaney and J. S. Martin, *Intercultural Business Communication*, 6th ed. (Upper Saddle River, NJ: Pearson, 2003).

16. W. B. Gudykunst (ed.), *Theories of Intercultural Communication, International and Intercultural Annual, 12*, 99–120.

17. M. L. Hecht, J. R. Warren, E. Jung, and J. L. Krieger, "The Communication Theory of Identity: Development, Theoretical Perspective, and Future Directions," in W. R. Gudykunst (ed.). *Theorizing About Intercultural Communication* (Thousand Oaks, CA: Sage, 2005).

18. G. Hofstede and G.J. Hofstede, *Cultures and Organizations*, 2nd ed. (New York, NY: McGraw-Hill, 2005).

19. http://www.who.int/mediacentre/factsheets/fs266/en/. Accessed July 10, 2016.

20. http://www.who.int/globalchange/health_policy/who_workplan/en/. Accessed July 10,2016.

21. http://www.who.int/bulletin/volumes/87/4/08-056713/en/. Accessed July 9, 2016.

CHAPTER 14

Professional Leadership Development

LEARNING OBJECTIVES

- Distinguish between *public health* and *population health*.
- Explore options for *giving back*.
- Determine differences between coaching and mentoring.
- Discuss the steps in developing a learning contract.
- Understand how to give a good speech.

The sixth level of leadership is special in that it relates not only to development of our leadership skills but also what we do to build a unified profession of public health. Credibility and trust are clearly a part of this process. Public health struggles each day with the issues of credibility and trust as perceived by our communities. Americans in general and our political leaders often still see public health as health care for the poor or the uninsured. Although this is partially true, public health is about health for all people. In recent years, there have been attempts to replace the name of the field of public health with a more clarifying name: *population health*.

Population health seems to expand on the definition of public health to include health outcomes for all people as well as the distribution of these outcomes within a specified population.[1] Kindig and Stoddard further argued that population health also includes patterns of health determinants and also policies and interventions that link these two. Population health includes both the measurement of health outcomes as well as the roles of the various physical, social, and environmental determinants. A management specialty has evolved with the population health approach. In testimony before the U.S. House of Representatives Ways and Means Committee in 2002, Hillman stated that this new management approach uses a variety of individual, organizational, and cultural interventions to aid in the improvement of morbidity patterns and healthcare use behavior by different populations.[2] In population health, leaders use a multiplicity of techniques with different models of prevention and care being used by individuals from different backgrounds.

This brief discussion of population health points to an ever-changing approach to public health. This redefinition of the field will have ramifications for leaders and for the profession as a whole. It will continue to be a concern for the working public health leader to share his or her experiences with the evolving models of health for all people.

The sixth level of leadership involves sharing our leadership experiences with others including model public health programs that worked—our best practices, how we have used leadership to create positive change in our communities, how we have created partnerships to enhance our work, what advocacy programs worked, and how we influenced policy. In this chapter, we explore some methods for using our leadership abilities to engage the public health profession.

GIVING BACK

Many of us are fortunate enough to get the opportunity to expand our leadership knowledge and to develop our personal talents into strengths through the opportunity to get training in areas that enhance our skills. Leadership development programs are an important mechanism for helping to make our work more effective in the real world. Thus, a leadership development program becomes a gift to ourselves. We get a chance to see the world in new and exciting ways.

However, it is important to use our gift wisely and in ways that benefit those with whom we work, our community partners, and people for whom we have strong affection. A gift of knowledge needs to be shared. Giving back is an important part of our responsibility to serve our organizations and communities. Leadership is not only about creating a vision; it is about improving the quality of life of all those with whom we work and whom we serve.

Training is for the mind. Leadership is to work with others for change. Giving is for the soul. Bolman and Deal discuss soul in the context of finding meaning in all parts of our lives.[3] Soul is not only about our faith; soul is what makes us human. Former President Clinton pointed out that giving changes the world.[4] There are many ways to give including money, time, things, and skills. The use of our talents and skills is what guides us as we practice our leadership. Bornstein discussed how new ideas come into being and how people create change to make their ideas a reality.[5] There are many individuals throughout the world who become social entrepreneurs an spend their lives in giving back to their communities, countries, and to the world at large. It is not as much about money as it is in sharing ourselves with our friends on this planet.

Leaders are committed to lifelong learning although leadership in practice is more about the applications of what we have learned to our field. For public health leaders, leadership is the ability to improve or provide direction for the improvement of the health of the public. In return for the gift of learning, there are at least 10 ways that we can give back our knowledge to our organization and our communities. First, we can share our knowledge with others through mentoring and coaching (see next section). Work with new colleagues to help them develop their management and leadership skills. Mentoring and coaching increases the value of ourselves and others. It is a return on investment in our own training and education. Mentoring and coaching are capacity builders for our organizations in that our personal commitment to others increases and spreads the knowledge around. Second, it is important that we consciously commit to doing things in a different way after we return to work after a training workshop. Although our organizations tend to be the same on our return, we need to be different if change is to occur. We must start with a change in behavior before values begin to change.

Third, leaders are often outliers. Gladwell has described outliers as individuals who have been given opportunities to lead and have grabbed these opportunities.[6] It is important for leaders to give opportunities to others. Leadership programs have been one important such opportunity in recent years. If you are fortunate enough to be the recipient, you may have the opportunity to give others a similar opportunity. Training is one of the things we can do for others. In addition to searching for new leaders, we can fourthly give training workshops in our own agency.

Most people are linear thinkers. Successful leaders tend to be systems thinkers. They tend to see beyond the narrow vision of today and concentrate on the big vision of tomorrow. They see their organization work in terms of its impact on the community that they serve. Leaders who give back teach others to appreciate the wider view. They concentrate on sharing the vision in language that others can understand. This is not an easy task and may take many explanations and refinements to make the system intelligible to others. It is critical to use the tools of leadership in a systems way. Many tools from strategic planning, conflict resolution and negotiation, and continuous quality improvement lend themselves to systems work.

Another way to give back is to tell stories that demonstrate your personal leadership or the leadership of others. Stories bring our fields of practice to life. People react strongly to personal as well as work-related stories. Leaders also have an obligation to discuss best practices at local and national professional meetings. It is important to document our work in local newspapers as well as in professional journals. Every time we write and publish, we give back to our field and our colleagues. Finally, we practice what we preach every time we return our leadership gift to our organization and community.

Whenever we take a training course, return to school for advanced education, or do any of the activities discussed here, we are using the gift of leadership to change the lives of others as well as ourselves. Leadership development and its impact are a gift that keeps on giving. **Exercise 14-1** gives you the opportunity to record your giving-back contributions.

EXERCISE 14-1   Giving Back

Purpose: to explore your own contributions

Key Concepts: giving back, journaling

Procedures: In your leadership journal or a new contributions book, record your giving-back activities. Continue to record these events over time.

MENTORING AND COACHING

Mentoring and coaching are critical leadership activities. Leadership development depends on experienced leaders acting as role models for novice leaders. Leader-mentors and coaches need to understand leadership and promote the development of leadership skills by others.[7] Mentoring and coaching novice and experienced leaders have become even more important in the past few years than in the previous century. An important aspect of the increase of interest in mentoring, coaching, and training is the acceptance of life-long learning by leaders and managers as well as young public health professionals. As leaders, we plan our actions as a key aspect of our work and nonwork lives. We often plan life projects related to family, work, recreation, creative activities, and social action and our contributions to our social justice values.[8] Life projects give us direction and motivation.

In general, mentoring is a form of one-to-one teaching, to be contrasted with training, which involves instructing more than one person. Public health leaders do engage in training as well, such as in team building.[9] A public health leader might facilitate the team-building process by presenting guidelines to the team as a whole and also acting as a mentor for each team member. (Peer mentoring is also possible in a team situation.) Mentors generally do not give formal instruction but instead teach by example.[10] They understand how public health works and can explain the written and unwritten laws to their mentees.[11]

Some authors use the term "coaching"[12] rather than "mentoring." This has become confusing. Coaching is more about how to do a specific job more effectively, and mentoring is more about career and career choices.[13] Leadership development is important in both mentoring and coaching situations. The relationship between the mentor and the mentee or the coach and the coachee are true partnerships, and each involved individual should gain something from it (in other words, it should be a win–win relationship). It should also be contractual, which means that the needs and expectations of both parties should be addressed when the relationship is first established.

Mentors can help in the training of a team by guiding the leadership learning of each team member. The challenge for the mentor in formal training situations is to help the team become a learning community. The mentor must be committed to the goals of the team and facilitate the learning process for the team members, including through direct one-on-one interaction related to the professional needs of a given member. It may also be beneficial to help the trainee address job-related issues, which means that a modified coaching relationship will be established in addition to the mentoring one. Thus, the boundary between mentoring and coaching becomes blurred.

The learning contract model has been used by both coaches and mentors to guide their development process with their protégés.[14] The learning contract has evolved from the literature on adult learning. In 1970, Knowles used the concept of andragogy to discuss the four assumptions of learning by adults.[15,16] The major assumption is that adult learners tend to move from a dependency model where they are passive learners to an approach that is more active and self-directed. Adult learning is also experiential in that adults incorporate their experiences into the learning process. Third, adults tend to accept that learning will be a part of all new jobs and activities in which they engage. Finally, adults learn new knowledge as required by new tasks. Leaders who accept adult learning approaches tend to become ecological leaders who tie their learning experiences to the contexts in which they work and play.

In developing a learning contract, several steps are followed:[17]

1. Diagnose personal learning needs.
2. Specify learning objectives.
3. Designate learning resources and strategies.
4. Determine target dates for completion.
5. Specify ways to determine that objectives are met.
6. Determine how evidence will be judged.
7. Review the contract personally and also with your mentor or coach.
8. Carry out the goals of the contract.
9. Monitor the process.
10. Evaluate the contract.

One way to translate these steps into a usable form is to create a chart with the objectives (step 2) on one axis and the remaining steps on the other axis as columns. Step 1 can be listed separately.

Friendship is an important element in mentoring and coaching, as is trust in a training situation. In discussing the importance of having vital friendships at work that are relationships benefitting both parties, Rath defined eight types of friendship roles: builder, champion, collaborator, companion, connector, energizer, mind opener, and navigator.[18] A friend at work may have a combination of the behaviors associated with each role. Mentors and coaches tend to be builders who are friends and who support your personal growth and are not threatened by your progress. When you appear valued by your organization, you enjoy the work more and become

PUBLIC HEALTH HEROES AND VILLAINS 14-1 Leo Levy, Hero

In 1965, I was finished with my graduate preliminary exams and began to search for a position where I hoped to complete my doctoral dissertation. One of the individuals who agreed to meet with me was Dr. Leo Levy, director of the Division of Planning and Evaluation of the Illinois Department of Mental Health and Developmental Disabilities. Levy was a psychologist with special training in the area of prevention studies. I met him and a colleague with a specialty in advanced statistical analysis. Levy informed me that he was putting together a high-powered research and program development team from the social sciences. He said he was impressed with my medical sociology background and wondered if I would consider a position as a social epidemiologist. The position would be located in the Chicago area, which was my hometown. I remember that I was intrigued at the time although I was not sure what a social epidemiologist does.

I decided to take the job thinking that a job in the practice world would provide me with excellent work experiences. Dr. Levy immediately began to work with me and guide my early work. He spent much time with me as we developed a work plan that would involve me in social epidemiologic concerns for 4 years. Levy also told me that one of the projects might serve me well as a doctoral dissertation. He nurtured me and gave me access to a major database that I could use. This database became my first book, which I coauthored with Levy.[20] My doctoral committee turned down my proposal related to this database saying it was not my own original set of data. I worked with Levy and other staff on a number of other research papers during this period from 1965–1969.

By 1970, Illinois had a new governor and the planning division was abolished, I spent the time working on a new dissertation topic on which Levy gave me advice. Levy left the department in 1970 and went to the University of Illinois Medical Center and in the early 1970s became one of the first faculty members of the new School of Public Health. Levy brought me to the university to join the new school as an assistant professor. Levy clearly was a hero to me and was always available to meet and coach me. After he retired from the university, I met him again a year before his death in New Mexico. At our last meeting, he still remained a good friend and colleague.

---

more committed to the work of the organization. In my last book, I told the story of a man who influenced me strongly in graduate school and remained a friend and mentor for many years afterwards.[19] I now want to tell the story of a second mentor in my professional life who also became my hero and my friend.

PUBLIC SPEAKING

An important part of giving back is talking to our professional colleagues through workshops, keynote addresses, speeches about our work, and poster sessions. In addition, many of us have attended numerous presentations by national leaders at conventions, conferences, luncheons, and other professional venues. As I was preparing to give a keynote address at a convention a few years ago, I noticed a pattern in the way that speakers gave their talk to a large professional group. Interesting characteristics of speaker styles could be seen. Perhaps a touch of humor will allow us to see how formal addresses are made and to allow us a chance to have some fun with ourselves. (The italics indicate more generally how not to give a talk). This section of the chapter perhaps creates a template for giving a formal group presentation.

Here are 10 rules to help you to give formal presentations:

1. *Stand behind the podium so that you look professional and clearly an expert.* The podium also gives the professional organization the chance to advertise themselves in front of the podium. Speakers tend to hold onto the sides of the podium to protect themselves from falling off the dais. The microphone is attached to the podium so that you cannot walk around the dais.

2. *Follow the dress code for speakers even if the clothes make you feel uncomfortable.* Men should wear suit jackets and conservative ties. Women do have some clothing options. A Hillary Clinton pantsuit would be appropriate or an unpatterned dress with a jacket would also work. Shorts and blue jeans are out for both men and women.

3. *Do not look at the audience when you read your paper, but if you do look outward make it a quick look.* Our presentations tend to be more and more complex these

days. Thus, many speakers write out their presentations in order to keep in the time frame for their presentation and also not to forget any critical content. However, audience members have reported that they forget many of the details of these presentations as soon as they leave the auditorium or large meeting room. Simplicity is still the best way to present.

4. *Put lots of numbers in your slide presentation so that nobody beyond the first three rows can see them.* Go through the slides with a slide commentary that does not relate to the slide presentation. Stories and anecdotes work better.

5. *Tell jokes and stories with no relevance to your talk.* Somebody has told the speaker that humor adds to the presentation and helps the audience to keep alert and not be concentrating on their cell phones. Humor is clearly beneficial if the speaker shows the relationship between the joke or story to the content of the talk.

6. *Talk about the theme of the meeting in as confusing a manner as possible.* The organizers of the meeting want the meeting theme to be part of the plenary sessions. However, many presenters have canned speeches that they have given at numerous conferences and meetings and often struggle to address the theme in their talks. Thus, the theme portion of the talk often seems unrelated to the speech being presented.

7. *Do not involve the audience in the presentation.* Plenary talks tend to be talking head experiences. We do not want audience members interrupting the flow of the presentations. We clearly do not want the audience involved in the presentation through exercises and dialogue. In order to show the dominance of the speaker in the process, they often run overtime. In actuality, a question and answer period helps in the resolution of this problem.

8. *Leave quickly after your presentation or do not leave time for questions that you may not be able to answer.* It also seems possible that many speakers have canned answers to potential questions that may be asked or answers that do not really address the question. Even when a question is asked that does not fit their planned answer, they give the answer anyway.

9. *Arrange the room, auditorium, in classroom style so that audience members can't see each other sleep.* It is important for the speaker to give the impression that everyone in the room loves every word that the speaker says. Seeing people sleep does not help the speaker to give an image of great expertise in the talk by the audience. Climate control can also help here.

10. *Mumble and speak in a monotone.* Because much of the talk is overly technical and complicated, mumbling helps to confuse the audience. Giving the audience a talk in a monotone seems to not interfere with the sleep patterns of the audience and the appearance that the speech is not even of interest to the speaker.

Although these 10 rules are presented in a humorous way, there are many clues to giving a speech in a dynamic and interesting way. The real challenge to the speaker who wants to involve the audience in a learning experience is to break as many of these rules as possible.

SUMMARY

The final level of public health leadership is a level on which the leader finds his or her place in the public health profession. Leaders struggle with the limitation of the words *public health* and the issues around the evolving idea of *population health*. An important part of this sixth level relates to our giving back. Public health leaders believe they have an obligation to share their experiences with other public health and health professions leaders and service providers. They also share their expertise with the communities that they serve. These are important characteristics of servant leaders. They also mentor and coach young leaders in the field of public health. Another way that leaders share their knowledge and experiences are through talks at professional meetings.

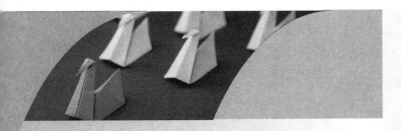

Discussion Questions

1. What are the similarities and differences between a public health approach and a population health approach to service?

2. Why is *giving back* important for a public health leader?

3. What are the differences between mentoring and coaching?

4. What are the lessons learned from this chapter about giving an oral presentation at a professional meeting?

REFERENCES

1. D. Kindig and G. Stoddard, "What Is Public Health," *American Journal of Public Health* 93, no. 3 (2003): 380–383.

2. M. Hillman, Testimony before the Subcommittee on Health of the House Committee on Ways and Means, hearing on promoting disease management in Medicare. http://waysandmeans.house.gov/Legacy/health/107cong/4-16-02/4-16hill.htm. Accessed October 12, 2008.

3. L. G. Bolman and T. E. Deal, *Leading with Soul*, new and revised (San Francisco, CA: Jossey-Bass, 2001).

4. B. Clinton, *Giving* (New York, NY: Knopf, 2007).

5. D. Bornstein, *How to Change the World*, updated ed. (New York, NY: Oxford University Press, 2007).

6. M. Gladwell, *Outliers* (New York, NY: Little, Brown, 2008).

7. R. Bell, *Managing as Mentors*, 2nd ed. (San Francisco, CA: Berrett-Koehler, 2002).

8. T. Fields, *Planning Life's Projects* (Tucson, AZ: Hats Off Books, 2001).

9. F. Wickman and T. Sjodin, *Mentoring* (Chicago, IL: Irwin Professional Publishing, 1996).

10. Bell, *Managing as Mentors*.

11. B. Nelson and P. Economy, *Managing for Dummies* (Foster City, CA: IDG Books Worldwide, 2010).

12. T. Peters and N. Austin, *A Passion for Excellence* (New York, NY: Random House, 1985).

13. Harvard Business Essentials, *Coaching and Mentoring* (Boston, MA: Harvard Business School Press, 2004).

14. M. S. Knowles, *Using Learning Contracts* (San Francisco, CA: Jossey-Bass, 1986).

15. M. S. Knowles, *The Modern Practice of Adult Education*, revised and updated ed. (Chicago, IL: Follett Publishing Co., 1988).

16. M. S. Knowles, R. A. Swanson, and E. F. Horton III, *The Adult Learner*, 7th ed. (New York, NY: Butterworth-Heinemann, 2011).

17. R. Hiemstra and B. Sisco, *Individualizing Instruction: Making Learning Personal, Empowering, and Successful* (San Francisco, CA: Jossey-Bass, 1990).

18. T. Rath, *Vital Friends* (New York, NY: Gallup Press, 2006).

19. L. Rowitz, *Public Health Leadership: Putting Principles into Practice*, 3rd ed. (Burlington, MA: Jones & Bartlett Learning, 2014).

20. L. Levy and L. Rowitz, *The Ecology of Mental Disorder* (New York, NY: Behavioral Publications, 1973).

Professional Public Health Organizations

Public health seems to have an ever-changing landscape. Leaders cannot always predict what tomorrow's public health challenges will be. We look to a number of governmental and professional organizations to work with us in addressing these new challenges. In order to use our adaptive leadership skills to address these challenges, we have to investigate whether our present tools will help us or whether we will have to adapt them in new ways or learn some new skills. Thus, we can say that the skills needed to be successful today and tomorrow are not the same as they were 50 years ago. Priorities in public health challenges also change. We also seem to have less respect for our political leaders as well as the decisions related to health and other issues. For example, as I write this Congress has so far voted down authorization for moving forward on addressing the problems associated with the Zika virus.

We can also see a number of skills needed for today's public health work as contrasted with other time periods. Here is a partial list of some new leadership skills for the work of today:

1. A sense of humor is critical. Humor often relieves stress.
2. Regardless of your position on critical and non-critical issues, ethical decision making should guide performance.
3. Science must take precedence over politics. Leaders must not discount scientific evidence—for example, regarding climate change. Science can be questioned but must still guide action.
4. Racial and religious dynamics are real. Leaders must find ways to deal with the result of these dynamics.
5. Respect our leaders even if we do not always agree with them. Demand respect in return.
6. Leaders should not distort facts in order to promote their private agendas.
7. Collaboration is the secret of success in today's world.
8. Develop your adaptive leadership skills. These skills are useful for most challenges.
9. Avoid toxic leaders if at all possible.

CENTERS FOR DISEASE CONTROL AND PREVENTION (CDC)

Public health leaders have several major resources in the Centers for Disease Control and Prevention, a source of information, data and surveillance on diseases, expert advice, collaboration on local and state public health work when needed, disaster information and alerts when available, and information on the spread of new diseases and threats around the world. The main goal of CDC is health protection and safety. The goal becomes realized through the control and prevention of disease, injury and disability. The attention of the agency is on infectious diseases, food-borne pathogens, environmental health, occupational health and safety health promotion, injury prevention, training of health professionals, leadership, and global health issues. CDC is clearly an important public health partner. In 2016,

CDC celebrated its 70th anniversary. During this time, the agency has been engaged in the control, containment and elimination of diverse health threats. Some specific examples of agency accomplishments include:[1]

1. Controlling malaria, polio, typhus, and cholera epidemics
2. Moving toward the eradication of smallpox
3. Leading toward the possible eradication of polio
4. Fighting malarial transmission in the United States
5. Addressing Middle East Respiratory Syndrome (MERS) and enterovirus outbreaks
6. Fighting Ebola in West Africa
7. Managing antibiotic-resistant infections, birth defects, diabetes management, and attention to other chronic diseases
8. Addressing challenges related to acquired immune deficiency syndrome (AIDS), the Zika virus, and other infectious diseases

On July 1, 1946, the Communicable Disease Center (first CDC name) opened its doors in a small building in Atlanta. Prior to 1946, the center was an Office of Malarial Control in war areas. This new center was charged with the prevention of the spread of malaria across the United States.[2] The new organization was founded by Dr. Joseph Mountin, a public health physician who advocated for public health throughout his life. He wanted the new agency to expand its responsibilities to include other communicable diseases. A controversial study of untreated syphilis in Black males (Tuskegee project) between 1932 and 1972 became associated with CDC in 1957 although there were staff at CDC who had been part of the Tuskegee study before that. The first director of the new center, Raymond Vonderlehr, had also been a director of the Tuskegee study. CDC has had negative reactions over the years in such areas as AIDS and ineffective communication, immunization concerns, and so on. On the whole, the agency has helped public health leaders do their work more effectively.

The agency became the Center for Disease Control in 1970 and the Centers for Disease Control in 1980. Congress added the words "and Prevention" to the agency's name in 1992. There have been 16 directors of the agency since its beginnings as an office in 1942. Most of these individuals had major contributions to public health during their tenure and afterward. The directors were:[3]

1942–1942 Louis L. Williams, MD
1944–1946 Mark D. Hollis, ScD

PUBLIC HEALTH HEROES AND VILLAINS 15-1 Joseph W. Mountin, MD, Hero[4]

Joseph W. Mountin (1891–1952) was an important public health leader of the first half of the 20th century. Mountin received his medical degree from Marquette University in 1914. In 1917, he entered the U.S. Public Health Service as a scientific assistant. He was involved in the management of safe and healthy zones around military camps that were constructed during World War 1 in several areas. In July 1918, he was commissioned as an assistant surgeon and received training involving quarantine duty, marine hospital service, and health administration. From 1922 to 1926, he worked with the Missouri State Health Department where he helped organize local health departments.

During the 1930s, Mountin worked in Washington in offices related to public health. In the late 1930s, he was director of the Office of Public Health Methods. He analyzed the nation's health resources and their relationship to public health. He engaged in a number of analytical studies on U.S. hospitals, which led in the 1940s to Hospital Survey and Construction Law (Hill-Burton). During World War I, he took responsibility for the direction of the national initiative for emergency health and sanitation. He became interested during the war in programs related to malarial control. His work on malaria led to his belief that a national center should be created to address concerns related to malaria and other infectious disease. This was the beginning of the Centers for Disease Control and Prevention in Atlanta, Georgia, in 1946. In 1947, Mountin initiated the Framingham Heart Study. He was also a supporter of the inclusion of public health and child health services as a member of the World Health Organization's Expert Committee on Public Health Administration. At the time of his death in 1952, he was still serving. He was clearly one of our public health heroes and definitely a leader.

https://en.wikipedia.org/wiki/Joseph_Walter_Mountin. Accessed July 23, 2016.

1947–1951 Raymond A. Vonderlehr, MD
1952–1953 Justin M. Andrews, ScD
1953–1956 Theodore J. Bauer, MD
1956–1960 Robert J. Anderson, MD, MPH
1960–1962 Clarence A. Smith, MD, MPH
1962–1966 James L. Goddard, MD, MPH
1966–1977 David J. Sencer, MD, MPH
1977–1983 William H. Foege, MD, MPH
1983–1989 James O. Mason, MD, MPH
1990–1993 William L. Roper, MD, MPH
1993–1998 David Satcher, MD, PhD
1998–2002 Jeffrey P. Koplan, MD, MPH
2002–2008 Julie Gerberding, MD, MPH
2009–2016 Thomas R. Frieden, MD, MPH

The founder of CDC provides us with an excellent public health story.

AMERICAN PUBLIC HEALTH ASSOCIATION (APHA)

For almost 150 years, the American Public Health Association has been the major voice of the public health professions. As an organization, APHA speaks with the voices of thousands of public health professionals. The first 25 years of the association saw major medical breakthroughs and discoveries including Koch's B. tuberculosis in 1882, Pasteur's vaccines against rabies in 1884, Loeffler's discovery of B. diphtheria in 1896 and its antitoxin by Behring in 1896.[5] Beginning in 1912, the association began its important journal, the *American Journal of Public Health*. In 1910, a series of papers was presented arguing that the state of education programs in public health was poor. Over the last century, this has led to the development of high-quality schools of public health and public health programs that all now go through an accreditation process. Annual APHA conventions now bring over 10,000 public health professionals together to address key public health concerns, advocacy initiatives, key advancements in research and service, and a meeting of public health and governmental leaders from all over the United States and other countries.

The executive director of the association currently is Dr. Georges C. Benjamin, who is also one of our public health heroes.

SOCIETY FOR PUBLIC HEALTH EDUCATION (SOPHE)

Most members of SOPHE are also members of APHA. The Society for Public Health Education was organized in 1950 to promote the health of all people in the United States through education.[7] The organization encourages research on the theory and practice of health education. It also seeks to promote performance standards for public health education programs

---

PUBLIC HEALTH HEROES AND VILLAINS 15-2   Georges C. Benjamin, Hero

Dr. Georges C. Benjamin has been the executive director of the American Public Health Association since 2002.[6] He began his career in Tacoma, Washington, in 1981 managing a 72,000-patient ambulatory care service as chief of the Acute Illness Clinic at the Madigan Army Medical Center. Later he served as chief of emergency medicine at Walter Reed Army Medical Center. After he left military service, he became chair of the Department of Community Health and Ambulatory Care for the District of Columbia General Hospital. In the 1990s, he became secretary of the Maryland Department of Health and Mental Hygiene. He has established a record of leadership as an excellent administrator, author, and speaker.

Over his 14 years as executive director of APHA, Dr. Benjamin has taken on many public health battles including:

1. Yearly battles over Congressional funding for public health

2. Fight for Congressional funding for Zika virus response (2016)
3. Education of policy makers on public health issues
4. Work on engaging the public around the nation on public health
5. Promotion of science as the foundation for public health practice
6. Support for the Affordable Care Act
7. Support for public health preparedness activities
8. Important research findings on climate changes and their impact on health

Dr. Georges C. Benjamin is clearly a public health hero. His work on behalf of public health professionals has been extensive. He constantly demonstrates his leadership through his advocacy initiatives and also his many writings.

and create standards for the practice of health education through the credentialing of health educators. Between 1952 and 1959, SOPHE began to have annual meetings, publish a newsletter, and develop a health education monograph. During the 1960s, many local chapters were formed. SOPHE contracted for administrative support from the International Union for Health Education for the Public. Many chapters and papers were published by members. The 1970s saw the appointment of an executive director (James Lovegren) and the passage of a code of ethics. Guidelines were also created for the development of baccalaureate programs in public health education. Growth continued through the 1980s and 1990s when graduate-level competencies were developed. Over the last 2 decades, Elaine Auld became executive director, a new textbook was published, and global competencies were developed.

Today, SOPHE has more than 4,000 members from all around the world. Elaine Auld has completed her 20th year as director. She is an excellent leader and manages a large portfolio of projects. She has been a major advocate for health education programs and has given testimony on these programs before Congress. Leadership development programs have been offered to members.

NATIONAL ASSOCIATION OF COUNTY AND CITY HEALTH OFFICIALS (NACCHO)

The local health department has many purposes.[8] The agency's main role is to determine policies and strategies for addressing ways to improve the health and prevent diseases within its geographic jurisdiction. The agency mission needs to be comprehensive enough to address all health-related problems that might arise. Problems may be associated with some subgroup of the population and not another. Health equity has to be the eventual goal for service. The health department also should look at all opportunities to develop health in its service area. This means that all community residents must be protected from health threats, communicable diseases, foodborne diseases, both natural and human-made disasters, toxic exposures, preventable illnesses and injuries, and services for people with chronic diseases. Social, economic, and physical determinants of health must be addressed.

The National Association of County and City Health Officials is an organization created to support the activities of the 2,800 member organizations. NACCHO has a vision to protect health, promote equity and health security for the individuals who live within the geographic area covered by the member organization.[9] At the mission level, NACCHO becomes the voice, advocate, health partner, coleader with the members, and champion for the members and for public health. As an organization, NACCHO concentrates on issues of community health, environmental health, public health infrastructure and systems, and public health preparedness. In addition to the annual meeting, which addresses cutting-edge issues in public health, there is a second meeting each year related to public health and preparedness. NACCHO came into being as an organization in the 1960s as an independent affiliate of the National Association of Counties. It later combined in 1994 with the United States Conference of Local Health Officers. In 2001 NACCHO added tribal public health agencies to the organization. The Association of State and Territorial Health Officials (ASTHO) serves a similar role for state health and deputy health officials.

NATIONAL ENVIRONMENTAL HEALTH ASSOCIATION (NEHA)

The National Environmental Health Association began in California in 1937.[10] The association was created to develop standards of excellence for the profession. This led to the creation of credentialing for Registered Environmental Health Specialists or Registered Sanitarians. NEHA also has a number of trainings and resources for the practicing professional. The association holds an annual conference that promotes networking and career growth and publishes an excellent environmental health journal.

NATIONAL ASSOCIATION OF LOCAL BOARDS OF HEALTH (NALBOH)[11]

In 1992, I met the Reverend Everett Hageman at a leadership program that I was running. I was impressed with his humanitarian spirit and his belief that leadership development in public health would be required if social justice was to guide public health professionals in their work. It turned out that the "Rev" was one of the founders of the National Association of Local Boards of Health. I spent many hours talking to him about partnership and the important relationship that needs to evolve between a local health department and its board. After Hageman's death, I put together a list of principles based on discussions with him. The following principles pertain to partnerships:

1. Allow time to get to know your community partners on a personal level.
2. Partnership is part of the human condition.
3. Working together is better than fighting.
4. Learn by listening to your partners.
5. True partnership is the gourmet approach to organization.

EXERCISE 15-1 Attend a
Professional Public Health Conference

Purpose: to begin networking as a public health leader

Key Concepts: leadership, professional organizations

Procedures: Over the next year, attend either a national or state professional organization conference to begin your work of becoming a professional public health worker and leader.

A committee was formed in 1991–1992 to discuss the formation of the National Association of Local Boards of Health. Ned Baker served as chair of the committee. Hageman was also on the committee. Baker became the first president of NALBOH in 1995. He then served as the association's first executive director and served in that role until his retirement in 1998.

NALBOH became the voice and advocate for both public health and for the citizens who served on local boards. Annual meetings have been held to discuss important public health issues of concern to board members. As the association has developed, public health professionals have come to annual meetings to work with boards on important issues. NALBOH has been involved in the development of performance standards for boards based on the public health essential services. **Exercise 15-1** above is important for those who will become public health leaders.

A NOTE ON ADVOCACY

An important responsibility for the public health leader and the public health organization is not only to advocate for public health but also to be a spokesperson for the role of public health. The Trust for America's Health has defined the advocate as an individual who defends and fights for the causes or petitions of others.[12] If you as a leader want to be an effective advocate, it is important to follow these five steps:

1. Identify whom you want to persuade.
2. Know the facts and do your homework.
3. Start to communicate with policy makers.
4. Begin to advocate this very day.
5. Always follow up.

Foundations have pointed out that it is important to evaluate the effectiveness of advocacy activities. In a report from the Annie E. Casey Foundation, it is argued that advocacy and policy change activities should be evaluated for effect.[13] Although the outcomes are numerous, leaders and organizations should determine whether the advocacy effort led to an increased awareness of the issue, more knowledge among elected officials of the severity of the issue or problem, clear determination of the actions to take to address the issue, salience of the issue, changes in the support of the issue, changes in voting on the issue, and passage of new legislation.

SUMMARY

The 21st century has required public health leaders to learn additional skills to address 21st century problems. Adaptive leadership skills have become critical for public health leaders. We need to work in partnership with a number of professional organizations to provide us with the information and training necessary for today and tomorrow. One of our key partners is the Centers for Disease Control and Prevention, which collects important health and disease information from around the world. CDC is also at the forefront of research and vaccines to help us address new health-related challenges. In addition, leaders get information, develop new skills, and work for changes and new legislation to aid in our public health work. A number of professional organizations were discussed. Finally, a brief discussion was given on the steps to advocacy.

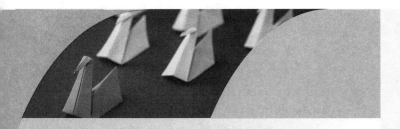

Discussion Questions

1. What type of skills do we need to work in public health today?

2. Why is CDC so critical to public health?

3. Why should we join public health professional organizations?

4. Who are the advocates for public health?

REFERENCES

1. http://www.cdc.gov/museum/history/7decades.html. Accessed July 23, 2016.
2. http://www.cdc.gov/mmwr/preview/mmwrhtml/00042732.htm. Accessed July 23, 2016.
3. http://www.cdc.gov/about/history/pastdirectors.htm. Accessed July 22, 2016.
4. https://en.wikipedia.org/wiki/Joseph_Walter_Mountin. Accessed July 23, 2016.
5. P. H. Bryce, "History of the American Public Health Association," *American Journal of Public Health* 8 (1918): 327–335.
6. http://www.apha.org/about-apha/executive-board-and-staff/apha-executive-board/georges-c-benjamin-md-facp-fnapa-facep-hon-frsph. Accessed July 24, 2016.
7. http://www.sophe.org/about.cfm. Accessed July 22, 2016.
8. J. E. Fielding, J. Freedman, and S. N. Caldwell, "Introduction and History of Public Health in Los Angeles County," In J. E. Fielding and S. M. Teutsch (eds.), *Public Health Practice: What Works* (New York, NY: Oxford, 2013).
9. http://archived.naccho.org/about/index.cfm. Accessed July 22, 2016.
10. http://www.neha.org/about-neha. Accessed July 22, 2016.
11. http://personal.bgsu.edu/~hermant/NALBOH/NedEBaker.htm. Accessed July 28, 2016.
12. Trust for America's Health, *You, Too, Can Be an Effective Public Health Advocate* (Washington, DC: TFAH, 2003).
13. J. Reisman, A. Gienapp, and S. Stachowiak, *A Guide to Measuring Advocacy and Policy* (Baltimore, MD: Annie E. Casey Foundation, 2007).

Epilogue: The Importance of Lifelong Learning

LEARNING OBJECTIVES

- Learn the advantages of lifelong learning for leaders.
- Describe the ladder of learning.
- Explore leadership learning content areas related to the leadership pyramid.

In 2009, I wrote the following blog posting:[1]

> As a biological species, we are programmed to learn. We are by our very natures lifelong learners. And yet, many of our species fight against the learning. In fact, as budgets tighten, as our elected officials fight for their causes, education and training initiatives end up on the cutting room floor. We have developed cultures that put rules, regulations, and protocols around us. We become ethnocentric by judging everyone else by our rules. We often close our minds to all the wonderful things that this world has to offer us. We often expect others to pay for all our learning, we do not think there is anything more for us to learn, or we do not often invest in ourselves. There is always more to learn. We become effective managers and leaders by building a toolbox full of wonderful things that enhance our skills and natural talents. I have spent my life with a commitment to my learning that I hope continues until my last day. Learning enriches my life and I hope the lives of those with whom I share my knowledge through action and discourse. That is the important message here. Sharing knowledge of ourselves and others will make our communities richer and stronger. Building social and human capital needs to be our goal. For us in public health and the human services field, social justice and servant leadership is our modus operandi. Every time we read a book, take a course, attend a conference, work collaboratively with others, use our creativity skills, solve a problem, resolve a conflict, improve the quality of our organizations, or communicate with others, we increase the return on investment in our personal growth and in the organizations for which we work. Knowledge management is cost effective and increases cost efficiency.
>
> I hear people say that they want to increase their skills, but their bosses or elected officials won't let them. It is true that training and educational dollars are often the first to go when budgets get cut. This is a very short-sighted view. Not only do we have lower salaries than those in the private sector, there is no money to help us grow and become more effective health professionals, managers, and leaders. It often seems that there is an expectation that we will fail, that government work is for those who will not survive in the private sector, or for those who don't want to work hard. The anti-intellectual stance that we seem to take in

our country works against us. Our value system needs to change if we are to remain a first-tier country in the world. Education and training are our key to success. If change is our modus operandi, then investment in lifelong learning models must become more highly valued than it is today. For every dollar that we invest in the growth of our governmental workforce, the returns will be significant. It is not only me that needs to grow in order to be a more effective professional and leader; we all need to grow and learn throughout our lives. When will our elected officials and agency bosses change their priorities to invest in our future? Maybe they need to learn and increase their skills as well. Trusteeship of our people and our future is an important concept that our elected officials need to practice.

As you prepare to end this course on the essentials of public health leadership and adopt a lifelong learning philosophy, the question of where to go next arises.

A LEADERSHIP LADDER OF LEARNING

Learning must be a lifelong process. Public health leaders live in a constantly changing environment, and the public health agenda is partly unpredictable. Public health leaders will require different training opportunities at different times in their professional lives, but it is clear that mentoring adds to virtually any learning experience. **Figure E-1** presents a lifelong learning agenda for leaders. As leaders move up the ladder, they begin to focus more on national or even global public health concerns rather than local ones and also begin to become aware of the abstract aspects of leadership and develop conceptual models to guide their leadership activities.

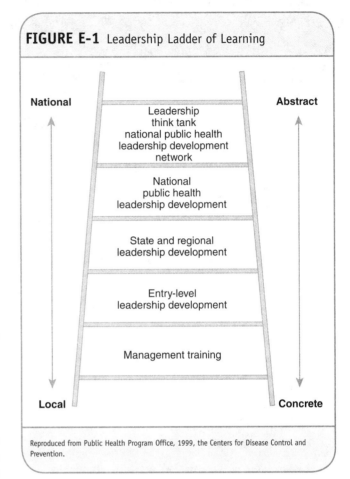

FIGURE E-1 Leadership Ladder of Learning

Reproduced from Public Health Program Office, 1999, the Centers for Disease Control and Prevention.

EXERCISE E-1 What's Next

Purpose: to discuss options for the next steps in leadership lifelong learning

Key Concepts: lifelong learning, leadership development

Procedures: With your classmates, have a discussion on what you think will be the areas for which you will need additional training.

On the first step of the ladder, where public health professionals initially take on supervisory or other administrative roles, they must learn how to use basic management and leadership tools. They need training in planning, organizing, monitoring, and administering.[2] They also should learn to distinguish clinical activities from management activities and develop leadership and adaptive skills that will help them advance to a more creative leadership role in the organization. There are numerous courses and training materials available for new leader-administrators. The foundation skills are fairly concrete and less conceptual than at the higher levels of leadership. Many of the skills needed are discussed throughout this book.

Entry-level leadership development can occur through involvement with a profession-specific group or a multidisciplinary group. After 3 to 5 years in an organizational leadership position, leaders will benefit from training at a state or regional public health leadership institute. Although many of these institutes have closed because of the loss of funding, some still exist. Such training is intended to integrate leadership concepts and public health governing paradigms.

National public health leadership institutes, such as the Public Health Leadership Academy funded by the Centers for Disease Control and Prevention, are useful for leaders in key state positions. Top-level leaders may also gain from specialized training programs that stress some major leadership functions.

At the highest step on the ladder, public health leaders can become involved in a think tank in order to explore public health issues with graduates of national leadership development programs and state and local public health leadership institutes. Public health think tanks are in the business of producing policy papers to guide public health action. The Trust for America's Health is an example of such a program.

THE LEADERSHIP PYRAMID

Effective leaders are lifelong learners. To put this lifelong learning approach into perspective, it is useful to look at education and learning in a sequential manner. The following discussion is based on a new approach to leadership development conceptualized by Lichtveld, Rowitz, and Cioffi.[3] Over the past 20 years, there has been increasing interest in developing a framework for training public health professionals in management and leadership under the assumption that

leaders help build a stronger public health system. Yet there is controversy about whether leaders differ in the realms of business and the governmental human services fields. Although it is true that leadership is a universal phenomenon, it takes different forms depending on the cultural and ecological context in which it takes place. There is clearly a difference between the profit motive in business and the social justice motive that drives much of the public health enterprise. As we view the public health system during the second decade of the new century with all the new challenges that public health now faces, it is necessary that the issue of leaders in public health be looked at from a new perspective. This model presents a perspective for a better understanding of leadership from the vantage points of leadership competencies, performance, capacity building, and best practices.

Public health leaders act within the core functions of public health and the essential services that drive the public health enterprise. In addition, the public health leader is prepared for any natural or abnormal crisis that might occur in the community. The leader is committed to lifelong learning and the need to develop competencies required to protect the health of the public.

Figure E-2 presents the leadership pyramid as an inverted triangle. Each level of the pyramid requires a determination

---

FIGURE E-2 New Leadership Pyramid

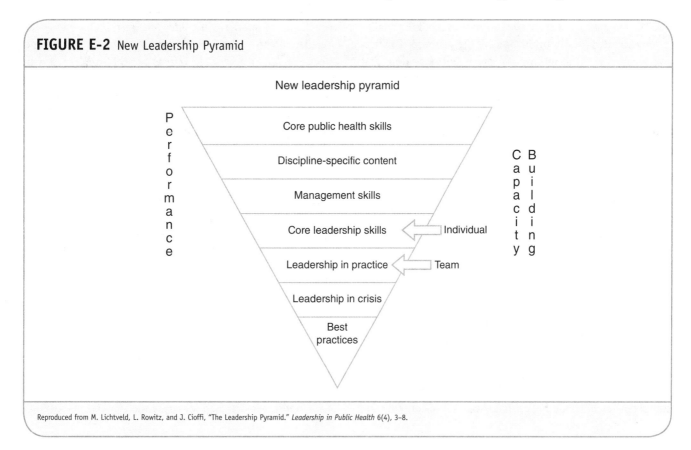

of the specific competencies necessary to master that level of the pyramid. The triangle is inverted to show that the broad set of core public health skills that public health professionals need to have acts as the foundation for all that follows. Each level of the inverted triangle becomes more specialized. There are numerous approaches these days to the learning competencies required to practice certain professional and administrative skills. The pyramid requires that we reorganize these competencies to fit each level of the leadership pyramid. As each public health workforce member masters each level of the pyramid, performance should improve and the infrastructure of public health should strengthen. Performance management systems and performance standards guided by a set of principles (e.g., essential public health services) would monitor this process.

Training is the key to mastering these skills, which are necessary to build infrastructure. If public health professionals improve their skills and become more effective as a result, they have increased their personal skills, which can then be translated into team-based and other collaborative processes. All of this would eventually improve the capacity of the total public health system. The bottom of the pyramid emphasizes the importance of best practices. The business community is not shy about discussing its best. Public health must begin to do the same.

We can look for clues to the understanding of the quality improvement approach in the body of the pyramid. The first layer emphasizes the importance of an understanding and mastery of a set of core public health skills. Public health must have a workforce that is trained in public health principles and practice. Too many of the people in our existing governmental public health workforce have no formal public health training. Recent discussions on credentialing have raised some of these issues, and proponents have argued that the public health system cannot be strengthened without this training. The set of competencies required for this level of the pyramid has been developed by a number of different organizations. All of this means that these skills will be required of all public health workers in the governmental public health sector.

Public health is a profession with a workforce from many different disciplines. Doctors, nurses, dentists, lawyers, business administrators, behavioral scientists, epidemiologists, biostatisticians, and many other discipline-specific experts are required if public health is to carry out its major responsibilities. The major message in level two of the pyramid is that the successful public health practitioner must blend the competencies of public health with discipline-specific competencies if public health is to function in an effective

manner. Business learned these lessons long ago and has been able to build profit enterprises through the combination of sound business practices with discipline-specific expertise in many different areas.

The skills necessary to achieve competence at the first two levels of the pyramid are somewhat technical in nature. When the public health professional moves to level three of the pyramid, the tasks to be performed relate to making an agency run effectively and efficiently. Thus, a shift occurs when an individual decides to move into a management role. New sets of skills are needed. In addition, many public health professionals find that during their professional education they were not trained to be managers. Although business schools have been involved in the development of competencies for work in commerce, adaptation of these skills to the public sector needs to become more formalized. Management competencies are quite complex and require training in such diverse topics as time management, performance appraisal, strategic planning, office management, budgeting, and so on. A few certification programs now exist for public health management that begin to build a public health competency-based management model.

The move from management to leadership is not as easy as it first appears. First, there is a shift from an agency focus to a systems and community focus affected by the complexity of modern life. The manager looks inside the organization to make sure it is functioning efficiently and effectively. The leader looks outward and is concerned with how public health functions at the community and national levels. In addition, the technical skills required at levels one and two and the administrative task-oriented skills of level three become secondary to people and relational skill competencies. The core skills required to be an effective leader are also not taught in most traditional health science curricula. The national, regional, and state-based public health leadership institutes have been trying to fill this gap from the early 1990s until about 2010 when funding ended for many programs. The National Public Health Leadership Network, in collaboration with the Centers for Disease Control and Prevention, developed a framework of core public health leadership competencies that have been integral to the training of public health leaders. Public health leaders throughout the country have gone through these training programs. The philosophy of these training programs has been that leaders exist throughout the public health system and that leadership can be taught.

Training without implementing the content of the training is nothing more than an academic exercise. Leadership development should be available for practicing public health professionals who can use these new leadership skills in the work and community context of their professional work. Leadership must be implemented to be effective. This may not be an easy task in environments that are resistant to change. Leaders need to be students of the cultural settings in which they work. Each new skill will undergo some transformation as it is applied in the work and community setting. These new challenges may require skills beyond those that occur in most leadership development programs. It is at this level that such skills as collaboration, team building, community building, assets planning and mapping, emotional intelligence, and others come to play a key role in effective leadership.

The events of September 11, 2001, changed the field of public health. Program priorities have changed. Bioterrorism and emergency preparedness specialists have become a critical component of the public health professional workforce. With these shifting priorities, it is clear that new leadership skills are needed to guide health departments. Public health preparedness and response have become a major priority for public health. Public health leaders require new skills for the types of collaboration required to deal with crisis events in communities, for risk management, and for health crisis communications. Forensic epidemiology has become a new specialty. Public health informatics is a new approach to the creation and use of data. Strategies are needed for working with families of the victims of a crisis event. New partnerships are required with the Federal Bureau of Investigation, police departments, fire departments, hospitals and other health facilities, crisis agencies, community partners, and elected officials. Communicating with people who use different jargon has also become a major leadership challenge. Higher levels of emotional intelligence skills have become more critical. Bioterrorism leadership competencies are different from traditional leadership skills. It is a new type of leadership with more complex skills required for working in environments of constant change. The leadership pyramid presents a start on the development of a complex, new approach to the training of public health leaders. Leaders themselves will need to move from level to level in the development of their personal, team, agency, community, global, and professional skills. Whereas technical skills are usually required to get a person a job in an agency, people skills become more critical to job performance over the long run. Leadership development becomes a lifelong learning activity that leaders must commit to if best practices are to occur and if the infrastructure of public health is to be strengthened.

PUBLIC HEALTH HEROES AND VILLAINS E-1 Tom Balderson, a Quiet Hero

This is the story of a leader who was also a champion for training public health professionals to take on leadership roles. Back in the early 1990s, Balderson was a public health advisor in the Public Health Practice Program Office (which no longer exists organizationally) at the Centers for Disease Control and Prevention in Atlanta. Balderson took on the responsibility for the promotion and development of a national public health leadership institute in the early 1990s. During the rest of his life, he attended all the National Public Health Leadership meetings to keep up with the latest knowledge and skills for leaders as well as enhance his own leadership as a lifelong learner.

In 1991, I met with Balderson to discuss an idea for a state-based leadership program. My argument was that local and state public health people did not often go to national meetings or undertake out-of-state work-related travel because of a lack of travel funds at their agency or restrictions on travel out of the state. I also argued that local and state public health professionals tended to be career oriented whereas state leaders tended to be in state government for shorter periods of time. Balderson was intrigued with the possibility of comparing the national program with a state program. I wrote a proposal to create the Illinois Public Health Leadership Institute (later the Mid-America Regional Public Health Leadership Institute), which was funded until 2010. The success of the Illinois program was the eventual development and funding of public health leadership programs around the country with the hero support of Tom Balderson. He did his championing from behind the scenes. He was a silent and quiet but steady leader. He never considered himself a leader although he was clearly one. He also became a good friend of mine. He was our hero and champion until his untimely death in 2001.

As Begun and Malcolm look forward to public health in the second decade of the 21st century and beyond, they envision five competency sets for lifelong learning for leaders:[4]

1. Strengthen a population health approach to the field.
2. Involve people from diverse backgrounds in public health work.
3. Learn power strategies to increase the impact of population health initiatives.
4. Recognize that public health is about the unexpected.
5. Promote a continuous quality improvement approach to public health programs and organizations.

One important hero was one of the first public health people to promote the development of leaders at the state and national level.

SUMMARY

Leaders need to continue their learning throughout their lives. Because public health challenges continue to occur, leaders will require new knowledge and skills after they leave school. Training and further educational opportunities will be needed. This book is only the beginning of a lifelong learning journey. Enjoy the journey.

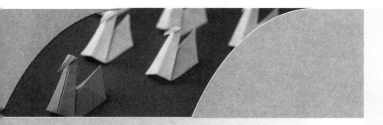

Discussion Questions

1. What are the learning needs of leaders at the six levels of leadership?

2. How can you advocate for leadership development programs for public health professionals?

3. Were my expectations for learning about leadership met?

REFERENCES

1. https://rowitzonleadership.wordpress.com/2009/11/. Accessed August 1, 2016.
2. S. P. Robbins and M. Coulter, *Management*, 11th ed. (Upper Saddle River, NJ: Prentice-Hall, 2011).
3. M. Lichtveld, L. Rowitz, and J. Cioffi, "The Leadership Pyramid," *Leadership in Public Health*, 6, no. 4 (2004): 3–8.
4. J. W. Begun and J. K. Malcolm, *Leading Public Health* (New York, NY: Springer, 2014).

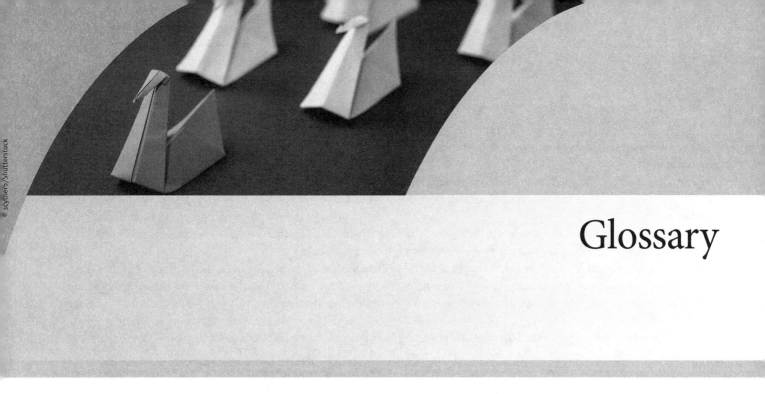

Glossary

Adaptive leadership A process of observing events and patterns without forming judgments or making assumptions, developing multiple hypotheses, and designing interventions based on observations and interpretations in order to address an adaptive challenge.

Adaptive organization An organization able to keep up with the rapid changes in its environment by entrusting more decision-making powers and associated resources to the employees.

Advisory board A group that provides nonbinding strategic advice to the management of an organization.

Advocacy Activity by an individual or group that aims to influence decisions within political, economic, and social systems and institutions.

AIM Leadership Model Depicts five building blocks of effective personal leadership: communication, the empowerment of followers, a focus on key issues, linkage to others, and life balance. Each block is affected by leadership style and practices as well as the systems approach to organizational change.

Assets-based approach A process of assessing the resources, skills, and experience available in a community; organizing the community around issues that mobilize its members; and determining and taking appropriate action.

Board of health A body of a municipal or state government that is responsible for coordinating public health activities in a specified city, county, or state.

Centers for Disease Control and Prevention An agency in the U.S. Department of Health and Human Services whose goal is to protect public health and safety through the control and prevention of disease, injury, and disability.

Coaching A form of development in which an experienced person supports another in achieving a specific personal or professional goal by providing training, advice, and guidance.

Coalition The coming together of people and organizations to influence outcomes related to a specific problem or set of problems.

Collaboration A mutually beneficial set of relationships that are well defined and that are entered into by two or more organizations in order to achieve some common goal.

Community building Practices directed toward the creation or enhancement of community among individuals within an area or with a common interest.

Community engagement A process in which individuals and community organizations promote programs that will benefit the community.

Community health alliance A group of healthcare and public health organizations that have combined forces to address key public health risks and problems for the population of a specific geographic area.

Continuous quality improvement A process of creating an environment in which management and workers strive to create constantly improving quality.

Core functions of public health The activities of assessment (identification of health problems), policy development (identification of possible solutions through policy), and assurance (the implications of the possible solutions) in a public health context.

Crisis An abnormal event or series of disruptive events that threatens the operation of an organization or the functioning of a community.

Crisis management The application of strategies designed to help an organization deal with a sudden and significant negative event.

Cross-cultural communication The ability to successfully form, foster, and improve relationships with members of a culture different from one's own, based on knowledge of the other culture's values, perceptions, manners, social structure, and decision-making practices and an understanding of how members of the group communicate.

Culture of health An ongoing set of activities to promote health and improve the quality of life for all community residents across geographic, demographic, and social sectors.

Ecological leadership The ability of an individual or group to guide positive change toward a vision of an environmentally better future.

Emergency preparedness Effective precautionary actions, rehabilitation, and recovery to ensure the timely, appropriate, and effective organization and delivery of relief and assistance following an emergency.

Emotional intelligence An ability and capacity to recognize one's own personal feelings and the feelings and emotional reactions of others.

Global health The area of study, research, and practice that places a priority on improving health and achieving equity in health for all people worldwide.

Global leadership The ability to adapt leadership and managerial skills to various economic and cultural environments.

Governance Administering programs and adjusting them to fit policies developed as part of the political process.

Governing board A group of individuals elected or appointed to direct the policies of an institution.

High-performing team A group of people with specific roles and complementary talents and skills, aligned with and committed to a common purpose, who consistently show high levels of collaboration and innovation, that produce superior results.

Human Sigma A process for improving relationships with community customers that involves viewing these relationships as primary, paying attention to the emotions involved, thinking globally and acting locally, recognizing the impact of relationships on finances, and using actions as the criterion for success.

Incident command system A standardized approach to the command, control, and coordination of a response to a community emergency that provides a well-defined structure for the coordination of the activities of community agencies and partners for dealing with the crisis.

Journaling A record of experiences, ideas, or reflections kept regularly for private use.

Knowledge management Efficient handling of information and resources within an organization.

Knowledge work Work involving the production and distribution of information with an emphasis on nonroutine problem solving that requires convergent, divergent, and creative thinking.

Leadership The activity of guiding a group of people or an organization by establishing a clear vision; sharing that vision with others so that they will follow willingly; providing the information, knowledge, and methods to realize that vision; and coordinating and balancing the conflicting interests of all stakeholders.

Leadership development Expansion of a person's capacity to be effective in leadership roles and processes such as communication, ability to motivate others, and management.

Leadership wheel A systems approach to organizational change that depicts the integration of planning, action, and evaluation.

Learning contract An agreement between a learner and an adviser or mentor that specifies learning objectives, activities to achieve them, and how learning will be verified.

Lifelong learning The use of both formal and informal learning opportunities throughout life in order to foster the continuous development of the knowledge and skills needed for employment and personal fulfillment.

Management-leadership continuum The range of styles and actions used by managers and leaders.

Matrix organization An organizational model in which program specialists from various functional units are brought together to work on a multidisciplinary team to carry out a project- or goal-based program.

Mentoring A relationship in which a more experienced or more knowledgeable person helps to guide a less experienced or less knowledgeable person, particularly in matters involving careers or career choice.

Mission statement A written declaration of an organization's core purpose and focus.

Paradigm An example, pattern, or model.

Paradigm shift A fundamental change in approach or underlying assumptions.

PERFORM model A model outlining characteristics of high-performing teams including Purpose, Empowerment, Relationships, Flexibility, Optimal productivity, Recognition, and Morale.

Personal leadership philosophy A system of guiding principles, core values, expectations, and perspectives on leadership.

Population health   An approach to health that aims to improve health outcomes for all people as well as the distribution of these outcomes within a specified population.

Professional association   An organization that seeks to further a particular profession, the interests of individuals engaged in that profession, and the public interest.

Quality of life   General well-being based on such factors as nutrition, exercise, income and employment status, sleep patterns, social integration into community life, physical and mental health status, educational level, recreation and leisure time, and the effects of retirement and aging.

Risk taking   The act of doing something that involves danger or risk in order to achieve a goal.

SCOPE model   A global leadership model with five stages: seeing differences in the practice of leadership in different cultures, closing the gap and building intercultural relationships, opening the system in order to expand the ownership and involvement in public health, preserving balance and knowing when to change and when not to, and establishing solutions and results that matter.

Shadowing   Following a leader for a period of time to explore how a leader practices leadership on a daily basis.

Stakeholder analysis   Determination of the services available, what each stakeholder resource can contribute to public health, and how stakeholders will perform relative to the goals and objectives for public health.

Starfish organization   A completely decentralized organization in which all participants share in the leadership of the organization.

Strategic planning   An organizational management activity that is used to set priorities, focus energy and resources, strengthen operations, ensure that employees and other stakeholders are working toward common goals, establish agreement around intended outcomes/results, and assess and adjust the organization's direction in response to a changing environment.

Teamwork   Cooperative or coordinated effort on the part of a group of persons acting together in the interests of a common cause.

Time management   The ability to use one's time effectively or productively.

Total quality management   A management approach to long-term success through customer satisfaction in which all members of an organization participate in improving processes, products, services, and the culture in which they work.

Transactional leadership   A form of leadership in which the leader engages others in the reciprocal activity of exchanging one thing for another.

Transformational leadership   A form of leadership in which the leader examines and searches for the needs and motives of others while seeking a higher agenda of needs; the interaction between leaders or between leaders and followers changes both parties.

Vision statement   An aspirational description of what an organization would like to achieve or accomplish in the midterm or long-term future intended to serve as a guide for choosing current and future courses of action.

Well-being   A good or satisfactory condition of existence.

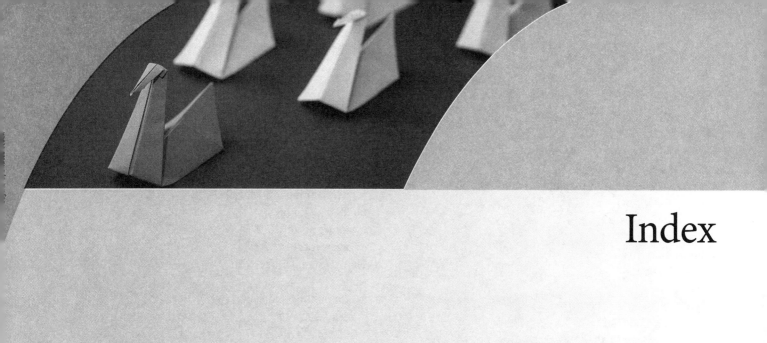

Index

Note: Page numbers followed by *f* and *t* refer to figures and tables, respectively.